Lesbian, Gay, Bisexual, and Transgender Aging

T0260343

This edited collection emphasizes the role of social work practice and research related to Lesbian, Gay, Bisexual, and Transgender (LGBT) aging. It highlights LGBT aging from a gerontological social work perspective by incorporating key values of the profession such as cultural competence, dignity, strengths, and resilience of the population while it offers an important contribution to the body of knowledge to the interdisciplinary field of aging.

This book was originally published as a special issue of the *Journal of Gerontological Social Work.*

Nancy Giunta is a John A. Hartford Geriatric Social Work Faculty Scholar, Assistant Professor at the Silberman School of Social Work, Hunter College, The City University of New York, USA. Her research explores collaborative interventions to improve culturally competent services for elders in community settings.

Noell L. Rowan is a John A. Hartford Geriatric Social Work Faculty Scholar, Associate Professor, and Coordinator of BSW Program at the School of Social Work, University of North Carolina Wilmington, USA. Her research focuses on LGBT populations and the intersection with aging and mental health and addiction, resiliency and quality of life.

Lesbian, Gay, Bisexual, and Transgender Aging

The Role of Gerontological Social Work

Edited by
Nancy Giunta and Noell L. Rowan

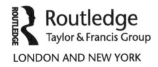

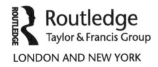**Routledge**
Taylor & Francis Group

LONDON AND NEW YORK

First published 2015
by Routledge

2 Park Square, Milton Park, Abingdon, Oxon OX14 4RN
711 Third Avenue, New York, NY 10017, USA

Routledge is an imprint of the Taylor & Francis Group, an informa business

First issued in paperback 2017

British Library Cataloguing in Publication Data
A catalogue record for this book is available from the British Library

ISBN 13: 978-1-138-84208-3 (hbk)
ISBN 13: 978-1-138-05715-9 (pbk)

Typeset in Garamond ITC
by RefineCatch Limited, Bungay, Suffolk

Publisher's Note
The publisher accepts responsibility for any inconsistencies that may have
arisen during the conversion of this book from journal articles to book chapters,
namely the possible inclusion of journal terminology.

Disclaimer
Every effort has been made to contact copyright holders for their permission to
reprint material in this book. The publishers would be grateful to hear from any
copyright holder who is not here acknowledged and will undertake to rectify
any errors or omissions in future editions of this book.

Contents

Citation Information

The chapters in this book were originally published in the *Journal of Gerontological Social Work*, volume 57, issue 2–4 (February–June 2014). When citing this material, please use the original page numbering for each article, as follows:

Chapter 1
Introduction: Building Capacity in Gerontological Social Work for Lesbian, Gay, Bisexual, and Transgender Older Adults and Their Loved Ones
Noell L. Rowan and Nancy Giunta
Journal of Gerontological Social Work, volume 57, issue 2–4 (February–June 2014) pp. 75–79

Chapter 2
Creating a Vision for the Future: Key Competencies and Strategies for Culturally Competent Practice With Lesbian, Gay, Bisexual, and Transgender (LGBT) Older Adults in the Health and Human Services
Karen I. Fredriksen-Goldsen, Charles P. Hoy-Ellis, Jayn Goldsen, Charles A. Emlet, and Nancy R. Hooyman
Journal of Gerontological Social Work, volume 57, issue 2–4 (February–June 2014) pp. 80–107

Chapter 3
Same-Sex Sexual Relationships in the National Social Life, Health and Aging Project: Making a Case for Data Collection
Maria T. Brown and Brian R. Grossman
Journal of Gerontological Social Work, volume 57, issue 2–4 (February–June 2014) pp. 108–129

Chapter 4
Hidden or Uninvited? A Content Analysis of Elder LGBT of Color Literature in Gerontology
Laurens G. Van Sluytman and Denise Torres
Journal of Gerontological Social Work, volume 57, issue 2–4 (February–June 2014) pp. 130–160

Chapter 5

Gender Transitions in Later Life: The Significance of Time in Queer Aging
Vanessa D. Fabbre
Journal of Gerontological Social Work, volume 57, issue 2–4 (February–June 2014) pp. 161–175

Chapter 6

Resilience in Attaining and Sustaining Sobriety Among Older Lesbians With Alcoholism
Noell L. Rowan and Sandra S. Butler
Journal of Gerontological Social Work, volume 57, issue 2–4 (February–June 2014) pp. 176–197

Chapter 7

Broadening Definitions of Family for Older Lesbians: Modifying the Lubben Social Network Scale
Marcena L. Gabrielson and Ezra C. Holston
Journal of Gerontological Social Work, volume 57, issue 2–4 (February–June 2014) pp. 198–217

Chapter 8

GayBy Boomers' Social Support: Exploring the Connection Between Health and Emotional and Instrumental Support in Older Gay Men
Jesus Ramirez-Valles, Jessica Dirkes, and Hope A. Barrett
Journal of Gerontological Social Work, volume 57, issue 2–4 (February–June 2014) pp. 218–234

Chapter 9

Acceptance in the Domestic Environment: The Experience of Senior Housing for Lesbian, Gay, Bisexual, and Transgender Seniors
Kathleen M. Sullivan
Journal of Gerontological Social Work, volume 57, issue 2–4 (February–June 2014) pp. 235–250

Chapter 10

The Highs and Lows of Caregiving for Chronically Ill Lesbian, Gay, and Bisexual Elders
Anna Muraco and Karen I. Fredriksen-Goldsen
Journal of Gerontological Social Work, volume 57, issue 2–4 (February–June 2014) pp. 251–272

Chapter 11

Older Lesbians and Bereavement: Experiencing the Loss of a Partner
Carol L. Jenkins, Amanda Edmundson, Paige Averett, and Intae Yoon
Journal of Gerontological Social Work, volume 57, issue 2–4 (February–June 2014) pp. 273–287

Chapter 18

"They Just Don't Have a Clue": Transgender Aging and Implications for Social Work
Anna Siverskog
Journal of Gerontological Social Work, volume 57, issue 2–4 (February–June 2014) pp. 386–406

Chapter 19

The National Resource Center on LGBT Aging Provides Critical Training to Aging Service Providers
Hilary Meyer and Tim R. Johnston
Journal of Gerontological Social Work, volume 57, issue 2–4 (February–June 2014) pp. 407–412

Chapter 20

Film Review: Transgender Tuesdays: A Clinic in the Tenderloin, *by Mark Freeman*
Reviewed by Debra Sheets
Journal of Gerontological Social Work, volume 57, issue 2–4 (February–June 2014) pp. 413–415

Please direct any queries you may have about the citations to clsuk.permissions@cengage.com

Introduction

Building Capacity in Gerontological Social Work for Lesbian, Gay, Bisexual, and Transgender Older Adults and Their Loved Ones

NOELL L. ROWAN

School of Social Work, University of North Carolina Wilmington, Wilmington, North Carolina, USA

NANCY GIUNTA

Silberman School of Social Work at Hunter College, The City University of New York, New York, New York, USA

We express our sincere gratitude to Dr. Amanda Barusch, former Editor-in-Chief, and Dr. Carmen Morano, Managing Editor, for their dedication and support of this special issue in the *Journal of Gerontological Social Work* *(JGSW)* on lesbian, gay, bisexual, and transgender (LGBT) older adults and aging. We are also immensely grateful to peer reviewers who contributed their time to review manuscripts; there was an enormous response to the call for papers for this issue. We are, therefore, pleased and grateful to the Editorial Board for their support in offering this triple issue focusing on LGBT aging. The volume of manuscripts received and accepted speaks to the quality of scholarship underway in the field of LGBT aging and to the timeliness of this publication as LGBT issues are gaining traction both in mainstream media and academic literature.

This issue sheds light on an often hidden and marginalized subset of aging persons. The contributing authors are considered experts in the field of LGBT aging, and provide a compelling argument for why the field of gerontological social work should actively include issues of LGBT aging in aging research, policy, education, and practice. We encourage readers to review each of the articles in this special issue in an effort to grasp the potential for the profession of social work to provide leadership with the LGBT aging population in all of these arenas, as well as in program development.

There is a swiftly growing literature on, and interest in LGBT people in the field of gerontology. The discipline of gerontological social work offers an excellent arena for building knowledge on how to support LGBT older adults as they experience the intersecting challenges of aging within a marginalized community.

The myriad research areas in the literature mirror the broad diversity in the aging LGBT population. Some pertinent areas of concern include human rights and policy; issues related to ageism, heterosexism, and gender identity; relations with families and relationships; social support networks; issues related to racial and multicultural identity; and health and mental health disparities. The changing policy arena, which includes, but is not limited to, state policies recognizing marital rights to same-sex couples, is one contextual factor that exemplifies the growing need to examine how LGBT older adults experience aging. Indeed, federal support of research and training to support LGBT elders has increased in the last decade through a variety of funding streams. The aim of this special issue is to provide an array of scholarly literature on LGBT aging in an effort to raise awareness of pertinent issues facing this population. The particular focus is to build capacity in the discipline of social work so that gerontological social work scholars and practitioners have a voice in the multidisciplinary dialogue.

This special issue serves a particular niche for *JGSW* readers, as it emphasizes the role of social work practice and research related to LGBT aging. This is the first social work journal to spotlight this issue. One advantage of highlighting LGBT aging within a gerontological social work perspective is the incorporation of cultural competence, strengths, and resilience of the population in the development of knowledge in this field. To ensure that there is a consistent social work theme throughout the special issue, all authors were encouraged to discuss implications and future directions for social work practice, research, or policy.

In the first article, Fredriksen-Goldsen, Hoy-Ellis, Goldsen, Emlet, and Hooyman (2014) aptly set the stage by proposing key competencies developed from results of the groundbreaking Caring and Aging with Pride study. The 10 competencies, as the authors posit, serve as a "blueprint for action" for social work scholars and practitioners to better meet the needs of our elders in LGBT communities. Brown and Grossman (2014) use data from the National Social Life Health and Aging Project to offer specific strategies, such as collecting sexual orientation data, to carry out more competent knowledge-building. Van Sluytman and Torres (2014) underscore that despite distinct cultural needs of sexual minorities of color, this population remains underrepresented in the LGBT aging literature. We move from building groundwork and a course of action to an examination of two populations through the construct of time. First, Fabbre (2014) offers a conceptual analysis of the notion of time with older transgendered persons; this is followed by Rowan and Butler's (2014) exploration of coping and resilience over time among older lesbians with alcoholism. After these two articles present inquiry through a temporal framework, we present a series of articles related to social networks and social support. Gabrielson and Holston (2014) carry the theme of building research capacity by presenting data for how the Lubben Social Network Scale may be refined to capture how families and social support networks are conceptualized in a sample of older lesbians. Ramirez-Valles, Dirkes, and Barrett (2014) present evidence that both instrumental and emotional social support from social networks is related to more positively perceived health and mental health among older gay men. In an examination of older adults' decisions to reside in LGBT senior housing, Sullivan (2014) discovered that residents enjoyed an increase in social network and emotional support, and identified acceptance as a driving construct to age-in-place in communities where elders feel safe being themselves.

There is a growing literature on caregiving and bereavement among LGBT elders. Muraco and Fredriksen-Goldsen (2014) contribute to this growth with their study of caregiver and care recipient experiences within the context of different types of relationships (i.e., committed partners or friends). We learn that relationship context may shape the narrative and perceived experiences of both caregivers and recipients in their "best" and "worst" times. Jenkins, Edmundson, Averett, and Yoon (2014) report on themes that reveal the unique needs of bereaved lesbians when a partner dies, and Fenge (2014) expands the view of same-sex bereavement among lesbian and gay elders in the United Kingdom. Fenge identifies this as an overlooked area of social work practice and education, thus supporting the argument for educating practitioners to deliver more culturally competent services. Portz and colleagues (2014) document such service delivery gaps in health and social service organizations and argue that social workers could play a key role in developing more culturally competent organizations. Moone, Cagle, Croghan, and Smith (2014) examine existing cultural competence trainings and preferences expressed by service providers who may participate in such trainings. Leyva, Breshears, and Ringstad (2014) investigated the efficacy of one such training, which resulted in promising outcomes such as increased knowledge, skills, and positive attitudes regarding LGBT elders.

The implications for practice and research are discussed by authors throughout the issue. Three articles, however, focus predominantly on such implications. Averett, Robinson, Jenkins, and Yoon (2014) offer common challenges of conducting research in lesbian and gay communities and strategies for addressing them. Erdley, Anklam, and Reardon (2014) discuss the role of social workers and their use of the strengths perspective as critical to building capacity for cultural competence in health care settings. Finally, Siverskog (2014) emphasizes through qualitative research findings the need for social work practitioners working with older transgendered adults to understand that each individual is unique and brings their own lived experiences within a historical legal and social context.

In the Brief Report, Meyer and Johnston (2014) describe the work of the National Resource Center on LGBT Aging (NRC), originally funded by the US Administration on Aging (now the Administration on Community Living, which continues to support some of the NRC programming). The NRC should be lauded for its work with a broad range of national partners, its extensive collection of online resources and large network of trainers conducting cultural competence trainings in communities throughout the United States. The film review by Debra Sheets (2014) exemplifies the use of a strengths-based perspective in working with trans elders through *Transgender Tuesdays*. This film could eloquently serve as an educational resource.

It is our intent that this special issue lays the groundwork to build capacity for continued scholarship on LGBT aging in social work as well as other disciplines. The need for multidisciplinary, interprofessional work is critical to ensure our LGBT elders are visible in practice, research, policy, and educational arenas. We hope you enjoy reading this special issue as much as we have enjoyed editing it.

REFERENCES

Averett, P., Robinson, A., Jenkins, C., & Yoon, I. (2014). "I want to know more about who we are": New directions for research with older lesbians. *Journal of Gerontological Social Work, 57,* 349–361. doi:10.1080/01634372.2013.860651

Brown, M. T., & Grossman, B. R. (2014). Same-sex sexual relationships in the National Social Life, Health and Aging Project: Making a case for data collection. *Journal of Gerontological Social Work, 57,* 108–129. doi:10.1080/01634372.2013.865695

Erdley, S. D., Anklam, D. D., & Reardon, C. C. (2014). Breaking barriers and building bridges: Understanding the pervasive needs of older LGBT adults and the value of social work in health care. *Journal of Gerontological Social Work, 57,* 362–385. doi:10.1080/01634372.2013.871381

Fabbre, V. D. (2014). Gender transitions in later life: The significance of time in queer aging. *Journal of Gerontological Social Work, 57,* 161–175. doi:10.1080/01634372.2013.855287

Fenge, L. (2014). Developing understanding of same-sex partner bereavement for older lesbian and gay people: Implications for social work practice. *Journal of Gerontological Social Work, 57,* 288–304. doi:10.1080/01634372.2013.825360

Fredriksen-Goldsen, K. I., Hoy-Ellis, C. P., Goldsen, J., Emlet, C. A., & Hooyman, N. R. (2014). Creating a vision for the future: Key competencies and strategies for culturally competent practice with lesbian, gay, bisexual, and transgender (LGBT) older adults in the health and human services. *Journal of Gerontological Social Work, 57,* 80–107. doi:10.1080/01634372.2014.890690

Gabrielson, M. L., & Holston, E. C. (2014). Broadening definitions of family for older lesbians: Modifying the Lubben Social Network Scale. *Journal of Gerontological Social Work, 57*, 198–217. doi:10.1080/01634372.2013.879683

Jenkins, C. L., Edmundson, A., Averett, P., & Yoon, I. (2014). Older lesbians and bereavement: Experiencing the loss of a partner. *Journal of Gerontological Social Work, 57*, 273–287. doi:10.1080/01634372.2013.850583

Leyva, V. L., Breshears, E. M., & Ringstad, R. (2014). Assessing the efficacy of LGBT cultural competency training for aging services providers in California's Central Valley. *Journal of Gerontological Social Work, 57*, 335–348. doi:10.1080/01634372.2013.872215

Meyer, H., & Johnston, T. R. (2014). The National Resource Center on LGBT Aging provides critical training to aging service providers. *Journal of Gerontological Social Work, 57*, 407–412. doi:10.1080/01634372.2014.901997

Moone, R. P., Cagle, J. G., Croghan, C. F., & Smith, J. (2014). Working with LGBT older adults: An assessment of employee training practices, needs, and preferences of senior service organizations in Minnesota. *Journal of Gerontological Social Work, 57*, 322–334. doi:10.1080/01634372.2013.843630

Muraco, A., & Fredriksen-Goldsen, K. I. (2014). The highs and lows of caregiving for chronically ill lesbian, gay, and bisexual elders. *Journal of Gerontological Social Work, 57*, 251–272. doi:10.1080/01634372.2013.860652

Portz, J. D., Retrum, J. H., Wright, L. A., Boggs, J. M., Wilkins, S., Grimm, C., . . . Gozansky, W. S. (2014). Assessing capacity for providing culturally competent services to LGBT older adults. *Journal of Gerontological Social Work, 57*, 305–321. doi:10.1080/01634372.2013.857378

Ramirez-Valles, J., Dirkes, J., & Barrett, H. A. (2014). GayBy Boomers' social support: Exploring the connection between health and emotional and instrumental support in older gay men. *Journal of Gerontological Social Work, 57*, 218–234. doi:10.1080/01634372.2013.843225

Rowan, N. L., & Butler, S. S. (2014). Resilience in attaining and sustaining sobriety among older lesbians with alcoholism. *Journal of Gerontological Social Work, 57*, 176–197. doi:10.1080/01634372.2013.859645

Sheets, D. (2014). [Review of the film *Transgender Tuesdays: A Clinic in the Tenderloin*, by M. Freeman]. *Journal of Gerontological Social Work, 57*, 413–415. doi:10.1080/01634372.2013.837308

Siverskog, A. (2014). "They just don't have a clue": Transgender aging and implications for social work. *Journal of Gerontological Social Work, 57*, 386–406. doi:10.1080/01634372.2014.895472

Sullivan, K. M. (2014). Acceptance in the domestic environment: The experience of senior housing for lesbian, gay, bisexual, and transgender seniors. *Journal of Gerontological Social Work, 57*, 235–250. doi:10.1080/01634372.2013.867002

Van Sluytman, L. G., & Torres, D. (2014). Hidden or uninvited? A content analysis of elder LGBT of color literature in gerontology. *Journal of Gerontological Social Work, 57*, 130–160. doi:10.1080/01634372.2013.877551

Creating a Vision for the Future: Key Competencies and Strategies for Culturally Competent Practice With Lesbian, Gay, Bisexual, and Transgender (LGBT) Older Adults in the Health and Human Services

KAREN I. FREDRIKSEN-GOLDSEN, CHARLES P. HOY-ELLIS,
and JAYN GOLDSEN

School of Social Work, University of Washington, Seattle, Washington, USA

CHARLES A. EMLET

Social Work Program, University of Washington, Tacoma, Washington, USA

NANCY R. HOOYMAN

School of Social Work, University of Washington, Seattle, Washington, USA

Sexual orientation and gender identity are not commonly addressed in health and human service delivery, or in educational degree programs. Based on findings from Caring and Aging with Pride: The National Health, Aging and Sexuality Study *(CAP), the first national federally-funded research project on LGBT health and aging, this article outlines 10 core competencies and aligns them with specific strategies to improve professional practice and service development to promote the well-being of LGBT older adults and their families. The articulation of key competencies is needed to provide a blueprint for action for addressing the growing needs of LGBT older adults, their families, and their communities.*

INTRODUCTION

By 2030, the number of lesbian, gay, bisexual, and transgender (LGBT) older adults in the United States will likely more than double, with 10,000 baby boomers turning 65-years old every day and continuing to do so for the next 17 years (Pew Research Center, 2010). LGBT adults are estimated to comprise between 3% and 4% of the general US adult population (Gates & Newport, 2012), and up to 11% when considering both sexual behavior and attraction (Gates, 2011). Yet, as a result of historical, social, and cultural forces, LGBT older adults have largely been invisible in the American landscape (Fredriksen-Goldsen & Muraco, 2010). Aging, combined with a history of marginalization and discrimination, increases the potential vulnerability of LGBT older adults, given heightened risks of discrimination and victimization, and the fear of and potential difficulty in accessing culturally responsive services.

LGBT older adults are an at-risk population, experiencing significant aging and health disparities (Fredriksen-Goldsen, Kim, et al., 2011). The first national and federally-funded research project, *Caring and Aging With Pride: The National Health, Aging and Sexuality Study* (CAP), was designed to better understand the risk and protective factors associated with aging, health, and well-being of LGBT midlife and older adults. In a comparison of key health indicators by sexual orientation, lesbian, gay, and bisexual older adults have higher rates of poor mental health and disability than their older heterosexual peers (Fredriksen-Goldsen, Kim, Barkan, Muraco, & Hoy-Ellis, 2013). The risk of cardiovascular disease and obesity is higher among older lesbians and bisexual women than for older heterosexual women; older gay and bisexual men are more likely than heterosexual men of similar age to have poor general health and to live alone (Fredriksen-Goldsen, Kim, Barkan, et al., 2013). Transgender older adults experience the highest rates of victimization as compared to nontransgender lesbian, gay, and bisexual adults, and have even higher rates of disability, stress, and poor mental and physical health (Fredriksen-Goldsen, Cook-Daniels, et al., 2013).

Despite the adversity experienced by many LGBT older adults, they display remarkable resilience. Many have built vibrant communities and a sensibility that they can count on each other, as exemplified during the height of the AIDS pandemic in the United States (Rofes, 1998). Many LGBT older adults have created close, intimate families of choice, comprised of loved ones, including current and former partners and friends (Heaphy, 2009). Yet, population estimates suggest that one-third to one-half of older gay and bisexual men live alone, without adequate services or supports (Fredriksen-Goldsen, Kim, Barkan, et al., 2013; Wallace, Cochran, Durazo, & Ford, 2011). In the CAP project, 61% of gay and 53% bisexual male participants reported experiencing loneliness (Fredriksen-Goldsen, Kim, et al., 2011).

Many in the LGBT community have been affected by the HIV/AIDS crisis. It is estimated that within 2 years, half of the 1.2 million Americans living with HIV will be 50 years old or older (High, Brennan-Ing, Clifford, Cohen, & Deeks, 2012). Even those who are not HIV-positive themselves have been affected by HIV, experiencing trauma and survivors' guilt through multiple cumulative losses from experiencing the deaths of friends, partners, and other loved ones (Rofes, 1998). This can have serious deleterious consequences for health and aging, which providers need to be aware of and be prepared to address (Wight, LeBlanc, de Vries, & Detels, 2012).

Need for LGBT-Specific Competencies

Social work students and practitioners often lack adequate knowledge and skills for competent practice with LGBT populations (Camilleri & Ryan, 2006; Fredriksen-Goldsen, Woodford, Luke, & Gutierrez, 2011; Logie, Bridge, & Bridge, 2007; Obedin-Maliver et al., 2011; Swank & Raiz, 2010), even though educational accreditation bodies address the need for preparedness for culturally competent practice. For example, the Council on Social Work Education (CSWE) prioritizes multicultural competency as an essential factor in both educational training and practice, with the inclusion of sexual and gender minority groups in definitions of multiculturalism (CSWE, 2008; National Association of Social Workers [NASW], 2008). The Patient Protection and Affordable Care Act mandates cultural competency in healthcare settings (Health Resources and Services Administration, 2012), with multiple initiatives intended to address health disparities and improve cultural competency with special populations, including LGBT and older adult populations.

Over the past several years, considerable efforts have also been made to increase the competence of both students and practitioners working with an aging population. Such competencies have been infused into social work curricula (Lee & Waites, 2006), as "social workers interact with older adults and their families in nearly all practice settings—child welfare, health and mental health, schools, domestic violence, and substance use to name a few—but are typically not formally prepared to do so" (CSWE Gero-Ed Center, 2013, para. 3). Additionally, efforts have been made to improve the competence of geriatric social work practitioners (Geron, Andrews, & Kuhn, 2005).

Knowledge, skills, and attitudes are three central components of culturally competent practice (Van Den Bergh & Crisp, 2004), which is foundational to removing barriers to accessing quality services and ensuring a qualified workforce in the health and human services. The identification of key competencies and content to support culturally competent practice is needed to provide a blueprint for action to address the growing social and health needs of LGBT older adults, their families, and their communities. The articulation and development of key competencies in this article is based on specific research findings with LGBT older adults and extant literature, as well as within the context of core competencies required by the CSWE (2008) Educational Policy and Accreditation Standards (EPAS), and the 2009 Geriatric Social Work Competency Scale II with Life-long Leadership Skills (GSW II). In this article, we outline key competencies and specific strategies to promote culturally competent practice with LGBT older adults and their families, and suggest specific strategies and resources to support these competencies.

METHODOLOGY

Competencies are composed of knowledge, attitudes, and values that are actualized through practice behaviors and assessable, measurable skills. The competencies articulated herein were developed based on a review of existing LGBT health and aging literature, CAP research findings, and an analysis of both CSWE's (2008) EPAS 10 core competencies, and the 2009 GSW II. The GSW II assesses micro and macro levels of practice via 50 skill-statements, utilizing a 5-point Likert scale (0 = *not skilled at all*, through 4 = *expert skill*). See CSWE (2010) for a full description of the iterative process used to establish these competencies.

In assessing each of the established sets of competencies, we asked, "What particular skills, knowledge, or attitudes are uniquely necessary for culturally competent practice with LGBT older adults at the required generalist level?" We also provide relevant background for each competency and suggest teaching content and resources to support attainment of students' and practitioners' competency at the generalist level. It is important to recognize that social work students engage in direct practice through foundational and advanced practica, and postdegree social work practitioners are required to engage in ongoing continuing education. Thus, the distinction between social work students and practitioners in regards to culturally competent practice and education is to some degree blurred.

Through the lens of LGBT aging, for this project we assessed the existing literature, the CAP findings, and both sets of competencies (i.e., EPAS, GSW II) for congruency and divergency for social work practice with LGBT older adults. Quotes from LGBT older adults who participated in the CAP study are included to highlight their voices and first-hand knowledge as they pertain to culturally competent practice. This process culminated with the 10 competencies recommended in this article, which are aligned with the the CSWE EPAS and the GSW II, and are summarized in Appendix A. These competencies are tailored to account for the unique circumstances, strengths, and challenges facing LGBT older adults.

1. Critically Analyze Personal and Professional Attitudes Toward Sexual Orientation, Gender Identity, and Age, and Understand How Factors Such as Culture, Religion, Media, and Health and Human Service Systems Influence Attitudes and Ethical Decision-Making

Heterosexism is the dominant culture's valuing of heterosexuality as the only natural, normal expression of human sexuality. When heterosexism is internalized, individuals, groups, and institutions hold and enact associated anti-LGBT stereotypes, beliefs, and attitudes. These may manifest in overt acts of victimization and discrimination, or covertly as attitudes existing below the level of awareness, inadvertently supporting discriminatory behaviors and conditions (Szymanski, Kashubeck-West, & Meyer, 2008).

Societal and internalized heterosexism also underlies ethical dilemmas in working with people with nonheteronormative identities. As a 66-year-old lesbian from the CAP study shared, "isolation, finding friend support, caregiving, and health are the biggest issues older gay persons face. Who will be there for us; who will help care for us without judgment?" Ageist stereotypes, beliefs, and attitudes operate in a manner similar to heterosexism (Cronin & King, 2010). Such biases embedded in personal and cultural beliefs are reinforced through religious doctrine, education, and the media.

Unaddressed biases can manifest in the form of micro-aggressions, "generally characterized as brief, daily assaults on minority individuals, which can be social or environmental, as well as intentional or unintentional" (Balsam, Molina, Beadnell, Simoni, & Walters, 2011, p. 163). Regardless of intent, these everyday experiences of assaults, insults, and invalidations can have profound and deleterious effects on LGBT older adults' mental and physical health, the helping relationship itself, and whether or not services are accessed and utilized.

The NASW Code of Ethics states that "social workers should obtain education about and seek to understand the nature of social diversity and oppression with respect to race, ethnicity, national origin, color, sex, *sexual orientation, gender identity* or *expression, age.* . ." (NASW, 2008, p. 1.05(c), italics added). Values related to serving those in need are reflected in the Hippocratic Oath, and in nursing (American Nurses Association, 2001). One of the challenges in applying ethics in social and health services settings that serve marginalized populations is that different cultures and groups often hold conflicting values (Kastrup, 2010). For example, religion has a long history of prescribing traditional gender norms and beliefs about heterosexuality. Such religious prescription has often been used to justify legal sanctioning of sexual and gender minorities (Tuck, 2012).

The NASW professional Code of Ethics mandates that professional values supersede personal values. Yet, some practitioners and students are instructed that if their moral or religious beliefs prevent them from treating sexual minorities with the same dignity and respect as any other client, they "should refer the client to someone who can" (Segal, Gerdes, & Steiner,

2013, p. 18). Such an approach creates unequal application and tensions in the prioritization of professional responsibilities, and is inconsistent with existing ethical standards.

Students and practitioners in the social and health services, regardless of their sexual orientation (Mulé, 2006), gender identity, or age, need to systematically and regularly assess their own attitudes and beliefs, and understand how these impact their ability to effectively deliver competent and unbiased care. Evidence-based self-assessment tools to support attainment of this competency include the Multicultural Counseling Inventory (Green et al., 2005); Age Is More, an online, self-scoring tool to assess ageism (Age Is More, 2013); and the Implicit Association Test, a self-administered, web-based assessment of implicit attitudes toward different cultural groups by characteristics such as sexual orientation, skin color, age, gender, and ability (Project Implicit, 2011).

Two online tools, *Ethics Framework: Overview* (Frolic et al., 2010), and *IDEA: Ethical Decision-Making Framework* (Trillium Health Centre, n.d.) can support achievement of the knowledge and skills to work through ethical dilemmas. Both provide overviews, rationales, detailed guidelines, and worksheets for dealing with ethical dilemmas. The key competency described here aligns with EPAS: Apply critical thinking to inform and communicate professional judgments and engage social work ethical principles to guide professional practice; and with GSW: assess and address values and biases regarding aging.

2. Understand and Articulate the Ways That Larger Social and Cultural Contexts May Have Negatively Impacted LGBT Older Adults as a Historically Disadvantaged Population

In culturally competent practice with LGBT older adults, it is important to understand not only the current contexts of their everyday lives, but also the continuing influence of historical, social, and cultural forces throughout the courses of their lives (Elder, 1994, 1998). Today's LGBT older adults constitute three different cohorts, including the Baby Boom Generation (b. 1946–1964), the Silent Generation (b. 1925–1945), and the Greatest Generation (b. 1901–1924); each cohort came of age during distinct historical periods. For example, the Silent Generation (those born prior to 1946) came of age during the McCarthy Era, a time when same-sex behavior and identities were severely pathologized and criminalized. The American Psychiatric Association considered homosexuality to be a "sociopathic personality disorder" until its removal from the *Diagnostic and Statistical Manual of Mental Disorders* (DSM) in 1973, with some LGBT people involuntarily committed and subjected to brutal treatments, including castration and lobotomy, in attempts to "cure" (Silverstein, 2009). Gender variance is still, even today, stigmatized in the DSM-5 (American Psychiatric Association, 2013), with gender dysphoria identified as a psychological disorder if gender nonconformity results in clinically significant distress. Given the historical circumstances of their lives, many LGBT older adults have spent years concealing their sexual orientation and gender identity from others, including health and human service providers.

Regardless of what point in the life course persons disclose their sexual orientation (e.g., adolescence, older adulthood), first awareness of same-sex sexual attraction often emerges in childhood, adolescence, or occasionally early adulthood, even if it is not acted upon (Floyd & Bakeman, 2006). Awareness of gender identity is evident even earlier, primarily during the preschool years (Halim, Ruble, & Amodio, 2011). That awareness is contextualized by the larger sociohistorical context, and is particularly salient during adolescence and early adulthood, when identity formation and individuation are critical. Hence, the consequences of a sexual or gender minority identity development during the McCarthy era may be quite different from today. For example, baby boomers, the current cohort of midlife adults, came of age during the civil rights and Stonewall gay liberation movements, and the beginning of the AIDS pandemic era, when same-sex behaviors and identities were becoming decriminalized. A gay male baby boomer who participated in the CAP project stated:

> I am trying to get my generation involved in the welfare and well-being of GLBT seniors. I was part of the first post-Stonewall generation that helped create gay communities and identities in the light of day, and feel it is extremely important for my generation to continue to create dialogue and programs for seniors—especially access to healthcare and affordable housing.

As they attend to LGBT people across the life course, health and human service providers must be cognizant of how different historical events, social structures, and cultural factors intersect with developmental trajectories to shape individual life experiences. Additionally, they must identify both the typical and unique normative experiences of LGBT people as they age, as well as distinct transitions over the life course, such as identity management (i.e., coming out or not), and how they influence service use. The growing body of literature on LGBT history and culture supports such knowledge development. Canaday (2009), and Knauer (2011) are two such examples. The documentary film *Gen Silent* is also an excellent resource that highlights the current and historical social and cultural contexts that have impacted older LGBT adults' lives; complimentary educational tools are also available (http://stumaddux.com/GEN_SILENT.html). This competency aligns with EPAS: Apply knowledge of human behavior and the social environment; and with GSW: Respect and promote older adult clients' right to dignity and self-determination.

3. Distinguish Similarities and Differences Within the Subgroups of LGBT Older Adults, as Well as Their Intersecting Identities (Such as Age, Gender, Race, and Health Status) to Develop Tailored and Responsive Health Strategies

Many LGBT older adults share a common history of discrimination, victimization, and marginalization, yet each of these subgroups (i.e., lesbians, gay men, bisexual, and transgender people) are increasingly being recognized as heterogeneous subgroups (Fredriksen-Goldsen, Kim, et al., 2011). For example, there are often important gender differences in health and service needs that require tailored responses. Despite having higher levels of education than their older heterosexual peers, older LGB adults do not have commensurate incomes (Fredriksen-Goldsen, Kim, Barkan, et al., 2013; Wallace et al., 2011); transgender older adults are at even greater risk of unemployment, underemployment, and poverty (Grant et al., 2011).

Just as LGBT people are silenced and marginalized in mainstream society, transgender and bisexual adults, regardless of age, are often obscured within the lesbian and gay communities, and older LGBT adults are often invisible within LGBT communities (Lyons, Pitts, Grierson, Thorpe, & Power, 2010). Bisexual and transgender older adults may feel a need to conceal their sexual orientation or gender identity in lesbian and gay communities (as well as in the larger society), which not only increases the risk of poor mental health outcomes, but may also preclude these groups from accessing important group and community level resources.

The ability to recognize the intersectional nature of social identities and oppression is a critical competency for health and human services providers. HIV-positive LGBT older adults, for example, experience at least three intersecting marginalized identities: being HIV positive, being older, and being a sexual and/or gender minority (Cahill & Valadéz, 2013). Their social networks may be constricted, compared to younger HIV-positive peers; HIV-positive older adults are significantly more likely to live alone and those of color may be even more socially isolated, impacting morbidity and mortality (Emlet, Fredriksen-Goldsen, & Kim, 2013).

Other LGBT individuals may experience additional obstacles due to other intersecting identities such as sexism, ableism, and socioeconomic bias. As a 76-year-old lesbian shared:

> I have been homeless, staying briefly on the streets, in car & [sic] in shelter . . . until my daughter began to help me. I am unable to get cataracts operated on as she cannot help me by paying for glasses and unable to get 2 [sic] hearing aides [sic] (medical pays for one).

The intersection of multiple identities along with the confluence of risk factors may mean that these older adults have unique and often unmet service needs.

The emerging literature on the distinct needs of subgroups of LGBT older adults, such as Addis, Davis, Greene, Macbride-Stewart, and Sheperd (2009), can support the attainment of this competency. Another learning resource is for practitioners to consult with specialists who have expertise in working with specific subgroups. Some states, such as Washington, require that mental health professionals obtain annual consultations with a certified specialist with expertise with certain designated special populations (e.g., LGBT, racial/ethnic minorities) to assure culturally competent services. The American Psychological Association provides a helpful overview of some of the important differences between lesbians, gay men, bisexual, and transgender individuals (DeAngelis, 2002). This competency aligns with EPAS: Engage diversity and difference in practice; and GSW: Respect diversity among older adult clients, families and professionals (e.g., class, race, ethnicity, gender and sexual orientation).

4. Apply Theories of Aging and Social and Health Perspectives and the Most Up-to-Date Knowledge Available to Engage in Culturally Competent Practice With LGBT Older Adults

Issues of aging are generally neglected in sexual and gender minority studies, just as sexual orientation and gender identity are largely absent in gerontological and health studies (Institute of Medicine, 2011). Health and human service providers must have knowledge of human behavior and the major theoretical approaches that facilitate an understanding of aging, sexual orientation, and gender identity. One unique aspect of the social work profession is its attention to the person-in-environment perspective (Segal et al., 2013), which maintains that the client-system (i.e., individual, family, group, community) can only be fully understood in the context of its environment. The life-course perspective posits that it is essential for providers to account for the historical eras in which lives are, and have been, linked and embedded (Elder, 1994, 1998). In addition to attention to intersectionality and the life-course perspective, the Institute of Medicine (2011) has suggested that the minority stress model (Meyer, 1995, 2003), and the social-ecological model (Centers for Disease Control and Prevention, 2009) are useful for understanding the complexities of LGBT lives.

The minority stress model explains the disparately high rates of psychological distress among LGBT populations relative to their heterosexual peers as being the result of stressors unique to sexual and gender minorities (Hendricks & Testa, 2012; Meyer, 1995, 2003). These stressors are in addition to general stressors (e.g., involuntary unemployment, bereavement). Minority stressors include external, objective discriminatory acts and conditions, and internal, subjective stressors, such as internalized heterosexism, concealment of minority identity, and expectations of rejection (Meyer, 2003).

The social-ecological model (Centers for Disease Control and Prevention, 2009) stresses the importance of attending to the dynamic interplay of factors at four levels across the life-span that place people at risk. The individual level attends to biological factors and personal histories, such as age, education, and minority status, that affect people's lives and outcomes. At the next level, relationships (e.g., partners/spouses, friends, family members) impact lived experiences and behaviors. At the community level, neighborhoods, employment, and other settings influence the dynamics of relationships. Finally, at the societal level are cultural and social standards, and social, health, and other policies that foster inequities and cultivate climates, which can either delimit or support human agency. An example of how these perspectives and theories could inform culturally competent practice with LGBT older adults is the selection of group work as a possible intervention. Although group work is often a useful intervention modality for older persons, LGBT older adults may not feel safe in groups that are composed primarily of heterosexual elders, which might harbor a climate hostile to sexual and gender minorities. A 71-year-old gay male CAP participant stated:

> Gay people do not choose to be gay. Could we try to make that common knowledge? Because all the bigotry (at least among adults) rests on the notion that we gays made the horrible choice to be attracted to people of the same sex or were somehow "recruited to the gay lifestyle." I believe we could try harder to dispel this myth.

Community-based organizations, such as the LGBT Aging Project of Boston (http://www.lgbtagingproject.org), National Resource Center on LGBT Aging (http://www.lgbtagingcenter.org/index.cfm), and Training to Serve in Minnesota (http://www.trainingtoserve.org) have successfully developed cultural competency trainings specific to LGBT aging. Such existing training models can be replicated or expanded to prepare health and human service providers to implement LGBT competent interventions. This competency aligns with EPAS: Apply knowledge of human behavior and the social environment; and with GSW: Relate social work perspectives and related theories to social work practice (e.g., cohorts, normal aging, and life course perspective).

5. When Conducting a Comprehensive Biopsychosocial Assessment, Attend to the Ways That the Larger Social Context and Structural and Environmental Risks and Resources May Impact LGBT Older Adults

Discrimination and victimization are chronic stressors that contribute to psychological distress. Lifetime experiences of discrimination and internalized heterosexism are significantly associated with poor mental health, physical health, and disability among older LGB (Fredriksen-Goldsen, Emlet, et al., 2013) and transgender adults (Fredriksen-Goldsen, Cook-Daniels, et al., 2013). More than 80% of CAP participants have been victimized at least once in their lives because of their sexual orientation or gender identity; over 60% have been three or more times (Fredriksen-Goldsen, Kim, et al., 2011). It is striking that a recent community-needs assessment of LGBT older adults living in San Francisco, known as a gay-friendly city, found that nearly half had been discriminated against during the past year because of their sexual orientation or gender identity (Fredriksen-Goldsen, Kim, Hoy-Ellis, et al., 2013).

Alienation can also emanate from within one's community. Bisexuality is often viewed as a nonlegitimate sexual orientation in lesbian and gay communities (Ochs, 1996; Weiss, 2003), and gender identity may be considered as alien among some LGB people (Lombardi, 2009). LGBT people of color experience racism within LGBT communities (Balsam et al., 2011; Stirratt, Meyer, Ouellette, & Gara, 2008). And, LGBT older adults are generally invisible in LGBT communities (Lyons et al., 2010), which often value and equate youth with beauty—just as the larger society does (Goltz, 2009; Jones & Pugh, 2005). As one older, HIV-positive man stated, "Yeah, ageism; it's a far mightier sword than HIV" (Emlet, 2006, p. 785). As part of a biopsychosocial assessment, an essential skill is to identify resources such as whether the person is connected to their respective LGBT community.

It is also critical that health and human services providers recognize the various structures of LGBT families, as well as the importance of families of choice in providing instrumental, emotional, and social support (Muraco & Fredriksen-Goldsen, 2011). Like the general population, LGBT individuals belong to an array of family structures: They may have a partner or spouse who may or may not be legally recognized across differing jurisdictions; they may have parents, siblings, and children; they may have a family of choice that provides needed support; or they may not have any family at all. LGBT families of choice are unique in that they often include former partners who remain friends, as well as other friends (Barker, Herdt, & de Vries, 2006). A 67-year-old lesbian CAP participant shared:

> My partner has two major diagnoses and I am the driver to the doctors. My sister and her husband and daughter are friendly but not caring, and not happy with me being gay, and will not allow us to stay there overnight. I have no real help should she get ill.

LGBT families-of-choice that are not related by blood or law are often unrecognized by providers, even though they provide consistent care, support, refuge, and nurturance to their members (Chapman et al., 2012). Although one in four LGBT older adults do have children (Fredriksen-Goldsen, Kim, et al., 2011) they are less likely to have children than their heterosexual peers (Fredriksen-Goldsen, Kim, Barkan, et al., 2013).

Among older adults in general, women provide the vast majority of informal care, primarily to legally or biologically related family members (Family Caregiver Alliance, 2003). However, in LGBT communities, men provide nearly as much care as women, with partners and friends primarily caring for one another (Fredriksen-Goldsen, Kim, et al., 2011). Although this social support provides essential resources, it also has its own set of challenges. As older LGBT adult peers reach older old ages, they may experience a diminished capacity to care for one another (Muraco & Fredriksen-Goldsen, 2011).

To effectively link clients to resources, providers should compile lists of both local and national resources relevant to the varying needs of LGBT older adults, their families, caregivers, and other supports. A good starting place is the National Resource Center on LGBT Aging (http://www.lgbtagingcenter.org/index.cfm), and Services and Advocacy for GLBT Elders (SAGE; http://www.sageusa.org/about/index.cfm). When providing such resources and referrals to LGBT older adults, it is important not to assume that what is salient to one group (e.g., lesbians) is salient to another (e.g., transgender). This competency aligns with EPAS: Engage, assess, intervene, and evaluate with individuals, families, groups, organizations and communities; and with GSW: Assess social functioning and social support of older clients.

6. When Using Empathy and Sensitive Interviewing Skills During Assessment and Intervention, Ensure the Use of Language Is Appropriate for Working With LGBT Older Adults to Establish and Build Rapport

Research indicates that individuals who hold negative attitudes, beliefs, and stereotypes regarding minority groups are likely to consciously or unconsciously convey those biases in their behavior (Shelton & Delgado-Romero, 2011), including their language. Those who work with LGBT older adults need to understand, and be comfortable with, the array of terms used to represent differing sexualities and gender identities. Sexual orientation and gender identity are distinct constructs, even though they are inextricably intertwined. *Sex* and *gender* are often used interchangeably, although the former relates to biology, and the latter refers to social constructions based on biology. Transgender identity refers an individual's innermost sense of self as female, male, or other sense of self that is incongruent with biological sex. Sexual orientation (i.e., lesbian, gay, bisexual, heterosexual) refers to an:

enduring pattern of emotional, romantic, and/or sexual attractions to women, men, or both sexes and also refers to a person's sense of identity based on those attractions, related behaviors, and membership in a community of others who share those attractions. (American Psychological Association, 2010, p. 74)

It is also important to remain cognizant of ascribed versus claimed identities. For example, researchers may ascribe a sexual minority identity to study participants (i.e., lesbian, gay, bisexual) based on same-sex attraction or behavior, but the participants themselves might not claim that identity; instead, they may identify differently (i.e., heterosexual).

LGBT older adults are often characterized as a homogenous group and even though the umbrella term *LGBT* is most often used, it can be exclusionary. Other terms are also used, such as *queer, questioning, intersex*, and *two-spirit*. There are also critical differences by age in the terminology used. Although *H* for *homosexuality* is typically not used in the LGBT acronym, it may be the preferred term used by some older gay men; some lesbians prefer to identify as gay. Likewise, although many LGBT people have embraced the term *queer* to regain and reclaim power, it still has enormously negative connotations for many older LGBT adults. It is also important to be cognizant of related terms. For example, *coming out* refers to disclosing one's sexual orientation or gender identity, and *closeting* means to conceal said orientation or identity or to pass as heterosexual or nontransgender. Equally important is the ability of health and human service providers to be aware of the language used by LGBT older adults, themselves, as those are the terms that most likely represent their lives and identities. A 58-year-old transgender bisexual woman who participated in the CAP project remarked:

> Long-term health care for trans people is a big, dark unknown. How long do we take hormones? How do trans people who don't "pass" get decent treatment and respect? And "passing" is all but impossible in some medical contexts. Where do trans people who do *not* identify as LBG fit into the picture?"

To support attainment of this competency and the use of culturally competent and appropriate language, the sixth edition of the *Publication Manual of the American Psychological Association* provides excellent guidelines for using language to reduce bias (American Psychological Association, 2010). As good rules of thumb, these guidelines highlight the importance of vocabulary in conveying respect while avoiding language that marginalizes (for example, avoid using *sexual preference*, as it implies choice).

Additionally, students and practitioners need to hone active listening skills, because many LGBT older adults welcome the opportunity to communicate their preferred terms and vocabulary. If disclosure as LGBT to a service provider is met with a neutral response, that response may well be interpreted as hostile (Harding, Epiphaniou, & Chidgey-Clark, 2012). Usage of appropriate language is a powerful way to convey empathy, understanding, and respect, as well as to facilitate the establishment of rapport. This competency aligns with EPAS: Assess with individuals, families, groups, organizations and communities; and with GSW: Use empathy and sensitive interviewing skills to engage older clients in identifying their strengths and problems.

7. Understand and Articulate the Ways in Which Agency, Program, and Service Policies Do or Do Not Marginalize and Discriminate Against LGBT Older Adults

In addition to discrimination in the larger society, LGBT older adults experience both overt and covert discrimination in health and human service settings. Discrimination within healthcare systems is a significant predictor of poor mental and physical health (Fredriksen-Goldsen & Muraco, 2010). Thirteen percent of CAP participants have been denied healthcare or received inferior care because of their sexual orientation or gender identity. Invisibility of LGBT older adults is pervasive across healthcare settings, and is a subtle form of discrimination (Brotman, Ryan, & Cormier, 2003).

Many providers are unaware that LGBT older adults are utilizing their services (Hughes, Harold, & Boyer, 2011). This can be especially damaging for LGBT older adults in long-term care facilities, where many may opt to go back into the closet due to fear and lack of support (National Senior Citizens Law Center, 2011). This invisibility leads to exclusion and marginalization, exacerbating feelings of loneliness and social isolation (LGBT Movement Advancement Project & SAGE, 2010). Unfortunately, such situations support nondisclosure of a stigmatized identity, which is a risk factor for poor health outcomes (Durso & Meyer, 2013).

Many health and human services adopt a *sexuality-blind* norm through avoiding the topic of sexuality and treating patients as asexual, especially older adults (Cronin, Ward, Pugh, King, & Price, 2011). As few as one in five healthcare providers routinely take a sexual history as part of new client intakes (Gay and Lesbian Medical Association, 2002). Thus, the importance of careful and in-depth examination of discriminatory and exclusionary behaviors among health care and human service professionals cannot be overemphasized. Although some healthcare organizations are committed to providing LGBT-centered patient care, only half of such organizations in one study expressed interest in including patients' sexual orientation or gender identity in their medical records (Snowden, 2013). As many as one in five LGBT older adults are concealing their sexual orientation or gender identity from their primary care physician (Fredriksen-Goldsen, Kim, et al., 2011). The American Medical Association (2009) has acknowledged that lack of attention to patients' sexual orientation can profoundly and negatively impact the delivery and quality of medical care. A 59-year-old transgender woman who participated in CAP commented, "The health care facility needs to revamp their policies on treatment of LGBT people. My partner and I are both [female] transsexuals but are treated as men when it comes to the services." It is imperative that health and human service organizations have explicit nondiscrimination policies in place, banning discrimination by sexual orientation and gender identity within the organization, as well as with agencies that provide contracted services.

To support the attainment of this competency, students and practitioners should begin with a review of all agency policies to determine if sexual orientation, sexual behavior, and gender identity are explicitly addressed. All assessment tools and standardized forms should be reviewed to ensure they are LGBT-inclusive. For example, clients should not have to select between inaccurate or inappropriate choices, such as between married or single. In addition, collection of patient-level data that includes sexual orientation and gender identity information can contribute to our understanding of LGBT older adults' health, social, and aging needs (Institute of Medicine, 2011).

A useful tool for assessing agency policies regarding LGBT clients is the Human Rights Campaign's Healthcare Equality Index (HEI; http://www.hrc.org/hei#.Um1UOoPn9LM). In addition to this annual online survey, available to healthcare organizations seeking to provide equitable, inclusive care to the LGBT community, it is also available to LGBT people looking for healthcare providers who have shown that they are proactive in providing culturally competent care (Snowden, 2013). In addition to being evaluated in four core areas with more than 30 best practices in LGBT culturally competent care, healthcare organizations that participate in the HEI are able to receive expert trainings for staff at no charge (http://www.hrc.org/hei/#.Uff51czn-po). This competency aligns with EPAS: Assess with individuals, families, groups, organizations and communities; and with GSW: Conduct a comprehensive geriatric assessment (bio-psychosocial evaluation).

8. Understand and Articulate the Ways That Local, State, and Federal Laws Negatively and Positively Impact LGBT Older Adults, to Advocate on Their Behalf

With the increasing acceptance of sexual and gender minorities in the United States, health and human service providers may assume that such discrimination is a thing of the past. However, discrimination based on sexual orientation is still legal in 29 states, and discrimination based on gender identity is legal in 33 states (Human Rights Campaign, 2013a). This is despite evidence that LGBT people that live in states that have passed antidiscrimination legislation and other legal protections experience significant decreases in psychological distress (i.e., mood, anxiety disorders), yet the opposite is true for those living in states that have passed anti-LGBT legislation (Hatzenbuehler, Keyes, & Hasin, 2009; Riggle, Rostosky, & Horne, 2010; Rostosky, Riggle, Horne, & Miller, 2009). Because LGBT older adults rely primarily on each other for social, emotional, and instrumental support, laws and policies that do not recognize the relationships of families of choice may also marginalize LGBT older adults economically.

There is a popular myth that LGBT individuals are affluent. Although some certainly are, research indicates that, despite significantly higher levels of education, LGBT people often earn less than heterosexuals. Because lifetime earnings have a significant impact on retirement age, LGBT older adults are at a distinct disadvantage economically (Grant, 2010). Older lesbian and bisexual women and transgender older adults are at particular risk for living in poverty (Fredriksen-Goldsen, Cook-Daniels, et al., 2013; Wallace et al., 2011).

Advocacy for justice (Killian, 2010) and the passing of laws in favor of equality is undeniably important to support the health and well-being of LGBT older adults. A 56-year-old lesbian CAP participant impacted by the lack of legal protections stated, "I worry a lot about my future, as I really age—not so much now. And if anything happens to my partner, I'll be in big trouble; my medical insurance and household income come through her." Because policies related to aging generally assume heterosexuality, they have historically discriminated against LGBT older adults and their partners and families. For example, Social Security provides significant economic benefits to older Americans, including spousal and survivors' benefits, that until recently were not available to same-sex couples. In *Windsor v. United States*, the Supreme Court struck down Section 3 of the Defense of Marriage Act as unconstitutional. Although the ruling extends federal recognition to legal same-sex marriages and provides access to Social Security spousal and survivors' benefits to LGBT older adults in legal marriages, it also left Section 2 intact, which recognizes states' right to refuse to recognize same-sex marriages performed in states where they are legal (Human Rights Campaign, 2013b). Although a growing number of states recognize same-sex marriage, LGBT older adults who live in states without legal same-sex marriage will not be able to access federal benefits unless they are able to travel to and be married in a state that sanctions same-sex marriages.

Health and human services providers who are culturally competent in LGBT issues are uniquely positioned to advocate for policies and laws that foster the dignity and worth of LGBT older adults, and the importance of their relationships. Organizations such as the Human Rights Campaign (http://

www.hrc.org/) and Lambda Legal (http://www.lambdalegal.org/) offer comprehensive and up-to-date information on laws, policies, and initiatives that impact the LGBT community. The Diverse Elders Coalition (http://www.diverseelders.org/) provides similar information specific to older adults who are racial, ethnic, sexual, or gender minorities. These resources can help health and human services providers understand the impact of laws and policies in LGBT older adults' lives, as well as assist LGBT older adults and their families. This competency aligns with EPAS: Engage, assess intervene, and evaluate with individuals, families, groups, organizations, and communities; and with GSW: Assess social functioning and social support of older clients.

9. Provide Sensitive and Appropriate Outreach to LGBT Older Adults, Their Families, Caregivers and Other Supports to Identify and Address Service Gaps, Fragmentation, and Barriers That Impact LGBT Older Adults

Past experiences of discrimination may make vulnerable older adults less likely to seek services from the very agencies that have historically marginalized them. In addition, some agencies may resist outreach efforts to not offend private donors (Knochel, Quam, & Croghan, 2010). Many LGBT older adults feel unwelcome in aging programs and services (LGBT Movement Advancement Project & SAGE, 2010), and feel they must conceal their sexual orientation (National Senior Citizens Law Center, 2011). Concealment of one's LGBT identity or orientation is associated with intensified psychological distress (Meyer, 2003), which, in turn, increases the risk of premature illness and death (Russ et al., 2012). A 63-year-old lesbian CAP participant shared:

> I work with a number of LGBT clients in nursing home environments and find them to be extremely isolated and actually have become "recloseted" due to community living with elderly heterosexual populations. Lack of transportation and outreach prohibit them from access to the LGBT community.

Even when agency staffs are open and affirming, other clientele (i.e., older heterosexual adults) may display anti-LGBT attitudes and behaviors. Cultural competency trainings should prepare staff and residents with strategies to respond effectively to such incidents.

Lack of adequate training may be an unacknowledged barrier that can impact the provision of appropriate services to LGBT older adults. Professional programs in various disciplines devote limited time and content to LGBT health, including medicine (Obedin-Maliver et al., 2011), nursing

(Eliason, Dibble, & Dejoseph, 2010), and social work (Logie et al., 2007). Three out of four social service directors in skilled nursing facilities report receiving no training in LGBT cultural competency in the preceding 5 years (Bell, Bern-Klug, Kramer, & Saunders, 2010). Only one in four healthcare organizations participating in the recent Health Equality Index survey indicated that they had reviewed their clinical services to identify gaps in the provision of services to LGBT patients, although another 54% indicated that they were interested in doing so (Snowden, 2013).

Recruiting LGBT older adults to serve on community advisory boards and other volunteer venues in LGBT and mainstream agencies will help to ensure that their voices are a central part of the mission and delivery of services; this can also provide expert insider perspectives regarding fragmentation of and gaps in existing programs and services, as well as how existing programs and services may be discriminatory. Such recruitment is likely to be challenging, especially in light of current and historic discrimination. An initial, yet critical, first step in this process is to communicate to LGBT older adults that the agency or program seeking their input is LGBT-affirming.

A resource for agencies and programs to communicate to LGBT older adults that they are LGBT affirming is the Safe Zone Project. Originally developed and implemented in university settings, the Safe Zone Project is "an adjunctive training module—one that signifies the acceptance and affirmation of LGBT individuals, and a commitment to training, recruitment, and retention of LGBT and LGBT-sensitive [staff]" (Finkel, Storaasli, Bandele, & Schaefer, 2003, p. 555), is becoming increasingly common in business and health and human service settings. Some Safe Zone training materials can be accessed online.[1] Posting Safe Zone signs and having other visible cues (e.g., LGBT magazines, posters) signal that the agency, service, or program is LGBT sensitive and affirming. In addition, LGBT services and programs should also provide visual cues that they are affirming of older LGBT adults, and whenever possible, develop programming specific to their particular issues. This competency aligns with EPAS: Respond to contexts that shape practice; and with GSW: Identify and develop strategies to address service gaps, fragmentation, discrimination and barriers that impact older persons.

10. Enhance the Capacity of LGBT Older Adults and Their Families, Caregivers, and Other Supports to Navigate Aging, Social, and Health Services

As older adults age, they are likely to experience an increased need for social and health services. The provision of human services in the United States has been historically bound with the profession of social work. Because of its

---

[1]   See for example: http://www2.webster.edu/shared/shared_selfstudyreport/documents/hlc1b1_safezone.pdf

complex and fragmented nature, navigating the system of social and health services can be daunting and frustrating at times.

Health and human service professionals can play a crucial role in helping LGBT older adults navigate the fragmented health and human services system, while advocating for the best possible solutions to the distinct challenges they face. As daunting as this system is, it is even more so for LGBT older adults because of discriminatory laws and policies, as well as agencies and programs failure to recognize and address the distinct needs of LGBT older adults. In addition, LGBT older adults may not have biologically or legally related family members to assist in navigating such systems, which older heterosexual adults often do (Brotman et al., 2003). Even when LGBT older adults do have friends or family-of-choice members to assist them, such assistance can be challenging not only because they, themselves, may also have aging- and health-related needs, but also because of confidentiality, legal decision-making authority, and other related issues (Muraco & Fredriksen-Goldsen, 2011).

It is also important to recognize that LGBT older adults have unique strengths that can be harnessed to empower them in navigating the complex array of social and health services. Some LGBT older adults continue to be socially and politically active, fighting for civil rights and social justice issues, which may enhance their resilience as they age (Ramirez-Valles, Kuhns, Campbell, & Diaz, 2010). Several studies have found that LGBT older adults are strengthened through "crisis competence," applying lessons learned from being a sexual minority to the aging process (Friend, 1991, p. 110). The biopsychosocial model for late life resilience (Smith & Hayslip, 2012) suggests that older adults can engage individual, interpersonal, and environmental resources to combat elements of risk and adversity. Professionals in the field need the knowledge, skills, and values to identify intrapersonal and interpersonal resources with older LGBT consumers, and to assist them in addressing their needs, those of their families, and other support systems. A 77-year-old gay male CAP participant affirmed:

> It makes sense to focus a lot of attention and work on educating mainstream senior service agencies and institutions to provide LGBT-sensitive and gay-friendly services. I know that there have been many advances already made in that direction, and I hope it continues. Educating mainstream services is also part of the larger movement toward integrating LGBT people of all ages and LGBT culture into the larger society.

In addition to educating LGBT older adults about available services and supports, asking for their expert knowledge can empower them to become advocates for themselves and others. The National Center on LGBT Aging also provides trainings free of charge that can help agencies and programs to be better able to enhance the capacity of LGBT older adults and their families, caregivers, and other supports to navigate aging, social, and health services. Two of these trainings are for general aging services providers; two others are for LGBT organizations (http://www.lgbtagingcenter.org/about/training.cfm). This competency aligns with EPAS: Engage in policy practice to advance social and economic well-being and to deliver effective social work services; and with GSW: Advocate on behalf of clients with agencies and other professionals to help elders obtain quality services.

DISCUSSION

Students and practitioners in the social and health services have generally not been well prepared to practice in a culturally competent manner with LGBT populations (Camilleri & Ryan, 2006; Fredriksen-Goldsen, Woodford, et al., 2011; Logie et al., 2007; Obedin-Maliver et al., 2011; Swank & Raiz, 2010). It should not be incumbent upon LGBT older adults to educate providers, services, and programs about their unique challenges and needs; this responsibility lies squarely on the shoulders of providers, educations, and other stakeholders. The competencies outlined herein can serve both educational and evaluative purposes; implementing them into practice, policy, and research will improve the effectiveness of each as they relate to LGBT older adults. Health and human service providers who are culturally competent in LGBT issues are uniquely positioned to advocate for practice modalities and policies that foster the dignity and worth of LGBT older adults, and the importance of their relationships and families.

It is time to more fully envelop the notion of inclusion, that is "including" LGBT older adults, through the notion of "nothing about us without us" (Charlton, 2000). This perspective highlights the importance of meaningfully engaging of community members in the process of practice, program, and policy development. Furthermore, the identification of successful programs and policies at the local, state, and federal levels that address the health and aging needs of LGBT older adults can be used as models and adapted for use in diverse urban, suburban, and rural communities.

The recommended competencies outlined here cover a wide range of issues and challenges in developing culturally relevant and sensitive practice modalities, yet they are by no means exhaustive. Future work will undoubtedly point to the need for additional competencies and require the refinement of what has been presented here. In the CAP study, participants were contacted though mailing lists maintained by agencies so the results are not generalizable or necessarily representative of LGBT older adults, and those who remain most hard to reach are likely underrepresented. The agencies are primarily located in major metropolitan areas so the needs and concerns of LGBT older adults living in rural areas need further investigation.

Although practitioners and educators have ethical mandates to be knowledgeable and competent in working with diverse populations, content relevant to the lives of LGBT older adults is largely absent in training and educational programs. Implementing standardized and comprehensive competencies will enhance the ability of social and health service providers to address both the needs and challenges facing LGBT older adults and their families, and, at the same time, acknowledge and support the resilience and many resources that exist within these communities. A 63-year-old CAP participant shared, "The LGBT community has stepped up in the past to address coming out, AIDS, and civil rights. The next wave has to be aging."

REFERENCES

Addis, S., Davies, M., Greene, G., Macbride-Stewart, S., & Shepherd, M. (2009). The health, social care and housing needs of lesbian, gay, bisexual and transgender older people: A review of the literature. *Health & Social Care in the Community, 17*, 647–658. doi:10.1111/j.1365-2524.2009.00866.x

Age Is More. (2013). *Quiz: Are you age aware?* Retrieved from http://ageismore.com/Ageismore/About/Age-Aware-Quiz.aspx

American Medical Association. (2009). *AMA policy regarding sexual orientation: H-65.973 Health care disparities in same-sex partner households.* Houston, TX: Author.

American Nurses Association. (2001). *Code of ethics for nurses with interpretive statements.* Retrieved from http://www.sfcc.edu/files/SFCC_NursingStudent Handbook_Fall2009-Spring2011.pdf

American Psychiatric Association. (2013). *Diagnostic and statistical manual of mental disorders* (5th ed.). Arlington, VA: American Psychiatric Publishing.

American Psychological Association. (2010). *Publication manual of the American Psychological Association* (6th ed.). Washington, DC: Author.

Balsam, K. F., Molina, Y., Beadnell, B., Simoni, J., & Walters, K. (2011). Measuring multiple minority stress: The LGBT People of Color Microaggressions Scale. *Cultural Diversity & Ethnic Minority Psychology, 17*, 163–174. doi:10.1037/a0023244

Barker, J. C., Herdt, G., & de Vries, B. (2006). Social support in the lives of lesbians and gay men at midlife and later. *Sexuality Research & Social Policy, 3*, 1–23.

Bell, S. A., Bern-Klug, M., Kramer, K. W. O., & Saunders, J. B. (2010). Most nursing home social service directors lack training in working with lesbian, gay, and bisexual residents. *Social Work in Health Care, 49*, 814–831. doi:10.1080/00981389.2010.494561

Brotman, S., Ryan, B., & Cormier, R. (2003). The health and social service needs of gay and lesbian elders and their families in Canada. *Gerontologist, 43*, 192–202.

Cahill, S., & Valadéz, R. (2013). Growing older with HIV/AIDS: New public health challenges. *American Journal of Public Health, 103*(3), e7–e15. doi:10.2105/AJPH.2012.301161

Camilleri, P., & Ryan, M. (2006). Social work students' attitudes toward homosexuality and their knowledge and attitudes toward homosexual parenting as an alternative family unit: An Australian study. *Social Work Education, 25*, 288–304. doi:10.5175/JSWE.2011.200300018

Canaday, M. (2009). *The straight state: Sexuality and citizenship in twentieth-century America.* Princeton, NJ: Princeton University Press.

Centers for Disease Control and Prevention. (2009). *The social-ecological model: A framework for prevention.* Retrieved from http://www.cdc.gov/violenceprevention/overview/social-ecologicalmodel.html

Chapman, R., Wardrop, J., Freeman, P., Zappia, T., Watkins, R., & Shields, L. (2012). A descriptive study of the experiences of lesbian, gay and transgender parents accessing health services for their children. *Journal of Clinical Nursing, 21*, 1128–1135. doi:10.1111/j.1365-2702.2011.03939.x

Charlton, J. I. (2000). *Nothing about us without us: Disability, oppression, and empowerment.* Berkeley: University of California Press.

Council on Social Work Education. (2008). *Educational policy and accreditation standards.* Retrieved from http://www.cswe.org/File.aspx?id=13780

Council on Social Work Education Gero-Ed Center. (2013). *About the Gero-Ed Center.* Retrieved from http://www.cswe.org/CentersInitiatives/GeroEdCenter/AboutGeroEd.aspx

Cronin, A., & King, A. (2010). Power, inequality and identification: Exploring diversity and intersectionality amongst older LGB adults. *Sociology: Journal of the British Sociological Association, 44*, 876–892. doi:10.1177/0038038510375738

Cronin, A., Ward, R., Pugh, S., King, A., & Price, E. (2011). Categories and their consequences: Understanding and supporting the caring relationships of older lesbian, gay and bisexual people. *International Social Work, 54*, 421–435.

DeAngelis, T. (2002). A new generation of issues for LGBT clients. *Monitor on Psychology, 33*(2), 45. Retrieved from http://www.apa.org/monitor/feb02/generation.aspx

Durso, L. E., & Meyer, I. H. (2013). Patterns and predictors of disclosure of sexual orientation to healthcare providers among lesbians, gay men, and bisexuals. *Sexuality Research and Social Policy, 10*(1), 35–42. doi:10.1007/s13178-012-0105-2

Elder, G. H. (1994). Time, human agency, and social change perspectives on the life-course. *Social Psychology Quarterly, 57*, 4–15.

Elder, G. H. (1998). The life course as developmental theory. *Child Development, 69*, 1–12.

Eliason, M. J., Dibble, S., & Dejoseph, J. (2010). Nursing's silence on lesbian, gay, bisexual, and transgender issues: The need for emancipatory efforts. *ANS: Advances in Nursing Science, 33*(3), 206–218. doi:10.1097/ANS.0b013e3181e63e49

Emlet, C. A. (2006). "You're awfully old to have *this* disease": Experiences of stigma and ageism in adults 50 years an older living with HIV/AIDS. *Gerontologist, 46*, 781–790.

Emlet, C. A., Fredriksen-Goldsen, K. I., & Kim, H. J. (2013). Risk and protective factors associated with health-related quality of life among older gay and bisexual men living with HIV disease. *Gerontologist, 53*, 963–972. doi:10.1093/geront/gns191

Family Caregiver Alliance. (2003). *Women and caregiving: Facts and figures*. Retrieved from http://www.caregiver.org/caregiver/jsp/content_node.jsp?nodeid=892

Finkel, M. J., Storaasli, R. D., Bandele, A., & Schaefer, V. (2003). Diversity training in graduate school: An exploratory evaluation of the Safe Zone project. *Professional Psychology-Research and Practice, 34*, 555–561. doi:10.1037/0735-7028.34.5.555

Floyd, F. J., & Bakeman, R. (2006). Coming out across the life course: Implications of age and historical context. *Archives of Sexual Behavior, 35*, 287–296. doi:10.1007/s10508-006-9022-x

Fredriksen-Goldsen, K. I., Cook-Daniels, L., Kim, H. J., Erosheva, E. A., Emlet, C. A., Hoy-Ellis, C. P., . . . Muraco, A. (2013). Physical and mental health of transgender older adults: An at-risk and underserved population. *Gerontologist*. Advance online publication. doi:10.1093/geront/gnt021

Fredriksen-Goldsen, K. I., Emlet, C. A., Kim, H. J., Muraco, A., Erosheva, E. A., Goldsen, J., & Hoy-Ellis, C. P. (2013). The physical and mental health of lesbian, gay male, and bisexual (LGB) older adults: The role of key health indicators and risk and protective factors. *Gerontologist, 53*, 664–675. doi:10.1093/geront/gns123

Fredriksen-Goldsen, K. I., Kim, H.-J., Barkan, S. E., Muraco, A., & Hoy-Ellis, C. P. (2013). Health disparities among lesbian, gay male and bisexual older adults: Results from a population-based study. *American Journal of Public Health, 103*, 1802–1809. doi:10.2105/AJPH.2012.301110

Fredriksen-Goldsen, K. I., Kim, H.-J., Emlet, C. A., Muraco, A., Erosheva, E. A., Hoy-Ellis, C. P., . . . Petry, H. (2011). *The aging and health report: Disparities and resilience among lesbian, gay, bisexual, and transgender older adults*. Seattle, WA: Institute for Multigenerational Health.

Fredriksen-Goldsen, K. I., Kim, H.-J., Hoy-Ellis, C. P., Goldsen, J., Jensen, D., Adelman, M., . . . De Vries, B. (2013). *Addressing the needs of LGBT older adults in San Francisco: Recommendations for the future*. Seattle, WA: Institute for Multigenerational Health.

Fredriksen-Goldsen, K. I., & Muraco, A. (2010). Aging and sexual orientation: A 25-year review of the literature. *Research on Aging, 32*(3), 372–413. doi:10.1177/0164027509360355

Fredriksen-Goldsen, K. I., Woodford, M. R., Luke, K. P., & Gutierrez, L. (2011). Support of sexual orientation and gender identity content in social work education: Results from national surveys of U.S. and Anglophone Canadian faculty. *Journal of Social Work Education, 47*, 19–35. doi:10.5175/JSWE.2011.200900018

Friend, R. A. (1991). Older lesbian and gay people: A theory of successful aging. *Journal of Homosexuality, 20*(3), 99–118.

Frolic, A., Flaherty, B., Fung, S., Jennings, B., Hutchinson, D., Green, L. T., & Cripps, D. (2010). *Ethics framework: Overview*. Retrieved from http://hamilton healthsciences.ca/workfiles/CLINICAL_ETHICS/HHSEthicsFramework.pdf

Gates, G. J. (2011). *How many people are lesbian, gay, bisexual, and transgender?* Los Angeles, CA: Williams Institute—UCLA School of Law.

Gates, G. J., & Newport, F. (2012, October 18). *Special report: 3.4% of U.S. adults identify as LGBT*. Retrieved from http://www.gallup.com/poll/158066/special-report-adults-identify-lgbt.aspx

Gay and Lesbian Medical Association. (2002). *MSM: Clinician's guide to incorporating sexual risk assessment in routine visits*. Washington, DC: Author.

Geron, S., Andrews, C., & Kuhn, K. (2005). Infusing aging skills into the social work practice community: A new look at strategies for continuing professional education. *Families in Society, 86*, 431–440. doi:10.1606/1044-3894.3442

Goltz, D. (2009). Investigating queer future meanings: Destructive perceptions of "the harder path." *Qualitative Inquiry, 15*, 561–586.

Grant, J. M. (2010). *Outing age 2010: Public policy issues affecting lesbian, gay, bisexual, and transgender elders*. Washington, DC: National Gay and Lesbian Task Force Policy Institute.

Grant, J. M., Mottet, L. A., Tanis, J., Harrison, J., Herman, J. L., & Keisling, M. (2011). *Injustice at every turn: A look at Black respondents in the National Transgender Discrimination Survey*. Washington, DC: National Center for Transgender Equality and National Gay and Lesbian Task Force.

Green, R. G., Kitson, G., Kiernan-Stern, M., Leek, S., Bailey, K., Leisey, M., ... Jones, G. (2005). The multicultural counseling inventory: A measure for evaluating social work student and practitioner self-perceptions of their multicultural competencies. *Journal of Social Work Education, 41*, 191–208.

Halim, M. L., Ruble, D. N., & Amodio, D. M. (2011). From pink frilly dresses to 'one of the boys': A social-cognitive analysis of gender identity development and gender bias. *Social and Personality Psychology Compass, 5*, 933–949. doi:10.1111/j.1751-9004.2011.00399.x

Harding, R., Epiphaniou, E., & Chidgey-Clark, J. (2012). Needs, experiences, and preferences of sexual minorities for end-of-life care and palliative care: A systematic review. *Journal of Palliative Medicine, 15*, 602–611. doi:10.1089/jpm.2011.0279

Hatzenbuehler, M. L., Keyes, K. M., & Hasin, D. S. (2009). State-level policies and psychiatric morbidity in lesbian, gay, and bisexual populations. *American Journal of Public Health, 99*, 2275–2281. doi:10.2105/AJPH.2008.153510

Health Resources and Services Administration. (2012). *Special populations: Culture, language, & health literacy resources*. Retrieved from http://www.hrsa.gov/culturalcompetence/specialpopulations.html

Heaphy, B. (2009). The storied, complex lives of older GLBT adults: Choice and its limits in older lesbian and gay narratives of relational life. *Journal of GLBT Family Studies, 5*(1–2), 119–138.

Hendricks, M. L., & Testa, R. J. (2012). A conceptual framework for clinical work with transgender and gender noncomforming clients: An adaptation of the minority stress model. *Professional Psychology: Research and Practice, 43*, 460–467. doi:10.1037/a0029597

High, K. P., Brennan-Ing, M., Clifford, D. B., Cohen, M. H. C., J., & Deeks, S. G. (2012). HIV and aging: State of knowledge and areas of clinical need for research. A report to the NIH office of AIDS research by the HIV and aging working group. *Journal of Acquired Immune Deficiency Syndromes, 60*(Suppl 1), S1–S18.

Hughes, A. K., Harold, R. D., & Boyer, J. M. (2011). Awareness of LGBT aging issues among aging services network providers. *Journal of Gerontological Social Work*, *54*, 659–677. doi:10.1080/01634372.2011.585392

Human Rights Campaign. (2013a). *Employment Non-Discrimination Act. Issue: Federal advocacy*. Retrieved from http://www.hrc.org/laws-and-legislation/federal-legislation/employment-non-discrimination-act

Human Rights Campaign. (2013b). *Respect for Marriage Act. Issue: Federal advocacy*. Retrieved from http://www.hrc.org/laws-and-legislation/federal-legislation/respect-for-marriage-act?gclid=CN665JXGt7oCFSU6QgodMBIA6Q

Institute of Medicine. (2011). *The health of lesbian, gay, bisexual, and transgender people: Building a foundation for better understanding*. Washington, DC: National Academies Press.

Jones, J., & Pugh, S. (2005). Aging gay men: Lessons from the sociology of embodiment. *Men and Masculinities*, *7*, 248–260.

Kastrup, M. (2010). Ethical aspects in providing care to marginalized populations. *International Review of Psychiatry*, *22*, 252–257. doi:10.3109/09540261.2010.484015

Killian, M. L. (2010). The political is personal: Relationship recognition policies in the United States and their impact on services for LGBT people. *Journal of Gay & Lesbian Social Services*, *22*, 9–21. doi:10.1080/10538720903332149

Knauer, N. J. (2011). *Gay and lesbian elders: History, law, and identity politics in the United States*. Burlington, VT: Ashgate.

Knochel, K. A., Quam, J. K., & Croghan, C. F. (2010). Are old lesbian and gay people well served? Understanding the perceptions, preparation, and experiences of aging services providers. *Journal of Applied Gerontology*, *30*, 370–379. doi:10.1177/0733464810369809

Lee, E.-K. O., & Waites, C. E. (2006). Innovations in gerontological social work education infusing aging content across the curriculum: Innovations in baccalaureate social work education. *Journal of Social Work Education*, *42*, 49–66.

LGBT Movement Advancement Project & SAGE. (2010). *Improving the lives of LGBT older adults*. Denver, CO: Author.

Logie, C., Bridge, T. J., & Bridge, P. D. (2007). Evaluating the phobias, attitudes, and cultural competence of master of social work students toward the LGBT populations. *Journal of Homosexuality*, *53*, 201–221.

Lombardi, E. (2009). Varieties of transgender/transsexual lives and their relationship with transphobia. *Journal of Homosexuality*, *56*, 977–992. doi:10.1080/00918360903275393

Lyons, A., Pitts, M., Grierson, J., Thorpe, R., & Power, J. (2010). Ageing with HIV: Health and psychosocial well-being of older gay men. *AIDS Care*, *22*, 1236–1244. doi:10.1080/09540121003668086

Meyer, I. H. (1995). Minority stress and mental health in gay men. *Journal of Health and Social Behavior*, *36*, 38–56.

Meyer, I. H. (2003). Prejudice, social stress, and mental health in lesbian, gay, and bisexual populations: Conceptual issues and research evidence. *Psychological Bulletin*, *129*, 674–697. doi:10.1037/0033-2909.129.5.674

Mulé, N. J. (2006). Equity vs. invisibility: Sexual orientation issues in social work ethics and curricula standards. *Social Work Education: The International Journal*, *25*, 608–622.

Muraco, A., & Fredriksen-Goldsen, K. (2011). "That's what friends do:" Informal caregiving for chronically ill lesbian, gay, and bisexual elders. *Journal of Social and Personal Relationships*, *28*, 1073–1092.

National Association of Social Workers. (2008). *Code of ethics of the National Association of Social Workers*. Retrieved February from http://www.naswdc.org/pubs/code/code.asp

National Senior Citizens Law Center. (2011). *LGBT older adults in long-term care facilities: Stories from the field*. Retrieved from http://www.lgbtlongtermcare.org/authors/

Obedin-Maliver, J., Goldsmith, E. S., Stewart, L., White, W., Tran, E., Brenman, S., . . . Lunn, M. R. (2011). Lesbian, gay, bisexual, and transgender-related content in undergraduate medical education. *JAMA*, *306*, 971–977. doi:10.1001/jama.2011.1255

Ochs, R. (1996). Biphobia: It goes more than two ways. In B. A. Firestein (Ed.), *Bisexuality: The psychology and politics of an invisible minority* (pp. 240–259). Newbury Park, CA: Sage.

Pew Research Center. (2010). Baby Boomers approach 65—Glumly. *Pew Social & Demographic Trends*. Retrieved from http://www.pewsocialtrends.org/files/2010/12/Boomer-Summary-Report-FINAL.pdf

Project Implicit. (2011). *IAT home*. Retrieved from https://implicit.harvard.edu/implicit/demo/

Ramirez-Valles, J., Kuhns, L. M., Campbell, R. T., & Diaz, R. M. (2010). Social integration and health: Community involvement, stigmatized identities, and sexual risk in Latino sexual minorities. *Journal of Health & Social Behavior*, *51*, 30–47.

Riggle, E. D. B., Rostosky, S. S., & Horne, S. (2010). Does it matter where you live? Nondiscrimination laws and the experiences of LGB residents. *Sexuality Research and Social Policy*, *7*, 168–175. doi:10.1007/s13178-010-0016-z

Rofes, E. (1998). *Dry bones breathe: Gay men creating post-AIDS identities and cultures*. New York, NY: Harrington Park Press.

Rostosky, S. S., Riggle, E. D. B., Horne, S. G., & Miller, A. D. (2009). Marriage amendments and psychological distress in lesbian, gay, and bisexual (LGB) adults. *Journal of Counseling Psychology*, *56*, 56–66.

Russ, T. C., Stamatakis, E., Hamer, M., Starr, J. M., Kivimäki, M., & Batty, G. D. (2012). Association between psychological distress and mortality: Individual participant pooled analysis of 10 prospective cohort studies. *British Medical Journal*, *345*, e4933. doi:10.1136/bmj.e4933

Segal, E. A., Gerdes, K. E., & Steiner, S. (2013). *An introduction to the profession of social work: Becoming a change agent* (4th ed.). Belmont, CA: Brooks/Cole, Cengage Learning.

Shelton, K., & Delgado-Romero, E. A. (2011). Sexual orientation microaggressions: The experience of lesbian, gay, bisexual, and queer clients in psychotherapy. *Journal of Counseling Psychology*, *58*, 210–221. doi:10.1037/a0022251

Silverstein, C. (2009). The implications of removing homosexuality from the DSM as a mental disorder. *Archives of Sexual Behavior*, *38*, 161–163. doi:10.1007/s10508-008-9442-x

Smith, G. C., & Hayslip, B. J. (2012). Resilience in adulthood and later life: What does it mean and where are we heading? In B. J. Hayslip & G. C. Smith (Eds.), *Emerging perspectives on resilience in adulthood and later life: Annual review of gerontology and geriatrics* (Vol. 32, pp. 3–28). New York, NY: Springer.

Snowden, S. (2013). *Healthcare equality index 2013: Promoting equitable & inclusive care for lesbian, gay, bisexual, and transgender patients and their families.* Washington, DC: Human Rights Campaign.

Stirratt, M., Meyer, I., Ouellette, S., & Gara, M. (2008). Measuring identity multiplicity and intersectionality: Hierarchical classes analysis (HICLAS) of sexual, racial, and gender identities. *Self and Identity*, *7*, 89–111. doi:10.1080/15298860701252203

Swank, E., & Raiz, L. (2010). Attitudes toward gays and lesbians among undergraduate social work students. *Affilia*, *25*, 19–29. doi:10.1177/0886109909356058

Szymanski, D. M., Kashubeck-West, S., & Meyer, J. (2008). Internalized heterosexism—A historical and theoretical overview. *Counseling Psychologist*, *36*, 510–524. doi:10.1177/0011000007309488

Trillium Health Centre. (n.d.). *IDEA: Ethical decision-making framework.* Retrieved from http://www.trilliumhealthcentre.org/about/documents/Trillium IDEA_EthicalDecisionMakingFramework.pdf

Tuck, R. C. (2012). *Parting the Red Sea: The religious case for LGBT equality.* Retrieved from http://ssrn.com/abstract=2101854

Van Den Bergh, N., & Crisp, C. (2004). Defining culturally competent practice with sexual minorities: Implications for social work education and practice. *Journal of Social Work Education*, *40*, 221–238.

Wallace, S. P., Cochran, S. D., Durazo, E. M., & Ford, C. L. (2011). *The health of aging lesbian, gay and bisexual adults in California.* Los Angeles, CA: UCLA Center for Health Policy Research.

Weiss, J. T. (2003). GL vs. BT: The archaeology of biphobia and transphobia within the U.S. gay and lesbian community. *Journal of Bisexuality*, *3*(3–4), 25–55.

Wight, R. G., LeBlanc, A. J., de Vries, B., & Detels, R. (2012). Stress and mental health among midlife and older gay-identified men. *American Journal of Public Health*, *102*, 503–510. doi:10.2105/AJPH.2011.300384

APPENDIX: COMPETENCY SCALE FOR WORKING WITH LGBT OLDER ADULTS

Please use the scale below to thoughtfully rate your current skill level:

0 = Not skilled at all (I have no experience with this skill)
1 = Beginning skill (I have to consciously work at this skill)
2 = Moderate skill (This skill is becoming more integrated into my practice)
3 = Advanced skill (This skill is done with confidence and is an integral part of my practice)
4 = Expert skill (I complete this skill with sufficient mastery to teach others)

Competency Scale for Working With LGBT Older Adults	Skill Level (0–4)
1. Critically analyze personal and professional attitudes toward sexual orientation, gender identity, and age, and understand how factors such as culture, religion, media, and health and human service systems influence attitudes and ethical decision-making.	
2. Understand and articulate the ways that larger social and cultural contexts may have negatively impacted LGBT older adults as a historically disadvantaged population.	
3. Distinguish similarities and differences within the subgroups of LGBT older adults, as well as their intersecting identities (such as age, gender, race, and health status) to develop tailored and responsive health strategies.	
4. Apply theories of aging and social and health perspectives and the most up-to-date knowledge available to engage in culturally competent practice with LGBT older adults.	
5. When conducting a comprehensive biopsychosocial assessment, attend to the ways that the larger social context and structural and environmental risks and resources may impact LGBT older adults.	
6. When using empathy and sensitive interviewing skills during assessment and intervention, ensure the use of language is appropriate for working with LGBT older adults in order to establish and build rapport.	
7. Understand and articulate the ways in which agency, program, and service policies do or do not marginalize and discriminate against LGBT older adults.	
8. Understand and articulate the ways that local, state, and federal laws negatively and positively impact LGBT older adults, in order to advocate on their behalf.	
9. Provide sensitive and appropriate outreach to LGBT older adults, their families, caregivers and other supports to identify and address service gaps, fragmentation, and barriers that impact LGBT older adults.	
10. Enhance the capacity of LGBT older adults and their families, caregivers and other supports to navigate aging, social, and health services.	

Same-Sex Sexual Relationships in the National Social Life, Health and Aging Project: Making a Case for Data Collection

MARIA T. BROWN

Aging Studies Institute, Syracuse University, Syracuse, New York, USA

BRIAN R. GROSSMAN

Department of Disability and Human Development, University of Illinois at Chicago, Chicago, Illinois, USA

This study describes the previously unexplored subsample of respondents who reported at least 1 same-sex sexual relationship (SSSR) in the National Social Life, Health, and Aging Project (NSHAP). The NSHAP collected data from 3,005 adults (aged 57–85). Approximately 4% (n = 102) of respondents reported at least one SSSR. These sexual minority elders were younger, more educated, were more likely to be working, had fewer social supports, and better physical health. Results may indicate crisis competence in sexual minority elders. Collecting sexual orientation and gender identity data in larger, US-based probability samples would inform the development of appropriate community-based services and supports.

INTRODUCTION

As the population of older adults grows over the next 30 years, the numbers of lesbian, gay, bisexual, and transgender (LGBT) older adults will also increase (Shankle, Maxwell, Katzman, & Landers, 2003). Historically, LGBT elders and others who have same-sex desires and/or engage in same-sex sexual behavior have been invisible in the field of gerontology (M. T. Brown,

34

2009; Butler, 2004). Recent research indicates that these older adults experience disparities in social supports and in health across the life course and in later life (Fredriksen-Goldsen et al., 2011; Wallace, Cochran, Durazo, & Ford, 2011). However, population-based health studies rarely collect information on sexual orientation or gender identity.

Specifically, few studies utilizing nationally representative samples gather data about older adults' sexual histories, and none collect information on gender identity. What limited sexual history data that is collected is generally not analyzed or examined (Waite, Laumann, Das & Schumm, 2009). Due, in part, to this lack of representative, population-based samples, LGBT elders and others with a history of same-sex sexual desire, behavior, or identity, remain invisible to policy-makers and, therefore, lack the policy protections available to other older adults (Cahill & South, 2002). Consequently, these older adults are at an increased risk for social isolation, certain chronic conditions and diseases, and living in poverty; all of which influence longevity and quality of life in old age (Cahill & South, 2002; Meyer & Roseamelia, 2007).

The National Social Life, Health, and Aging Project (NSHAP; Waite et al., 2010) is the only probability-based nationally representative study of older Americans that captures data on the sexual behavior of older adults. Despite the array of data collected via the NSHAP, there were no questions about respondent gender identity or sexual identity or desire. Consequently, it is not possible to identify any transgender older adults in the sample, and the only way to identify older adults who might be described as sexual minority elders is to examine the data on sexual behavior. In an operational sense, this requires analyzing the subsample who reported a history of at least one same-sex sexual relationship (SSSR). Approximately 4% of the NSHAP sample, with a slightly higher percentage of women than men, reported SSSRs (Waite et al., 2009). These data on SSSRs have not been examined in previous published analyses of the NSHAP data.

The limited data collected via the NSHAP do not allow us to make explanatory claims about the health and well-being of self-identified LGBT older adults. However, they do provide a potential source for describing social and health disparities between some sexual minority (SSSRs) and sexual majority elders (respondents with no history of SSSRs). Although this study originally involved inferential analyses, the results were inconclusive due to the very small size of the SSSR subsample; therefore, the study was refocused on bivariate descriptive analyses. The results of the bivariate analyses of this subsample highlight the need to use data collected about sexual minority older adults, and to design and develop new instruments and enhance existing ones to generate this type of data.

These descriptive analyses examine the following research questions: (a) What is known about the population of NSHAP respondents with a history of SSSR? and (b) How do these respondents compare to their sexual majority counterparts? The study addresses these questions with a descriptive analysis of the sample, and a comparison of respondents reporting a history of SSSRs with the remainder of the sample on selected demographic, social support, health behavior, physical health, and mental health variables.

BACKGROUND

Insufficient Data About Sexual and Gender Minority Adults

As the population of older adults grows over the next 30 years, the numbers of sexual and gender minority[1] older adults will also increase (Shankle et al., 2003). To date, the limitations of gerontology research on these groups[2] have meant that the growth of this knowledge base is not keeping pace with the growth of the population itself (Healthy People 2020, 2011; Sell & Becker, 2001). Researchers studying sexual and gender minority older adults face multiple challenges in recruiting representative samples. The majority of this research conducted over the last 3 decades has included relatively small, local convenience samples (Fredriksen-Goldsen & Muraco, 2010). Most of these studies have focused exclusively on one part of the LGBT population, and did not include heterosexuals in their sample, limiting the ability to draw comparisons against the majority population. Furthermore, researchers have had difficulty recruiting certain sexual and gender minority older adults, who may be more likely to experience multiple forms of oppression and marginalization, including transgender people, lesbians, people of color, and low-income elders.

A valid criticism of the body of work in LGBT aging is that the majority of samples are overwhelmingly White, middle-class, and male (Shankle, et al., 2003). Transgender aging is frequently studied under the umbrella of LGBT aging, with a small minority of subjects actually claiming a trans identity (Finkenauer, Sherratt, Marlow & Brodey, 2012). Due, in part, to the lack of representative, population-based samples, LGBT older adults remain invisible to policy-makers and, therefore, lack the policy protections available to other older adults (Cahill & South, 2002). Consequently, LGBT older adults

---

[1]   Throughout this article, the terms *sexual minority* and *gender minority* are purposefully used to differentiate between the power positions of those in the dominant position and those on the margins. The term *sexual minority* refers to a broader umbrella of people than just those who identify as lesbian, gay, or bisexual, reflecting a nuanced understanding of sexual orientation as more than just behavior or identity (Institute of Medicine [IOM], 2011). Similarly, the term *gender minority* recognizes the broad spectrum of people who are not adequately served by the binary categories of male or female; here, too, the conceptualization of gender is greater than identity alone and encompasses desire, behavior, and trajectory.

[2]   Gerontology research on sexual or gender minority older adults is often referred to as *LGBT aging research* because most studies tend to focus on sexual minorities or specific types of sexual minorities (lesbians or gays, men who have sex with men, bisexuals) or on specific gender minorities (like individuals who identify as transgender).

are at an increased risk for social isolation, certain chronic conditions and diseases, and living in poverty; all of which influence longevity and quality of life in old age (Cahill & South, 2002; Meyer & Roseamelia, 2007).

Measuring Sexual Orientation

Regardless of age, generating national estimates of the number of sexual and gender minority adults is challenging, given current data collection systems. Most US-based population surveys suffer from both a lack of questions about gender identity and/or sexual orientation, and great variability in the measures employed to capture LGBT people. Although questions about sexual orientation allow lesbians, gay men, or bisexual men or women to identify themselves, transgender identity is a product of gender identity and presentation, and should, therefore, be measured separately (IOM, 2011).

Social scientists describe sexual orientation as encompassing three potentially distinct dimensions: desire, behavior, and identity (IOM, 2011). *Sexual desire* has been defined as "an enduring pattern of experiencing sexual or romantic feelings" (IOM, 2011, p. 28) for one or more sexes or genders, and *sexual behavior* has been defined as an "enduring pattern of sexual or romantic activity" (IOM, 2011, p. 28) with one or more sexes or genders. *Sexual identity* has been defined in terms of both personal and social identity: how an individual sees himself or herself based on his or her history of sexual and romantic attractions to one or more sexes or genders, and how the individual sees himself or herself as a member of a social group formed around a shared sexual orientation (IOM, 2011).

Of these three dimensions, sexual desire is least likely to be addressed. Sexual behavior is most likely to be directly assessed, and although sexual identity is generally not ascertained directly, individuals with limited knowledge about, or experience with, sexual minorities may presume that one's sexual identity can be defined based on responses to questions about the sex/gender of the respondent and the sex/gender of their relationship partner(s). Although all three dimensions of sexual orientation have been identified as important in appropriately estimating the number of lesbian, gay, or bisexual (LGB) people in a given sample, the few population-based surveys that include questions about sexual orientation do not include questions about all three dimensions, and none include questions about gender identity (Sell, Wells, & Wypij, 1995; Wallace et al., 2011).

Currently, the only national survey that includes any information related to sexual orientation for all ages of Americans, including older adults, is the US Census (Gates & Cooke, 2010). The Census identifies couples in cohabitating, same-sex relationships, which is one way to study sexual orientation. Although this method successfully counts the number of people willing to acknowledge that they are currently involved in same-sex cohabitating relationships, the drawback is that there is no way to identify a respondents as

LGB if they are currently single or do not live with a partner. Surveys that only allow for the identification of same-sex cohabiting couples reproduce, perhaps unintentionally, the invisibility of both bisexual and transgender people. Additionally, these surveys capture current relationship status but miss the life course trajectory of sociosexual experiences that are so critical when studying aging and older adults.

In terms of sexual identity, social science researchers have historically believed, based on an overgeneralization of Kinsey's research on human sexuality, that 10% of the population would identify as LGB (Savin-Williams, 2009). However, recent Gallup surveys measuring LGBT identity indicate that the proportion of Americans claiming these identities vary by state, with a low of 1.7% in North Dakota to a high of 10% in the District of Columbia (Gates & Newport, 2013).

Studies comparing sexual behavior and sexual identity report greater proportions of people who have engaged in same-sex sexual behavior than who identify as LGB, and both measures identify larger proportions of LGB respondents in younger samples (Savin-Williams, 2009). The 4% of the NSHAP sample who reported at least one SSSR (Waite et al., 2009) is consistent with other studies of same-sex behavior in the United States, New Zealand, and Great Britain, in which between 4% and 6% of adults reported same-sex sexual behavior (Baumle, Compton, & Poston, 2009; Hayes et al., 2012; Michael, Gagnon, Laumann, & Kolata, 1994; Wells, McGee, & Beautrais, 2011).

The NSHAP sexual history questions allow for the collection of historical information on one dimension of sexual orientation: sexual behavior. Respondents are able to acknowledge any history of same-sex sexual behavior over the course of their life (Waite et al., 2009), rather than limiting them to identifying only current, cohabiting same-sex relationships. However, the instrument does not collect information on same-sex desire or sexual identity, resulting in a rather narrow definition of sexual minority elders in this sample, including only individuals reporting a history of SSSR. Nor does the instrument collect data on gender identity, effectively erasing gender minority elders in this sample.

How Do LGBT Elders Differ From Other Older Adults?

The limited research (small, nonprobability samples) that has been conducted on LGBT adults indicates that they experience a variety of disparities in both health access and health outcomes across the life course and in later life (Healthy People 2020, 2011). Transgender individuals have less access to health insurance; lesbians underutilize preventive services for cancer, and bisexual individuals are frequently invisible to healthcare (J. P. Brown & Tracy, 2008; Clements-Nolle, Marx, & Katz, 2006; Koh & Ross, 2006; San Francisco Human Rights Commission, 2011). Sexual and gender minority adults, in comparison with their sexual and gender majority peers, report higher rates of tobacco, alcohol use, and drug use (Healthy People 2020, 2011). Gay men and transgender individuals experience greater risk of sexually transmitted diseases, including HIV, and transgender individuals live with a greater prevalence of victimization, mental health problems, and suicide (Clements-Nolle et al, 2006; Healthy People 2020, 2011). Lesbians and bisexual women have higher rates of obesity, emotional stress, and mental health problems (Cochran et al., 2001; Healthy People 2020, 2011).

In addition to differences in health outcomes, LGBT older adults report differences in their social networks; relying much more on the support of friends than family (Dorfman et al., 1995; Grossman, D'Augelli, & Hershberger, 2000). LGBT older adults face additional barriers due to physical and social isolation and due to the lack of culturally competent social service providers (Healthy People 2020, 2011; Kuyper & Fokkema, 2010). Some of these smaller studies have been confirmed by probability-based studies of American adults, like the 2003, 2005, and 2007 California Health Interview Surveys (Wallace et al., 2011). However, the continued invisibility of sexual and gender minority older adults in population-based samples of older adults in the United States limits the understanding of these social and health disparities and the ability to address them. To develop a comprehensive understanding of the differences between sexual and gender minority older adults and their majority counterparts, population-based surveys must include measures of sexual orientation and gender identity. The inclusion of these measures in national studies, as well as in local and regional studies, would enhance our understanding of the lives of all older adults.

Previous NSHAP Analyses

The NSHAP dataset offers a unique opportunity to compare the social networks, physical and mental health outcomes, and chronic disease conditions of older adults with different sexual histories. Although the majority of articles using the NSHAP dataset do not directly address the subsample of older adults with a history of SSSR, many of these articles address outcomes that have been found to disproportionately affect sexual minority older adults in smaller, convenience samples. Of the existing NSHAP publications, only Waite and colleagues (2009) indicated the proportions of the sample reporting a history of sex with male or female partners over the course of their lifetime. However, the authors do not compare the outcomes in their analyses by sexual history nor do they address the implications of their research findings for LGBT older adults or other older adults with a history of same-sex sexual relationships, indicative of sexual behavior.

Analyses of the NSHAP data have linked social isolation to poorer physical and mental health outcomes, and identified living arrangements as a key factor influencing patterns of social contact among older adults

(B. Cornwell, 2011; E. Y. Cornwell & Waite, 2009a, 2009b). Researchers have also compared self-reported quality of life; measures of anxiety, stress, and self-reported emotional health; smoking and drinking behaviors; and biometric and self-report data on chronic conditions by sex and age category (Drum, Shiovitz-Ezra, Gaumer, & Lindau, 2009; Shiovitz-Ezra, Leitsch, Graber, & Karraker, 2009; Williams, Pham-Kanter, & Leitsch, 2009).

In each of these NSHAP publications, the analyses focus exclusively on heterosexual or sexual majority older adults. Consequently, these analyses do not engage the findings from other studies about sexual and gender minority older adults. For example, previous research on LGBT older adults has identified social and physical isolation as barriers to physical and emotional wellbeing in LGBT older adults, who are more likely to live alone than their heterosexual peers (Healthy People 2020, 2011; Wallace et al., 2011). The NSHAP data represent a unique opportunity to compare the social supports and aging experiences of older adults who reported one or more SSSRs with their sexual majority peers. Given work that has already been completed on the heterosexual respondents to the NSHAP and the extant literature on LGBT older adults, this study attempts to examine these data for differences in emotional and physical health, and health behaviors, between these two groups.

METHODS

NSHAP Data

This project analyzes data from Wave 1 ($N = 3,005$) of the NSHAP survey. The NSHAP is a community-based multistage area probability sample of older adults, which oversamples men, Hispanics, Blacks, and individuals aged 75 to 85 (O'Muircheartaigh, Eckman, & Smith, 2009; Waite & Das, 2010). Among nationally representative studies of older adults, the NSHAP is the only study to gather specific information on sexual behavior and attitudes, including information on the sex of past sexual partners. The NSHAP data is a restricted-access dataset housed at the University of Michigan Inter-University Consortium for Political and Social Research.

Wave 1 of the NSHAP was collected from 3,005 adults aged 57 to 85 between July 2005 and March 2006, using in-home interviews and a self-administered postinterview questionnaire (Waite & Das, 2010). The NSHAP interview and leave-behind questionnaire collected data on sexuality and health. Questions addressed a variety of social factors, including social networks and support and romantic partnerships and sexual activity. The survey also collected information on physical health, mental health, and selected biomarkers (Waite et al., 2007). Measures include social disconnectedness and perceived isolation (E. Y. Cornwell & Waite, 2009a), intimate relationships (Waite & Das, 2010), quality of life and psychological health indicators (Shiovitz-Ezra, Leitsch, Graber, & Karraker, 2009), self-rated health and selected chronic conditions and diseases (Williams et al., 2009).

Sample

Cases were excluded from this sample if they did not complete the sexual history questions, due to either incomplete interview or failure to return the leave-behind survey, or if they were missing data on any of the social support or physical or mental health variables. The amount of missing data on several of these variables (10% or greater) necessitated the use of a complete case sample, which reduced the sample by 18.6% from 3,005 to 2,446 respondents, ages 57–85. For this analysis, respondents across the full age spectrum were included to retain meaningful sample sizes for the sexual minority subsample. Excluding respondents between the ages of 57 and 64 would have eliminated 34% of the sexual minority subsample.

Variables

This study utilizes several measures from the NSHAP instrument to describe the sexual minority elders in this sample, and to compare them to their sexual majority counterparts. These variables include sexual history, demographics, employment status, level of physical activity, social supports, health behaviors, and physical and mental health.

Sexual history. Sexual history variables were constructed from two questions[3] to indicate each respondent's number of lifetime male partners (0–699) and number of lifetime female partners (0–1005). These variables were coded into four dichotomous variables: men who have ever had sex with a man (MSM, $n = 45$) or with a woman (MSW, $n = 992$); women who have ever had sex with a woman (WSW, $n = 57$) or with a man (WSM, $n = 1083$).[4] Two dichotomous variables represent sexual history, regardless of respondent sex: any SSSR ($n = 102$) and a pattern of more than two SSSR ($n = 40$).

Demographics. The demographic variables were constructed from several items in the NSHAP dataset. Respondent age was an interval variable, and respondent ages were also combined into three age groups (57–64, 65–74, and 75–84). Respondents were asked to identify as either male or

---

[3] The two sexual history questions are: "In your entire life so far, how many men have you had sex with, even if only one time?" and "In your entire life so far, how many women have you had sex with, even if only one time?" (Waite et al., 2007).

[4] These are proportions of the weighted sample. Approximately 11% of the weighted sample ($n = 266$) responded with a 0 to both questions.

female.[5] A nominal variable combined the race and ethnicity variables from the data, creating four categories (White non-Hispanic, Black non-Hispanic, other non-Hispanic, and Hispanic). All respondents identifying as Hispanic were assigned to the Hispanic category, regardless of their racial identification. Job status was constructed as a dichotomous variable, indicating whether or not a respondent was working at the time of the survey.

Social supports. Several variables were constructed from social support measures in the NSHAP instrument. *Partnership status* is a dichotomous variable indicating if respondents are married or living with a partner. *Number of children* is an interval variable summing the number of sons and daughters. A dichotomous variable indicates if respondents have at least one child. Interval variables were constructed from respondent reports of the number of friends they had, the number of people they considered close family members, and the number of alters or network members in their social network.

Health and health behaviors. The health and health behavior variables were constructed from several measures in the NSHAP instrument. Self-rated physical health and mental health were based on individual Likert scales. Each was coded as a dichotomous variable indicating whether respondents report good, very good, or excellent health, or fair or poor health. Physical activity is a dichotomous variable, indicating whether or not respondents are physically active one or more times a week. Self-reports on health behaviors were coded as dichotomous variables: currently smoking or, if they do not currently smoke, ever having smoked in the past; currently drinking or, if they do not currently drink, ever drinking in the past; and having ever been tested for HIV.

Happiness was coded based on a Likert scale of general self-rated happiness, and was coded as a dichotomous variable (1 = *pretty happy to extremely happy*). Loneliness was coded based on a Likert scale indicating how often respondents felt lonely, and was coded as a dichotomous variable (1 = *rarely or none of the time*).

Analysis Plan

Bivariate analyses were employed to compare social supports and the physical and mental health outcomes of those who report a history of SSSR with those who did not. In an attempt to distinguish between sexual minority adults whose relationship patterns are indicative of a gay or lesbian lifestyle and those individuals whose relationship patterns are indicative of heterosexual or bisexual lifestyles, sexual minority elders were broken into two

---

[5]   We did not want to reinscribe the erasure of the trans population by defining gender as a dichotomous variable; however, the NSHAP survey forces trans respondents to choose either male or female as their gender identity, thereby erasing their trans identity.

additional subgroups: (a) those who reported one or two SSSRs and (b) those who reported more than two SSSRs. Descriptive statistics were generated for both sexual minority and sexual majority respondents, and for all respondents in the sample ($n = 2446$). Bivariate analyses were then run to identify differences between groups based on sexual minority status for demographic variables, social supports, physical health and health behaviors, and mental health variables. These two groups were compared with each other, and with the rest of the sample, via cross-tabulations and difference of the means t-tests. Cross-tabulations were run to compare social supports and physical and mental health across age groups and types of sexual history, but there were not enough elements in the subsample to support the analysis of any of these variables by both sexual history and age group. The statistical significance of the cross-tabulations was determined using the Rao-Scott chi-square (χ^2) test.

All analyses were run in SAS, using survey procedures (i.e., surveyfreq). These survey procedures accommodate the complex survey design, which involved strata and clusters, and allow for the use of weighted or unweighted models.

RESULTS

Table 1 displays the proportions of respondents in the original NSHAP Wave 1 sample ($n = 3,005$) who reported a history of SSSRs, by sex and age group. In the younger age groups (57–64 and 65–74), both men and women were more likely to report having had any SSSRs in their lifetime than those in the oldest age group (75–85). In the two older age groups (65–74 and 75–85), men were more likely to report a pattern of more than two SSSRs than those in the youngest age group (65–74).

The demographic characteristics of the complete case sample are displayed in Table 2. The mean age of the sample was 67.82 ($SD = 7.9$). The sample was predominately White, non-Hispanic (81.69%), and female (52%). Over half of the sample (55.9%) had at least some education beyond high school. The majority of respondents was not working (65%), was married (69.6%), and had at least one child (91.7%).

Bivariate analyses reveal that sexual minority elders in this sample, particularly those reporting a pattern of more than two SSSRs in their lifetime, differed from their sexual majority peers in several ways (see Table 2). Sexual minority elders, and those with a pattern of more than two SSSRs, were younger on average ($p < 0.05$), were more likely to be in the younger age groups (57–64 and 65–74; p=0.06), and reported higher levels of educational attainment ($p < 0.05$).

Sexual minority elders also reported different family structures and social supports than their sexual majority peers (see Table 3). More than half of sexual minority adults in this sample were unmarried or were not living with

TABLE 1 Lifetime History of Sexual Partners, by Sex and Age Group, National Social Life, Health, and Aging Project (NSHAP) 2005–2006 (n = 3005)

	Women (n = 1550)				Men (n = 1454)			
	Ages 57–64 (n = 492)	Ages 65–74 (n = 545)	Ages 75–85 (n = 513)	All Women	Ages 57–64 (n = 528)	Ages 65–74 (n = 547)	Ages 75–85 (n = 380)	All Men
Lifetime male sex partners								
0 male partners	79 16.1%	117 21.5%	129 25.1%	325	509 96.4%	525 96.0%	370 97.4%	1404
1–2 male partners	201 40.9%	242 44.4%	278 54.2%	721	12 2.3%	10 1.8%	5 1.3%	27
> 2 male partners	212 43.1%	186 34.1%	106 20.7%	504	7 1.3%	12 2.2%	4 1.1%	23
Total	492	545	513	1550	528	547	379	1454
Lifetime female sex partners								
0 female partners	473 96.1%	518 95.0%	497 96.9%	1488	105 19.9%	118 21.6%	90 23.7%	313
1–2 female partners	9 1.8%	19 3.5%	12 2.3%	40	116 22.0%	118 21.6%	109 28.7%	343
> 2 female partners	10 2.0%	8 1.5%	4 0.8%	22	307 58.1%	311 56.9%	180 47.4%	798
Total	492	545	513	1550	528	547	379	1454

Note. These categories were compiled from the two sexual history questions in the NSHAP instrument: "In your entire life so far, how many men have you had sex with, even if only one time?" and "In your entire life so far, how many women have you had sex with, even if only one time?" (Waite et al., 2007).

TABLE 2 Sample Demographics, Complete Case Sample, Weighted, National Social Life, Health, and Aging Project 2005–2006

	Total Sample (N = 2446)	No SSSRs (N = 2344)	Any SSSRs (N = 102)†	χ²	≤ 2 SSSRs (N = 2406)	> 2 SSSRs (N = 40)†	χ²
Sexual history (%)							
Men who had sex with men	1.77	0	39.97		0.93	46.05	*
Women who had sex with women	2.65	0	60.03		1.69	53.95	~
1–2 same-sex sexual relationships	4.42	0	58.18		2.62	0	
> 2 same-sex sexual relationships	1.85	0	41.82		0	100	
Demographics							
Age (mean)	67.82	67.86	66.89	*	67.87	65.30	~
Age group (%)							
57–64	41.77	41.98	37.41		41.64	48.69	
65–74	35.59	35.04	47.45		35.43	43.61	
75–84	22.64	22.99	15.14		22.92	7.70	
Sex (%)							
Male	47.92	48.29	39.97		47.96	46.05	
Female	52.08	52.12	60.03		52.04	53.95	
Race/Ethnicity (%)							
White non-Hispanic	81.69	81.35	88.76		81.52	90.72	*
Black non-Hispanic	8.87	9.09	4.23		8.98	2.97	
Other non-Hispanic	2.58	2.61	1.97		2.58	2.59	
Hispanic	6.86	6.95	5.04		6.92	3.70	
Education (%)				~			
Did not graduate from high school	16.93	17.30	9.02		17.22	1.61	
High school diploma or equivalent	26.94	27.18	21.76		26.97	25.70	
Vocational/Some college/Associate's degree	30.50	30.46	31.51		30.47	32.41	
Bachelors degree or higher	25.62	25.06	37.70		25.35	40.28	
Employment status (%)							
Not working	64.90	64.99	62.37		65.20	47.50	*
Working	35.10	35.01	37.63		34.80	52.50	**

Note. SSSR = Same sex sexual relationship. †These subsample sizes reflect the 18% reduction in sample size that resulted from the creation of the complete case sample.

$*p < .05.$ $**p < .01.$ $***p < .001.$ $\sim p = .05.$

TABLE 3 Social Supports, by Sexual History, Complete Case Sample, Weighted, National Social Life, Health, and Aging Project 2005–2006

	Total Sample (N = 2446)	No SSSRs (N = 2344)	Any SSSRs (N = 102)†	χ^2	≤ 2 SSSRs (N = 2406)	> 2 SSSRs (N = 40)†	χ^2
Marital status (%)							
Married/partnered	69.61	70.12	41.60	*	70.16	40.73	**
Unmarried/not living with partner	30.39	29.88	58.40	*	29.85	59.27	**
Children in family (%)							
Number of children	2.89	2.92	2.33	*	2.92	1.71	**
No children	8.29	7.65	22.07	***	7.63	43.08	***
Number of alters in social network (mean)	3.65	3.65	3.72		3.65	3.60	**
Number of friends (mean)	3.34	3.34	3.31		3.34	3.27	
Number of close relatives (mean)	2.90	2.91	2.62	*	2.91	2.38	*

Note. SSSR = Same sex sexual relationship. †These subsample sizes reflect the 18% reduction in sample size that resulted from the creation of the complete case sample.

*p < .05. **p < .01. ***p < .001. ~p = .05.

an intimate partner ($p < 0.01$). Sexual minority elders reporting a pattern of more than two SSSRs were nearly twice as likely to be childless than those reporting one or two SSSRs, and six times as likely to be childless than those reporting no SSSRs. Those sexual minority elders who did have children had fewer children on average ($p < 0.01$) than their sexual majority peers. Sexual minority elders did not have significantly more friends or alters in their social networks, but they did have fewer people they identified as close relatives ($p < 0.05$). In addition, sexual minority elders with a pattern of more than two SSSRs were more likely to be working ($p = 0.05$) and to be physically active ($p < 0.01$) than respondents without this sexual history.

In this sample, there was no difference in smoking behavior between sexual minority elders and their sexual majority counterparts (see Table 4). Sexual minority elders were more likely to report ever having been tested for HIV ($p < 0.05$). Respondents reporting a pattern of more than two SSSRs were more likely to report currently drinking alcohol ($p < 0.05$) or having drunk alcohol in the past ($p < 0.05$). More sexual minority elders reported good or excellent self-rated physical health ($p < 0.05$). However, there were no significant differences in terms of reporting good mental health, less loneliness, more happiness, or high self-esteem.

DISCUSSION

Because the NSHAP is one of the only surveys of older Americans that include a measure of sexual orientation, even one that is problematic, it is important that these data be used to explore the disparities that have previously been identified in sexual minority older adults. Until now, however, the sexual history data in the NSHAP has received very little attention in the literature.

The results of these bivariate analyses support some findings from some previous community-based studies of LGBT elders (Dorfman et al., 1995; Grossman et al., 2000). There is evidence that the social supports, and types of relationships within social networks, are different for respondents defined as sexual minority elders in this sample. Sexual minority elders in this sample are younger, are less likely to have children, and, if they have children, they have fewer than their heterosexual counterparts. They also have higher levels of education, report fewer sources of social support and/or potential informal caregivers in their networks, and are more likely to be working. These differences were greater for sexual minority respondents who reported a pattern of more than two SSSRs. These data do not reveal why sexual minority elders are more likely to be working—nor do they elucidate the relationship between their higher level of physical activity and greater likelihood to work. Sexual minority elders may be working more because they are

TABLE 4 Health and Health Behaviors, by Sexual History, Complete Case Sample, Weighted, National Social Life, Health, and Aging Project 2005–2006

	Total Sample (N = 2446)	No SSSRs (N = 2344)	Any SSSRs (N = 102)[†]	χ^2	≤ 2 SSSRs (N = 2406)	> 2 SSSRs (N = 40)[†]	χ^2
Health behaviors							
Physical activity one time a week or more (%)	79.00	78.92	80.63	*	78.65	97.44	*
Smoking (%)							
Smokes tobacco	14.82	14.92	12.57		14.84	14.05	
Has smoked in the past	45.51	45.45	46.80		45.46	48.37	
Drinking alcohol (%)							
Drinks alcohol	60.51	60.12	68.94	*	60.14	80.03	*
Has drunk alcohol in the past	25.87	25.96	24.01		26.08	14.80	*
Has been tested for HIV (%)	14.39	13.85	26.00	*	14.10	29.67	
Physical health							
Good self-rated physical health (%)	76.05	75.65	84.82	*	75.86	86.45	
Mental health							
Good self-rated mental health (%)	90.60	90.42	94.44		90.49	96.43	
Pretty happy or more (%)	91.93	91.95	91.47		91.84	96.98	
Rarely or never lonely (%)	70.87	70.98	68.43		70.92	68.34	
Have high self-esteem (%)	86.66	86.56	88.82		86.56	91.92	

Note. SSSR = Same sex sexual relationship. [†]These subsample sizes reflect the 18% reduction in sample size that resulted from the creation of the complete case sample.

$*p < .05.$ $**p < .01.$ $***p < .001.$ $\sim p = .05.$

younger, or they could be working because they are experiencing income and asset shortfalls as they approach retirement age.

However, other results from this analysis do not support other findings from previous studies, specifically in relation to health disparities for LGBT older adults (Clements-Nolle, Marx, & Katz, 2006; Cochran, et al., 2001; Fredriksen-Goldsen et al., 2011; Healthy People 2020, 2011). Sexual minority elders in this sample do not seem to have experienced poorer mental health or physical health outcomes. Sexual minority elders were more likely to report good physical health, and there were no statistical differences between sexual minority and sexual majority elders in terms of mental health. These findings may indicate that sexual minority elders are experiencing healthy aging in spite of the disparities they experience in social supports; however, there is insufficient data in wave I to test this hypothesis.

The similarities in physical and mental health outcomes seen in the NSHAP data among sexual minority and majority elders may reflect what Kimmel (1978) referred to as "crisis competence" (p. 117). Kimmel posited that older gay men may develop some degree of crisis competence after a lifetime of dealing with adversity (e.g., interpersonal and structural homophobia) resulting from their sexual minority status. The survival strategies gained by managing these experiences may be transferable to the experiences of aging, thus enabling these elders to age successfully, even with fewer social supports and often with lower income levels. In the MetLife survey, *Out and Aging*, 38% of LGBT baby boomers reported that they thought being LGBT had helped prepare them for aging (Met Life Mature Market Institute, 2006). Although it is tempting to interpret the results of these NSHAP analyses as evidence that sexual minority elders are aging successfully, more data is needed before we can make these assertions and before we can determine if the successful aging framework is an appropriate framework for evaluating the LGBT aging experience (Rowe & Kahn, 1987). Researchers at the Fenway Institute's Center for Population Research on LGBT Health have begun exploring successful aging among LGBT older adults in Massachusetts. Their findings suggest that modifying the successful aging framework to include coping would more accurately reflect the experiences of LGBT older adults (Van Wagenen, Driskell, & Bradford, 2013).

There are efforts underway to generate data that will allow researchers and policy makers to assess the degree to which LGBT older adults are aging successfully. Fredriksen-Goldsen and colleagues (2011) recently conducted the first federally funded study of LGBT elders, recruiting LGBT elders through community-based agencies in several major metropolitan areas across the country. This broadened recruitment effort resulted in a larger convenience sample than historically seen in LGBT aging research. Although these research efforts make significant contributions to the knowledge base, researchers will continue to be limited in their ability to examine the health and economic disparities faced by sexual minority adults without a nationally representative sample.

The federal government has recognized the need for a better understanding of the issues affecting the health and well being of LGBT Americans across the life course (IOM, 2011; National Institutes of Health, 2012; Sebelius, 2011). In response to the IOM's (2011) recommendation that federally funded surveys should collect data on sexual orientation and gender identity, the National Institutes of Health LGBT Research Coordinating Committee has stated, "the DHHS is committed to working toward increasing the number of federally funded health and demographic surveys that collect and report sexual orientation and gender identity data" (2013, p. 11). This commitment holds great potential for generating data that allows for a clearer understanding of the experiences of aging for LGBT older adults and other older adults who experience same-sex desire and behavior, as well as the broader field of gerontology.

Limitations

This study reports on same-sex sexual relationship data previously neglected in publications of NSHAP analyses. Although this study makes a unique contribution to the literature on sexuality and aging, there are several limitations to this analysis. Many of these limitations are related to the reality that this was a secondary data analysis.

Although the original sample size in Wave 1 ($N = 3,005$) was large enough to lend statistical power to most analyses, the subset of the sample reporting a history of SSSR was substantially smaller ($n = 112$). As a result of the high rates (approximately 10%) of missing cases on sexual history and several outcome measures, the potential sample was reduced by 18.6% from 3,005 to 2,446, and the subset of respondents with a history of SSSRs was reduced by 9% from 112 to 102. The size of this subset may be affecting our ability to identify associations between sexual minority status and selected physical and mental health outcome variables. Additionally, the SSSR subsample is predominantly White and more educated, as well as younger, which limits our ability to generalize these findings to the broader population.

The sexual history measures in the NSHAP data indicate which respondents have a history of SSSR, but do not provide information on desire, sexual orientation/identity, or gender identity. It is impossible to know which respondents with this history identify as gay, lesbian, or bisexual, or heterosexual, or to identify gender minority elders (across the trans spectrum) in this sample. Questions of sexual or gender identity may not be predictive of sexual behavior, but identity matters in terms of policy protections and access to family caregivers and community-based services and supports (Cahill & South, 2002; Hughes, Harold, & Boyer, 2011). Without data on sexual identity, we cannot determine which respondents in this sample have lived their lives as gay men or lesbians, and were therefore vulnerable to economic and social disparities caused by these policy failures. Measuring only one facet of sexual orientation inevitably provides a limited picture of the variations in sexual orientation among respondents in any sample.

The NSHAP sample was intended to be a nationally representative sample, but there were some issues with undercoverage due to the exclusion of institutionalized adults, and the fact that some potential respondents were out of the country during data collection (O'Muircheartaigh et al., 2009). The link between the NSHAP and the Health and Retirement Study was a substantial source of undercoverage, as the Health and Retirement Study (HRS) eligibility rules prevented some eligible individuals from participating in the NSHAP because they were living with nonpartners who were eligible for the HRS study (O'Muircheartaigh et al., 2009).

These data contain very limited economic information, and the income and wealth data that is available is missing for approximately 30% of cases, which meant that economic measures could not be included in the analyses. Therefore, it was not possible to explore the role of economic status in the relationship between sexual history and the physical or mental health in these data. Other surveys of older adults, such as the HRS, collect stronger and more comprehensive economic information, including data on employment and intergenerational transfers (University of Michigan, 2013). The larger sample sizes and broader range of measure collected in these national surveys allow researchers to analyze an array of demographic and life course factors for their influence on health and economic outcomes. These probability-based surveys, which do not collect information on sexual behavior, desire or identity, are untapped opportunities to collect comprehensive data on sexual orientation and gender identity. The data generated from these instruments hold the promise for meaningful comparisons between sexual and gender minority elders and their majority counterparts.

Implications for Future Research and Practice

To fully understand the aging experiences of all adults, surveys need to capture the complexity of their identities, including sexual orientation and gender identity. The utility of the NSHAP data are limited by the size of the subsample with a history of SSSRs, by the demographics of the subsample, and by the NSHAP instrument itself, which does not allow respondents to identify their gender identity. Possible solutions to this problem in future NSHAP waves could include the oversampling of individuals reporting a history of one or more SSSRs and the addition of questions measuring sexual desire, sexual identity, and gender identity. To better understand the social, health, and economic differences among older adults with different sexual and gender identities, the complexities of these constructs need to be captured in larger probability-based studies, like the HRS, by including questions about sexual desire, sexual behavior, sexual identity, and gender identity.

These larger studies, which already oversample Blacks and Hispanics and the oldest old, would enhance researchers' ability to collect data on more diverse subsamples of sexual minority older adults.

Studies of the aging population in the United States would be enhanced by the inclusion of comprehensive questions on sexual orientation and gender identity (Shankle et al., 2003). Enhancing current high-quality, nationally representative systems of data collection to include questions that allow gender and sexual minority adults to identify themselves is imperative to generating enough data to ensure that all aspects of aging research recognize the significance of addressing and including these populations. As Baumle and colleagues (2009) advocated, "Demographers must 'bring sexuality in.' . . . Sexual orientation results in differential outcomes on a number of issues that are fundamental to population study, supporting the additional exploration of sexuality in this field" (p. 4).

Furthermore, inclusion of these questions would allow for a more comprehensive understanding of the social support resources available to, and coping mechanisms employed by, LGBT older adults. This data is essential for both empirical comparisons and theoretical exploration.

Collecting gender identity and sexual orientation data in larger, US-based probability samples of older adults would address the rhetorical silencing of LGBT older adults that has historically been an issue in gerontological theory, research, and practice (M. T. Brown, 2009). Increasing the visibility of these gender- and sexual-minority elders would give policy makers and service providers the information necessary to identify different levels of need for formal, community-based services and supports, and to develop appropriate programs for vulnerable gender and sexual minority elders.

FUNDING

This study was funded by a 2012 Research Seed Grant from Syracuse University's David B. Falk College of Sport and Human Dynamics and a training fellowship at the 2012 Summer Institute in LGBT Population Health at the Fenway Institute and the Boston University School of Public Health.

REFERENCES

Baumle, A. K., Compton, D. R., & Poston, D. L. (2009). *Same-sex partners: The demography of sexual orientation*. Albany: State University of New York Press.

Brown, J. P., & Tracy, J. K. (2008). Lesbians and cancer: An overlooked health disparity. *Cancer Causes and Control, 19*, 1009–1020.

Brown, M. T. (2009). LGBT aging and rhetorical silence. *Sexuality Research & Social Policy, 6*(4), 65–78.

Butler, S. S. (2004). Gay, lesbian, bisexual, and transgender (GLBT) elders: The challenges and resilience of this marginalized group. *Journal of Human Behavior in the Social Environment*, *9*(4), 25–44.

Cahill, S., & South, K. (2002). Policy issues affecting lesbian, gay, bisexual, and transgender people in retirement. *Generations*, *26*(2), 49–54.

Clements-Nolle, K., Marx, R., & Katz, M. (2006). Attempted suicide among transgender persons: The influence of gender-based discrimination and victimization. *Journal of Homosexuality*, *51*(3), 53–69.

Cochran, S. D., Mays, V. M., Bowen, D., Gage, S., Bybee, D., Roberts, S. J., . . . White, J. (2001). Cancer-related risk indicators and preventive screening behaviors among lesbians and bisexual women. *American Journal of Public Health*, *91*, 591–597.

Cornwell, B. (2011). Age trends in daily social contact patterns. *Research on Aging*, *33*, 598–631.

Cornwell, E. Y., & Waite, L. J. (2009a). Measuring social isolation among older adults using multiple indicators from the NSHAP study. *Journal of Gerontology: Social Sciences*, *64B*(S1), i38–i46.

Cornwell, E. Y., & Waite, L. J. (2009b). Social disconnectedness, perceived isolation, and health among older adults. *Journal of Health and Social Behavior*, *50*, 31–48.

Dorfman, R., Walters, K., Burke, P., Hardin, L., Karanik, T., Raphael, J., & Silverstein, E. (1995). Old, sad and alone: The myth of the aging homosexual. *Journal of Gerontological Social Work*, *24*(1/2), 29–44.

Drum, M. L., Shiovitz-Ezra, S., Gaumer, E., & Lindau, S. T. (2009). Assessment of smoking behaviors and alcohol use in the National Social Life, Health, and Aging Project. *Journal of Gerontology: Social Sciences*, *64B*(S1), i119–i130.

Finkenauer, S., Sherratt, J., Marlow, J., & Brodey, A. (2012). When injustice gets old: A systematic review of trans aging. *Journal of Gay & Lesbian Social Services*, *24*, 311–330.

Fredriksen-Goldsen, K. I., Kim, H.-J., Emlet, C. A., Muraco, A., Erosheva, E. A., Hoy-Ellis, C. P., . . . Petry, H. (2011). *The aging and health report: Disparities and resilience among lesbian, gay, bisexual, and transgender older adults*. Seattle, WA: Institute for Multigenerational Health.

Fredriksen-Goldsen, K. I., & Muraco, A. (2010). Aging and sexual orientation: A 25-year review of the literature. *Research on Aging*, *32*, 372–413.

Gates, G. J., & Cooke, A. M. (2011). *United States–Census snapshot 2010*. Los Angeles, CA: Williams Institute. Retrieved from http://williamsinstitute.law.ucla.edu/wp-content/uploads/Census2010Snapshot-US-v2.pdf

Gates, G. J., & Newport, F. (2013). *LGBT percentage highest in D.C., lowest in North Dakota*. Los Angeles, CA: Williams Institute. Retrieved from http://www.gallup.com/poll/160517/lgbt-percentage-highest-lowest-north-dakota.aspx

Grossman, A. H., D'Augelli, A. R., & Hershberger, S. L. (2000). Social support networks of lesbian, gay, and bisexual adults 60 years of age and older. *Journal of Gerontology: Psychological Sciences*, *55B*, P171–P179.

Hayes, J., Chakraborty, A. T., McManus, S., Bebbington, P., Brugha, T., Nicholson, S., & King, M. (2012). Prevalence of same-sex behavior and orientation in England: Results from a national survey. *Archives of Sexual Behavior*, *41*, 631–639.

Healthy People 2020. (2011). *Lesbian, gay, bisexual and transgender health: Overview*. Retrieved from http://www.healthypeople.gov/2020/topicsobjectives 2020/overview.aspx?topicid=25

Hughes, A. K., Harold, R. D., & Boyer, J. M. (2011). Awareness of LGBT aging issues among aging services network providers. *Journal of Gerontological Social Work, 54*, 659–677.

Institute of Medicine. (2011). *The health of lesbian, gay, bisexual, and transgender (LGBT) people: Building a foundation for better understanding*. Washington, DC: National Academies Press.

Kimmel, D. C. (1978). Adult development and aging: A gay perspective. *Journal of Social Issues, 34*, 113–130.

Koh, A. S., & Ross, L. K. (2006). Mental health issues: A comparison of lesbian, bisexual, and heterosexual women. *Journal of Homosexuality, 51*(1), 33–57.

Kuyper, L., & Fokkema, T. (2010). Loneliness among older lesbian, gay, and bisexual adults: The role of minority stress. *Archives of Sexual Behavior, 39*, 1171–1180.

Met Life Mature Market Institute. (2006). *Out and aging: The MetLife study of lesbian and gay baby boomers*. Retrieved from https://www.metlife.com/assets/ cao/mmi/publications/studies/mmi-out-aging-lesbian-gay-retirement.pdf

Meyer, M. H., & Roseamelia, C. (2007). Emerging issues for older couples: Protecting income and assets, right to intimacy, and end-of-life decisions. *Generations, 31*(3), 66–71.

Michael, R. T., Gagnon, J. H., Laumann, E. O., & Kolata, G. (1994). *Sex in America: A definitive survey*. New York, NY: Little, Brown.

National Institutes of Health. (2012). *Funding opportunities: Research on the health of LGBTI populations*. Retrieved from http://www.nia.nih.gov/research/funding/ 2012/02/research-health-lgbti-populations-r21

National Institutes of Health LGBT Research Coordinating Committee. (2013). *Consideration of the Institute of Medicine (IOM) report on the health of lesbian, gay, bisexual, and transgender (LGBT) individuals*. Retrieved from http://www. nih.gov/about/director/01032013_lgbt_plan.htm

O'Muircheartaigh, C., Eckman, S., & Smith, S. (2009). Statistical design and estimation for the National Social Life, Health, and Aging Project. *Journal of Gerontology: Social Sciences, 64B*(S1), i12–i19.

Rowe, J. W., & Kahn, R. L. (1987). Human aging: Usual and successful. *Science, 237*(4811), 143–149.

San Francisco Human Rights Commission. (2011). *Bisexual invisibility: Impacts and recommendations*. Retrieved from http://www.sf-hrc.org/Modules/ ShowDocument.aspx?documentid=989

Savin-Williams, R. C. (2009). How many gays are there? It depends. In D. A. Hope (Ed.), *Nebraska Symposium on Motivation: Vol. 54: Contemporary perspectives on lesbian, gay, and bisexual identities* (pp. 5–41). New York, NY: Springer.

Sebelius, K. (2011). *U.S. Department of Health and Human Services recommended actions to improve the health and well-being of lesbian, gay, bisexual, and transgender communities*. Retrieved from http://www.hhs.gov/secretary/about/ lgbthealth.html

Sell, R. L., & Becker, J. B. (2001). Sexual orientation data collection and progress toward Healthy People 2010. *American Journal of Public Health, 91*, 876–882.

Sell, R. L., Wells, J. A., & Wypij, D. (1995). The prevalence of homosexual behavior and attraction in the United States, the United Kingdom and France: Results of national population-based samples. *Archives of Sexual Behavior, 24,* 235–248.

Shankle, M. D., Maxwell, C. A., Katzman, E. S., & Landers, S. (2003). An invisible population: Older lesbian, gay, bisexual, and transgender individuals. *Clinical Research and Regulatory Affairs, 20,* 159–182.

Shiovitz-Ezra, S., Leitsch, S., Graber, J., & Karraker, A. (2009). Quality of life and psychological health indicators in the National Social Life, Health, and Aging Project. *Journal of Gerontology: Social Sciences, 64B*(S1), i30–i37.

University of Michigan. (2013). *About the Health and Retirement Study.* Retrieved from http://hrsonline.isr.umich.edu/index.php

Van Wagenen, A., Driskell, J., & Bradford, J. (2013). "I'm still raring to go": Successful aging among lesbian, gay, bisexual, and transgender older adults. *Journal of Aging Studies, 27,* 1–14.

Waite, L., & Das, A. (2010). Families, social life, and well-being at older ages. *Demography, 47,* S87–S109.

Waite, L. J., Laumann, E. O., Das, A., & Schumm, L. P. (2009). Sexuality: Measures of partnerships, practices, attitudes, and problems in the National Social Life, Health, and Aging Project. *Journal of Gerontology: Social Sciences, 64B*(S1), i56–i66.

Waite, L. J., Laumann E. O., Levinson, W., Lindau, S. T., McClintock, M. K., O'Muircheartaigh, C. A., & Schumm, L. P. (2007). *Wave I: In-Person Interview & Leave-Behind Questionnaire.* Retrieved from http://www.icpsr.umich.edu/icpsrweb/NACDA/studies/20541?q=%22National+Institute+on+Aging%22&paging.rows=25&sortBy=4&paging.startRow=26

Waite, L. J., Laumann, E. O., Levinson, W., Lindau, S. T., McClintock, M. K., O'Muircheartaigh, C. A., & Schumm, L. P. (2010). *National Social Life, Health, and Aging Project (NSHAP).* Ann Arbor, MI: Inter-University Consortium for Political and Social Research. doi:10.3886/ICPSR20541.v5

Wallace, S. P., Cochran, S. D., Durazo, E. M., & Ford, C. L. (2011). *The health of aging lesbian, gay and bisexual adults in California.* Los Angeles, CA: UCLA Center for Health Policy Research.

Wells, J. E., McGee, M. A., & Beautrais, A. L. (2011). Multiple aspects of sexual orientation: Prevalence and sociodemographic correlates in a New Zealand national survey. *Archives of Sexual Behavior, 40,* 155–168.

Williams, S. R., Pham-Kanter, G., & Leitsch, S. A. (2009). Measures of chronic conditions and diseases associated with aging in the National Social Life, Health, and Aging Project. *Journal of Gerontology: Social Sciences, 64B*(S1), i67–i75.

Hidden or Uninvited? A Content Analysis of Elder LGBT of Color Literature in Gerontology

LAURENS G. VAN SLUYTMAN

School of Social Work, Morgan State University, Baltimore, Maryland, USA

DENISE TORRES

Graduate School and University Center, City University of New York, New York, New York, USA

As longevity increases and marginalized communities achieve greater visibility in the United States, a content analysis of 64 articles in social work, health, medicine and nursing, and gerontology/psychology examined the extent to which the literature examines the needs and concerns of lesbian, gay, bisexual, and transgender (LGBT) seniors of color (SOC). We found recognition of the distinct cultural needs of sexual orientation and gender minorities. However the distinctive needs of LGBT SOC remains underexplored and poorly documented. Gerontologists, social workers, policymakers, and advocates must support research that values the experience and multiple vulnerabilities of LGBT seniors and questions the structures preventing inclusion and participation.

Increased attention has been given to the issues facing seniors who identify as lesbian, gay, bisexual, and transgender (LGBT). A growing and diverse body of literature has emerged from the various fields working within gerontology. This study was undertaken to determine the extent to which the literature examined and addressed the needs and concerns of older LGBT persons of color (POC), with the central question being, "What has been written about people of color LGBT seniors?" Although their numbers are comparatively small, as compared to their White counterparts, or even as compared to their sexual orientation and gender minority peers, the anticipated growth among non-White communities is greater than among the White population. Holders of multiple minority statuses—age, ethnic and/or racial, and sexual orientation and/or gender identity—LGBT seniors of color may have distinct concerns following from and reflecting the intersection of multiple vulnerabilities. Given these potentially interactional dynamics and the expected increase in the population's size, the authors conducted a content analysis of articles addressing LGBT older adults published in the English language within the past decade to ascertain the visibility of LGBT seniors of color.

AN "INVISIBLE/HIDDEN" POPULATION WITHIN AN UNSEEN MINORITY

Little over 30 years ago, Berger (1982, p. 236) described the senior lesbian and gay community as "an unseen minority" that was "ignored" by professionals. Almost 20 years later, Barranti and Cohen (2001) reaffirmed that this community remains invisible. And there is little national-level health data in the United States for LGBT populations, given that most national and state surveys do not ask sexual orientation and gender identity questions (Gay and Lesbian Medical Association, 2001). The National Gay and Lesbian Task Force (NGLTF) suggests that LGBT senior populations represent anywhere between 3.8 and 7.6% of the total elder population (Grant, 2010), which according to 2012 revised estimates, was 41.4 million Americans (Administration on Aging [AoA], 2012). Using these estimates, there are presently between 1,573,200 and 3,105,000 LGBT seniors in the United States.

Of all seniors, 21% are persons of color, with 9% African American, 7% Latino, 4% Asian or Pacific Islander, 1% American Indian or Alaskan Native, and 0.6% identifying as two or more races. Greater increases are anticipated among minority populations as compared to Whites: Based on recent US Census revisions, the White senior population is projected to increase by 54%, as compared with 124% for older minorities, with Latino seniors quadrupling, Asians and Pacific Islanders and American Indian/Alaskan Natives tripling, and African Americans doubling in size by 2030 (AoA, 2012) Combining these increases with the midpoint of the NGLTF estimate of LGBT seniors (i.e., 5%), we calculated the potential LGBT POC elder population to make the invisible visible: If current estimates are accurate, almost 3.5 million seniors will identify as LGBT, with just under a million of these also a member of a racial or ethnic group.

INTERSECTIONALITY: WHO HEARS THE INVISIBLE?

Individual lives and the history of the United States are intertwined. To discuss gender and gender identity, sex and sexual orientation, race, ethnicity, class, and (dis)ability without recognizing these as socially constructed categories ignores that they are negotiated and reified in "written material and to lived contexts, daily situations and activities through which meanings and identities are produced, reproduced, and contested" (Danforth & Rhodes, 1997, p. 358). Understanding the experience of LGBT seniors of color requires examining the historical forces that contribute to differences in the perception and performance of identities marked by race, gender, and class designations (Knapp, 2005) that potentially create dominant–subordinate relations and that shape how individuals experience and are experienced by others.

Identity categories are frequently treated as analytically distinct aspects of an individual's or groups' lived experience, so that the needs of POC LGBT are "ignored" by "separating out and ranking oppression" (Matsuda, 1991, p. 1191) or "by identifying the community solely on same-sex partner choice, ignoring the class, race, ethnicity, sexual and gender identity diversity of the queer community" (Rosenblum, 1994). Of late, *intersectionality* proliferates much of the social science literature, creating opportunities for rich discussion and exploration of issues meaningful to identity, difference, and power (Davis, 2008), as well as generating engagement in difficult dialogues (Nash, 2010; Watt, 2007). Part of these dialogues is to confront the multiple forms of discrimination that inform and shape the lives of LGBT seniors of color.

Heterosexism in the Aged Community

A significant part of the problem has been that LGBT individuals are often invisible to mainstream senior serving organizations. The elder, in turn, eschews the agency for fear of discrimination: In 1994, almost all of the 24 senior centers in 15 metropolitan areas, or 96%, did not outreach to or provide targeted services and 46% reported LGBT seniors would not be welcome at their center (Behney, 1994). It was not surprising, then, that 72% of LGBT seniors interviewed admitted they avoid presenting to Area Agencies on Aging for services. More recently, 320 agencies from 45 states were queried, and the researchers found limited progress: Although more than a third of agencies provided training to staff on LGBT issues for seniors ($n = 109$ for LGB; $n = 101$ for T), only roughly 12% conducted outreach to LGB ($n = 40$) or T ($n = 39$) persons, with 7.8% offering services targeted to LGB seniors and 7.2% targeting T older adults (Knochel, Croghan, Moone, & Quam, 2012).

Ageism in the Queer Community

Seniors are often isolated from the larger LGBT community. Brotman, Ryan, and Cormier (2003) noted that many LGBT groups in Canada are youth focused, making intergenerational connections difficult as youth have negative attitude towards their older peers, and seniors have difficulty relating to younger persons who have had very different experiences with, and attitudes around, identity and disclosure. Others suggest that this youth focus and generational divide are salient issues in the United States (Barker, Herdt, & de Vries, 2006; LGBT MAP & SAGE, 2010) with researchers finding such differences (Hostetler, 2004), especially among gay men (de Vries, 2011; Schope, 2005) who may perceive *old* as 39 years and older (Schope, 2005). Although others reported that some older LGBT men found growing older exciting and satisfying, these men still couched aging in terms of surviving (Kertzner, 1997; Quam &Whitford, 1992).

Ethnocentrism in the United States

Although "ageism within the LGBT community and homophobia within the mainstream senior community combine to alienate LGBT elders from these two natural constituencies" (Knauer, 2009, p. 304), LGBT seniors of color are also alienated by ethnocentrism, racism, and xenophobia. In fact, race, ethnicity, and culture continue to be after-the-fact considerations, rather than part of an integrated approach to service delivery and research (Bass, Bolton & Murray, 2007). For example, in 2011, the National Academy on An Aging Society, a policy institute of The Gerontological Society of America, dedicated an entire issue to the need to integrate sexual orientation and gender minority individuals into the field's discussions, research, and policy efforts. Yet, discussions in the special issue left unaddressed the unique difficulties in reaching and working with this population although three of the nine articles mentioned the need to see LGBT issues across the oppressions they may experience (de Vries, 2011; Fredriksen-Goldsen, 2011; Meyer, 2011). This oversight has implications for practice, as research has clearly demonstrated that POC LGBT may retreat from the larger LGBT community due to experiences of discrimination associated with race (Beam, 1983, 1986; Bonilla & Porter, 1990; Boykin, 1996; Harper, 1992; Herek & Capitanio, 1995; Riggs, 1991; Simmons, 1991). Our analysis was specifically undertaken to determine the extent to which the gerontological literature has grappled with the complex issues faced by LGBT seniors of color.

METHODS

Content analysis is a research methodology that systematically and objectively considers the nature of content (Allen-Meares, 1984) and communication influenced by cultural transformations over time (Holsti, 1969; Tripodi & Epstein, 1980). In content analyses, researchers describe the procedures they used to select texts and code the material for others to replicate this research, a critical factor to ascertaining validity in social science research (Babbie, 2004; Krippendorff, 2004).

Literature Search and Selection Criteria

For inclusion and retrieval in this review, we used the following selection criteria: (a) published in an English-language peer-reviewed journals; (b) published between 2002 to 2012; (c) a research or literature review; (d) included the terms *LGBT, homosexual, gay, lesbian, bisexual, transgender, elder, aging, senior, people of color (POC), Black, African American, Latino, Hispanic*, and *Asian*; and (e) excluded the terms *youth, adolescent*, and/or *teen*. Relevant articles were identified using 10 computerized databases, traditionally used in the social sciences by social workers: Academic Search Complete, CINAHL Plus with Full Text, Health Source: Nursing/Academic Edition, JAMA, the Journal of the American Medical Association, MEDLINE with Full Text, PsycARTICLES, PsycINFO, Social Sciences Full Text (H. W. Wilson), and SocINDEX with Full Text. Specifically, we retrieved all peer-reviewed scholarly articles published from 2002 to 2012 that discussed LGBT seniors, using the following search terms: LGBT OR Homosexual OR gay OR Lesbian OR Gay OR bisexual OR transgender AND elder OR aging OR senior OR gero* NOT youth OR adolescent OR teen AND "social work" OR "social services" OR nursing OR medicine. The initial review yielded 67 articles.

We defined POC within the sample as those we identified as Black/African American, Hispanic/Latino, Asian/Pacific Islander, American Indian/Native American or Alaskan Native," or mixed/multiracial. Individuals identified as *other race or urban* were not included, as other race was not reported as belonging to any of the racial/ethnic categories previously mentioned. Using the same databases and time frame, we searched for articles that examined POC using the following terms: LGBT Homosexual gay Lesbian Gay bisexual transgender AND elder OR aging OR senior AND "people of color" OR POC OR black OR "African American" OR Latino OR Hispanic OR Asian NOT youth OR adolescent OR teen. We identified 56 articles using these terms. When we limited the search to articles with samples that included people 60+ there were four articles. Of these, one article, Farley, Golding, Young, Mulligan, and Minkoff (2004), had both African Americans and people 60+, but it did not focus on LGBT elders. It was removed from the sample. Similarly, DeMuth (2004) did not examine elder LGBT POC and was removed from the sample. As such, we retained only two articles. For both searches, the database reported overlap between journals: for example, the articles that appeared in *Journal of Gay & Lesbian Social Services: The Quarterly Journal of Community & Clinical Practice* and the

Journal of Gay & Lesbian Social Services: Issues in Practice, Policy & Research. Thus, of the 67 articles initially identified, three articles were removed as they did not address LGBT issues or were duplicates, leaving 64 articles for analysis.

Coding and Analysis

A spreadsheet was created to manage the coding and analysis. The initial content analysis examined easily observable or manifest content, such as a written word or phrase in a text (Potter & Levine-Donnerstein, 1999). After recording the full citation of each article in the first cell, separate columns were created for journal name, year of publication, professional discipline, type of article, methodology, sample, country, geographic location, and density. The total number of articles from each journal was recorded to obtain percentages and frequencies of the occurrence of LGBT seniors and LGBT POC seniors journal articles. Articles were examined closely to determine the methodology employed. These were limited to literature reviews, qualitative, quantitative, and mixed methods. After reading the article, the researcher documented authors and their professional affiliation. Discipline was defined as the authors' professional credential (e.g., MD or RN) or their academic affiliation. In cases where there was no professional or academic affiliation, we used the journal's discipline. Data regarding the discipline of the author were presented qualitatively. Next, the articles' samples were coded according to demographic composition by gender/orientation identity and race/ethnicity and, where discussed, the geographic location and density.

The next wave of coding examined both manifest and latent content. Babbie (2004) described latent content as the fundamental meaning of the text. Each article was read and analyzed considering the primary research question, "What has been written about LGBT POC seniors in selected scholarly journals?" This inductive category development attempted to stay as close to the material as possible by using the article authors' identified key words and phrases concerning outcomes and recommendations. We approached the content in a step-by-step process with each type—key words, outcomes, and recommendations—presented qualitatively. Labels for each phrase and/or text chunk were pulled directly from the articles and served as thematic descriptors. We maintained the themes as global descriptions and in analyzing the outcomes and recommendations identified and created categories to capture the particular sub-themes an article examined. Once the inductive categories were formulated, the researchers reviewed category definitions and, where necessary, modified existing categories and formulated new categories to ensure each was conceptually distinct until all relevant content was captured (saturation).

Deductive categories were applied following from the formulation of categories and were used to manage and systematize coding. For example, in discussing outcomes many of the articles were concerned with the types and nature of health services (i.e., theme) that were available. Within this theme, the specific types of services mentioned were captured as categories (e.g., outreach, gay-friendly, intergenerational, long-term care, end-of-life care). Similarly, the articles addressed the psycho-emotional needs and concerns of seniors: One such theme, fear and discrimination, was discussed in different ways by various authors so that categories included internalized homonegativity, ageism, abuse, family rejection, work discrimination, homophobia, and rejection from service providers or primary care physicians. Thus, we used the deductive categories of *instrumental* and *social* concerns to thematically organize the content. This analytic process resulted in two coding worksheets, Outcomes and Recommendations (Appendix 1), which served as a data reducing aid allowing the authors to create representation units, identify important content, and to guide analysis (Krippendorff, 2004). To insure validity of the coding process, each coder read and analyzed 32 articles, identifying emergent primary and latent content themes and completing a worksheet for each article. We discussed the results until we were in agreement with emerging themes and did not have additional recommendations or changes to the process or the coding worksheet.

We used the IBM SPSS Statistics 20 software to conduct exploratory analyses. The statistical analysis of data included univariate analysis to measure the prevalence of sample demographics of the articles used in this study and bivariate correlations, *t*-test, and Chi square. P-values under 0.05 were considered to indicate statistical significance.

RESULTS

Disciplines and Approach to Investigating LGBT POC Seniors

Based on selection criteria, 64 articles were identified, retrieved, and reviewed. From a disciplinary standpoint, the majority of articles grappling with gerontological issues among the LGBT POC population were social workers with 35 (54.7%) articles. Close to two-fifths of the articles (*n* = 25, 39.1%) were from *health, medicine, and nursing*, with the remaining four articles (4.6%) representing gerontology/psychology. Methodologically, researchers tended to equally employ quantitative and qualitative methods, with 28 articles (43.1%) using the former and 31 (48.4%) employing the latter. Of the remaining five articles, two (3.1%) used a mixed-methods design and three (4.6%) were literature reviews. Table 1 provides a summary of the articles by discipline and methodology employed.

Population Demographics

Given that only English language articles were included in our criteria, the locality or country of origin of the studies was limited. The vast majority

TABLE 1 Article Discipline and Methodological Approach

	N	%
Discipline		
Social work	35	54.7
Medicine/Nursing/Health	25	39.1
Gerontology/Psychology	4	4.6
Methods		
Quantitative methodology	28	43.1
Qualitative methodology	31	48.4
Mixed methodology	2	3.1
Literature review	3	4.6

described US populations, with 43 (67.2%) articles. The remaining third of articles ($n = 21$) investigated populations in Australia ($n = 7$, 10.8%), Canada ($n = 5$, 7.8%), New Zealand ($n = 2$, 3.1%), Sweden (n = 1, 1.6%) and the United Kingdom ($n = 6$, 9.4%). In terms of the representativeness of samples and their inclusion of POC or indigenous populations, 39 articles (60.9%) reported racially mixed samples, whereas three articles (4.7 %) reported only White participants and two articles (3.1%) examined the nexus of race/ethnicity and LGBT aging. Almost a quarter of articles ($n = 15$) did not report the racial composition of the sample. Regarding gender identification, 16 articles (25%) sampled only female participants; two (3.1%) male only; and 33 (51.6%) used a mixed-gender sample. Of the articles employing a mixed-gender sample, seven (11%) included individuals identified as transgender in the sample. Table 2 captures the demographic compositions of the samples within the articles reviewed, including racial/ethnic, gender, and national identification.

Types of Outcomes

Given that the articles examined various issues in their reviews of the literature and discussion sections, we specifically attended to the types of outcomes the articles described during coding. Outcomes were classified as instrumental or social. Outcomes categorized as instrumental dealt with issues such as health access, health status, and health care services. Social outcomes addressed issues such as identity, fear and discrimination, isolation, networks, mental health, and locus of control. The majority of articles ($n = 35$, 54.7%) reported both instrumental and social concerns, 16 articles (25%) reported only social outcomes, and 13 articles (20%) reported only instrumental outcomes.

Instrumental outcomes. Among those articles reporting instrumental outcomes, the majority ($n = 48$, 75%) discussed research as part of their outcomes, followed by health services ($n = 17$, 26%) and financial legal services ($n = 17$, 26.6%). Those discussing health services predominantly

TABLE 2 Article Population Descriptions by Race, Gender, and Location

	N	%
Sample race		
White only	3	4.7
Persons of color only	2	3.1
Racially mixed	39	60.9
Unknown*	15	23.4
Literature review	5	7.8
Sample gender*		
Female only	16	25
Male only	2	3.1
Transgender only	0	0
Mixed gender sample	33	51.6
Unknown	8	12.5
Literature review	5	7.8
Sample location		
Australia	7	10.9
Canada	5	7.8
New Zealand	2	3.1
Sweden	1	1.6
United Kingdom	6	9.4
United States	43	67.2

*Race/Ethnicity not reported.

focused on long-term care with eight articles (12.5%) and four articles (6.3%) discussing outreach and training outcomes, respectively.

Social outcomes. Among articles with social outcome findings, 24 (37.5%) discussed identity, 22 (34.4%) fear and discrimination, and 23 (35.9%) discussed isolation. Articles describing identity outcomes predominantly focused on sexuality ($n = 13$, 20.3%) and disclosure ($n = 12$, 18.8%) with only two (3.1%) specifically discussing identity diversity. Outcomes focused on fear and discrimination predominantly discussed fears of homophobia and rejection by organizations/providers or primary care ($n = 11$, 17.2% each). Only one article (1.6%) discussed fear and discrimination associated with race within its outcomes. Among those articles discussing social isolation, 14 articles (21.9%) discussed social networks and 13 articles (20.3%) discussed caregiver networks.

Focus of Outcomes by Discipline

Analysis by discipline revealed no significant differences between or among articles in terms of outcomes discussed. The majority of articles in *social work* and *Medicine, Nursing, and Health* attended to both social and instrumental outcomes; only in the gerontology/psychology articles were social outcomes given greater attention. As reported in Table 3, bivariate analysis revealed that of the 35 social work articles, 12 (75%) discussed only social outcomes; six (46.2%) discussed only instrumental outcomes; and close to

TABLE 3 Number and Percentage of Articles Discussing Outcomes by Discipline and Recommendation Themes

	Social Outcomes		Instrumental Outcomes		Both Social and Instrumental Outcomes	
	N	%	N	%	N	%
Social work	12	75	6	46.2	17	48.6
Medicine, nursing & health	2	12.5	6	46.2	17	48.6
Gerontology/Psychology	2	12.5	1	7.7	1	2.9

half, or 17 articles (48.6%), discussed both instrumental and social outcomes. Among the 25 *medicine, nursing, and health* articles, two (12.5%) discussed only social outcomes, six (46.2%) discussed only instrumental outcomes and 17 (48.6%) discussed both. Within the four gerontology/psychology articles, two (12.5%) discussed social outcomes, and one each discussed instrumental or social outcomes (7.7%), and one discussed both social and instrumental outcomes (2.9%). These findings were not statistically significant.

Recommendations

We examined the types of recommendations made by the studies and categorized these as practice, staff, policy, organizational, educational, and research (Table 4). Of the recommendations made within the 64 articles reviewed, they can be captured as follows (in descending order):

- 47 articles (73.4%) encouraged further research (e.g., exploration of family constellations);
- 27 articles (42.2%) made organizational recommendations (e.g., more inclusive language);
- 14 articles (21.9%) made recommendations concerning practice (e.g., changes to assessment);

TABLE 4 Number and Percentage of Articles Proposing Recommendation by Discipline and Recommendation Themes*

	Practice		Staff		Policy		Organization		Education		Research	
	N	%	N	%	N	%	N	%	N	%	N	%
Social work	8	22.9	1	2.9	7	20.0	14	40.0	4	11.4	24	68.6
Medicine, nursing & health	6	24.0	1	4.0	4	16.0	11	44.0	3	12.0	19	76.0
Gerontology/ Psychology	0	0.0	1	25.0	1	25.0	2	50.0	0	0	4	100.0

*Article may propose more than one theme.

- 12 articles (18.8%) recommended addressing policy (e.g., LGBT legal recommendation and rights);
- 7 articles (10.9%) recommended education for the workforce (e.g., LGBT content in schools or discipline specific curricula); and,
- 3 articles (4.7%) made recommendations concerning staff sensitivity training (e.g., respect for differences).

These recommendations can be framed by traditional areas of specialty/practice, as follows:

- *Research*: Of the 47 articles that made recommendations concerning future research, the majority cited the need to explore social networks (12 articles or 18.8%). Other recommendations included: future research on racial diversity (11 articles/17.2%); the need to explore diversity (11 articles/17.2%); the need to collect more data concerning sexual orientation (7 articles/10.9%); examination of family constellations (6 articles/9.4%); the need for more large scale studies (4 articles/6.3%); and research on caregivers, isolation, discrimination and long term care and end of life planning (3 articles/4.6%).
- *Organizational and direct practice*: Among the 27 articles that made recommendations concerning organizational policies and procedures, 10 (15.6%) addressed the need for increased organizational awareness and another 11 (16.9%) reinforced the need to create safety and safe spaces for LGBT seniors. Ten articles (15.6%) recommended greater culturally appropriate and sensitive engagement; two articles (3.1%) each recommended use of more inclusive language and greater outreach. Only one article (1.6%) recommended intergenerational services. Of the 14 articles (21.9%) making practice recommendations, four (6.2%) recommended greater emphasis on assessment, four addressed alcohol abuse treatment (6.3%), and two (3.1%) dealt with exercise. Practice recommendations reported by only one article (1.6%) included aging services, coping skills, financial support, and health services.
- *Education and training*: Overall, seven articles (10.9%) encouraged education of the workforce with three (4.7%) recommending more LGBT content in schools, four (6.2%) encouraging specific workforce training in LGBT issues, and two (3.1%) more general workforce development in this area. Only three articles (4.6%) made recommendations concerning staff, which included LGBT content in schools. Among those articles making recommendation for staff, two (3.1%) discussed recommendations for caregiver support, and only one (1.6%) made recommendations concerning the need for respect of difference.
- *Policy and advocacy articles:* In the articles recommendations concerning policy addressed targeted advocacy (4 articles/6.3%) and caregivers

(3 articles/4.7%). Across disciplines most articles made recommendations concerning transforming organizations: 14 in social work (40%); 11 in medicine, nursing, and health (44%); and two in gerontology/psychology (50%).

DISCUSSION

As the demographic shift known as *the graying of America* unfurls, the health and human services sectors must contend with the implications of an aging populace. In our analysis of 64 articles spanning a decade of studies (2002–2012), we found that the unique needs and concerns of LGBT seniors are being examined. Of the 10 articles specifically encouraging the use of LGBT culturally appropriate and/or sensitive approaches (15.6% of the sample), the majority have been written in the latter part of the decade (Gabrielson, 2011a, 2011b; Hash & Netting, 2007; A. K. Hughes, Harold, & Boyer, 2011; M. Hughes, 2009; Landers, Mimiaga, & Krinsky, 2010; Lovejoy et al., 2008; Persson, 2009; Richard & Brown, 2006; Zaritsky & Dibble, 2010), suggesting that progress is being made in recognizing the distinct cultural needs of sexual orientation and gender minority communities.

Equally instructive is that many of the articles spoke to the differences within the LGBT community itself and the need to identify and explore the needs and experiences of lesbian, gay, bisexual, and transgender persons that fall under the larger LGBT umbrella. In point of fact, when the articles in this review spoke to the need for more research diversity, the majority addressed the diversity of LGBT identities (Averett, Yoon, & Jenkins, 2011; Fredriksen-Goldsen & Hooyman, 2007; Fredriksen-Goldsen, Kim, Muraco, & Mincer, 2009; Goldberg, Sickler, & Dibble, 2005; M. Hughes, 2009; Jacobs & Kane, 2012; Jones & Nystrom, 2002; Scherrer, 2009). Goldberg et al. (2005) captured this perspective, stating:

> It is important to stress diversity. LGBT people are not one 'community' and likewise lesbians themselves do not constitute one sub population with identical needs, desires, and wants. The importance of building this body of literature cannot be overemphasized in order to explore the diversity of lesbian 'communities' and create a range of services geared to address different needs. (p. 210)

Hence, this analysis revealed an increased understanding that the LGBT community is not monolithic, but comprises multiple communities.

Although a body of literature that identifies the needs of sexual orientation and gender minority seniors is emerging, among the articles reviewed cultural competence referred solely to the capacity to attend to issues related to sexual orientation with little discussion of how these are further influenced by race, ethnicity, and class, so that the experience and distinctive needs of elders of color who identify as LGBT remains underexplored and poorly documented. One article specifically examining issues for African American lesbians noted, "Intersections of race, class, gender, sexual orientation, and body size have rarely been studied" (Dibble, Eliason, & Crawford, 2012, p. 834). Although the majority of articles included a racially/ethnically mixed sample ($n = 39$, 60.9%), given the small sample sizes of many of the studies, analysis based on race or ethnicity would yield statistically insignificant results. Thus, although some articles highlighted ethnic/racial concerns in their reviews of the literature and drew attention to the need for inclusion of racial and ethnic minority elders in LGBT samples, few addressed their needs.

As well, even when studies obtained large samples, too few persons of color or indigenous respondents were reached making use of race/ethnicity as a variable of analysis inappropriate. In addressing this, M. Hughes (2009, p. 371, emphasis added) noted, *"the small number of people reporting as having a non-Anglo Australian background meant that cultural background* could not be used as a variable in statistical analysis." In fact, of the 39 articles with mixed samples, only nine had samples wherein racial/ethnic minorities or indigenous populations exceeded 21%. Hence, researchers' continued encouragement of larger sample sizes (Dibble & Roberts, 2002; Jessup & Dibble, 2012) and more inclusive studies to ascertain how concerns may differ among POC, indigenous peoples, and more impoverished and less educated LGBT persons (Fritsch, 2005; Hash & Cramer, 2003; McFarland & Sanders, 2003; Orel, 2004; Stein, Beckerman, & Sherman, 2010). Lamentably, based on these findings, the answer to the question "What has been written about LGBT POC seniors in selected scholarly journals?" is, very little.

IMPLICATIONS

Given that the particular needs and concerns of LGBT seniors of color were largely unaddressed by the articles in this review, we explore some of the major themes in the context of LGBT POC. We use direct quotes from the reviewed articles, as appropriate, to highlight key concerns or issues.

Hidden and Invisible?

The analysis makes clear that LGBT seniors, in particular POC, are rendered invisible because providers, organizations, and policymakers are not looking. Hughes, Harold, and Boyer (2011) offered that the "results about agency or organizational service . . . tell . . . of a system that is paying little attention to this community. This systematic negligence begins when sexual orientation is not addressed at intake" (p. 671). From an organizational per-spective, a number of articles underscored the need to assess their policies and procedures and make changes to their intake and other documents to assure multiple opportunities are available for disclosure. Furthermore, the assumption that an individual is straight based on documentation in the record of a prior history of heterosexual marriage and/or of offspring needs to be examined and dichotomous conceptualizations of orientation contested. Organizations need to create safe and accepting spaces where there is awareness of the historical, political, and social forces that make dis-closure conflictual for LGBT seniors. In discussing provider willingness and perceived capacity to provide service to LGBT seniors, A. K. Hughes et al. (2011) also offered that the "perception of invisibility likely contributes to the concerns related to fear and prejudice" (p. 670). Thus, the suggestion that LGBT seniors are hidden and/or invisible is unfair—providers are not looking or seeing this aspect of identity, as demonstrated by their failure to ask the question—and this unfairness diminishes LGBT seniors' sense of safety in disclosing their identity.

Identity and Discrimination

As LGBT individuals of color age, they must not only contend with ageism, but age-based discrimination in the context of complex histories and experi-ences with racism and hetero-sexism. As discussed earlier, LGBT seniors of color must confront hetero-sexism in the aged community, ageism within the queer community, and ethnocentrism more generally. Although many of the articles discussed identity in terms of managing disclosure, visibility, and per-formance (Almack, Seymour, & Bellamy, 2010; Averett et al., 2011; Brotman et al., 2003; Cronin, Ward, Pugh, King, & Price, 2011; M. Hughes, 2007, 2008; Jones & Nystrom, 2002; Jönson & Siverskog, 2012; Knochel et al., 2012; McFarland & Sanders, 2003; Persson, 2009; Politi, Clark, Armstrong, McGarry, & Sciamanna, 2009; Stein et al., 2010), no article examined specifically how seniors of color who identify as LGBT enact or refrain from performing aspects of their identities. For example, many of the articles examining dis-crimination focused on fear and discrimination as it related to heterosexist views within organizations/providers or primary care settings ($n = 11$, 17.2% each). In speaking to this issue from the Australian perspective, M. Hughes (2008) noted:

> The findings suggest a complex relationship between identity and com-munity in the lives of older lesbians and gays. The two appear to be intertwined, and contingent upon and constantly negotiated in interac-tions with friends, groups, organizations, and neighbourhoods. Effective planning and delivery of health and aged care for lesbian and gay people will need to accommodate this complexity and diversity. Services reliant

upon assumed uniform and essentialist notions of identity and assumed positive engagement with imagined lesbian and gay communities may not reach all who might benefit from the care and support of these agencies. (p. 183)

Given that this "complex relationship between identity and community" for American seniors of color includes negotiating interactions based on race-ethnicity, service providers and researchers are well advised to heed the warning about essentialist notions of identity.

Caregiving and Natal Networks

Similarly, despite the body of literature (Shippy, 2007) that LGBT individuals may not be estranged from their biological families and may, in fact, participate in caregiving responsibilities for parents, the focus appears to remain on families of choice, or the social networks that LGBT create beyond their families of origin. In those articles discussing the resilience found in biological family networks and intergenerational health services, the need to explore natal networks more fully emerged from histories of previous heterosexual marriages, including children (Averett, Yoon & Jenkins, 2012; Jones & Nystrom, 2002; Goldberg, Sickler & Dibble, 2005; Hash, 2006; Brotman et al., 2007), dependence on families of origin and natal networks (Almack, Seymour & Bellamy, 2010; Averett, Yoon & Jenkins, 2011; Fredriksen-Goldsen & Hooyman, 2007; Fredriksen-Goldsen, Kim, Muraco & Mincer, 2009; Owen & Catalan, 2012; Persson, 2009; Porter, Russell & Sullivan, 2004; Richard & Brown, 2006), and from the reality that regardless of their experience in disclosing to families many LGBT seniors provide caregiving to family members (Cronin, Ward, Pugh, King & Price, 2011; Gabrielson, 2011b). Thus, Fredriksen-Goldsen & Hooyman (2007) offered that "most current family and caregiving programs and policies simply do not recognize the changing nature of the family and the important role of informal caregiving with historically marginalized communities" (p. 143). Within communities of color, this is a particularly important issue as reliance on family-of-origin networks buffer the stress associated with discrimination (Ajrouch, Reisine, Lim, Sohn, & Ismail, 2010; Cohen & Wills, 1985; Kawachi, & Berkman, 2001).

Health and Health Care Access

Given that POC experience significant health disparities, including barriers to care and discrimination, the lack of attention to this issue within the articles analyzed is concerning: Like their LGBT peers, POC anticipate discriminatory responses from health providers (Kessler, Mickelson, & Williams, 1999). Although a number of articles addressed health-seeking behaviors within the context of fear and discrimination related to sexual orientation, they fail to acknowledge how this is compounded by negative experiences based on racial and sexual identities for LGBT POC (Malebranche, Peterson, Fullilove & Stackhouse, 2004). Moreover, although health care status inequalities were often recognized because of *triple minority* status for women (i.e., LGBT, women, and senior) the fourth intersection of race and ethnicity is not discussed. This is critical as LGBT seniors of color have been found to perceive themselves as less healthy than their White counterparts: 42.8% of noninstitutionalized White seniors reported excellent or very good health, whereas only 26% of African American, 28.2% of Latino, 24.3% of American Indian/Alaskan Natives, and 35.3% of Asians reported their health as excellent or very good (AoA, 2012).

Education, Training, and Cultural Competence

Recommendations to improve the capacity of health, social service, and other providers to more competently serve LGBT older adults were made by a number of articles. In addition to workforce training (4), the articles emphasized the integration of LGBT content into the curricula in schools of medicine, social work, nursing, and other professions to better prepare the emerging workforce that will serve seniors (3). Yet, it is equally important to note that "training programs have contributed to stigma through the invisibility of sexual and gender identities in the curriculum except for mention as pathologies, diseases, or "exotic" forms of human sexuality" (Eliason, Dibble, & Robertson, 2011, p. 1357). Although progress is being made in training professionals in LGBT aging issues, these efforts have generally been local and opportunistic (LGBT MAP & SAGE, 2010), sending the "implicit message" that such expertise is "optional for health care providers and that only those who are so inclined need to seek out this knowledge" (Hanssmann, Morrison, & Russian, 2008, p. 6). It also has implications for care-seeking as agencies that trained staff are more likely to conduct targeted outreach and to elicit service requests (Knochel et al., 2012).

Inclusive Sampling and Research Strategies

The two articles addressing LGBT older adults of color dealt with POC seniors within the context of known health risks or disparities suggesting that, as with training efforts, their inclusion is deficit based. Indeed, one of the articles captured this issue well with a study participant's own words: "I am not a disease. I am not an experimental animal" (Kidd & Witten, 2008, p. 55). Moreover, the articles suggested the need to conduct further research on diversity and discrimination primarily focused on sexual orientation, rather than fear and discrimination related to sexual orientation as being contributory to, and impacting, fear and discrimination related to other aspects of identity. As Lanehart (2009) noted,

> Our parts are many—gender, region/locale, nationality, religion, skin color, phenotype, education/schooling, ability, sexuality, race, ethnicity, age/generation, socioeconomic class, physiology, language, variety, sex, etc.—but we are more than the sum of them. All that makes us who we are intersects multiplicatively, not additively. (p. 2)

Hence, more diverse research is needed on the intersectionality of class, (dis)ability, gender, location, ethnicity, and race in sexual orientation, as well as the multiple stress associated with these categories and their relationship to disparities in health outcome and inequities in access to services.

Among those articles that were able to penetrate into communities of color, the sampling strategies and lessons learned may prove instructive for future research. Those who successfully reached LTBG older adults of color also engaged community members in generating questions and in other phases of the research process. In particular, Smith, McCaslin, Chang, Martinez, and McGrew (2010) were able to obtain a 26% non-White sample (i.e., 10 of 38 respondents) by specifically engaging African American and Latino students to field their survey. The Latino students were able to translate face-to-face interviews, allowing individuals with limited English proficiency to participate in the study, emphasizing how consideration of linguistic and cultural issues can increase access to populations deemed hidden.

Many of the more successful studies used varied recruitment strategies, including use of affinity groups such as advocacy organizations, houses of worship, fellowship and mutual aid groups, and online communities and listservs. Notably, some researchers used faith communities to identify LGBT seniors (e.g., Averett et al., 2011: Dibble et al., 2012; Kidd & Whitten, 2008; McFarland & Sanders, 2003), recognizing that spirituality contributes to well-being and remains an important aspect of identity regardless of a particular faith's stance (Dibble et al., 2012; Fredriksen-Goldsen et al., 2009; Jenkins, Walker, Cohen, & Curry, 2010; Jones & Nystrom, 2002; Kidd & Whitten, 2008; Orel, 2004). However, as noted by Dibble et al. (2012) church-based recruitment may be challenging. And we suggest, given the role of faith among POC, it must be seen intersectionally when outreaching to LGBT seniors of color: In a study where recruitment was conducted solely using churches, researchers were able to reach 59 LGBT identified seniors, but racial/ethnic identification was left completely unaddressed (McFarland & Sanders, 2003).

Social Work Practice and Pedagogy

The attention to both social and instrumental issues and outcomes among the majority of social work articles is encouraging, as it suggests that researchers employ a dual perspective of practice competence with minority populations and attend to the interplay between micro- and macro-level forces (Van Den Bergh & Crisp, 2004). Similarly, the articles were well rounded in their recommendations for practice, policy organization, and research. However, the issues surfaced speak to the need in social work practice and education to see the full complexity of clients' lives and identity construction by asking questions, engaging in difficult dialogues, and developing culturally competent knowledge and skills. Although the recent publication of the National Resource Center on LGBT Aging's (2013) guide to inclusive questioning may assist in regards to identifying LGBT seniors, a central concern is social workers' capacity to competently address any issues following from their disclosure: Although MSW students did not hold stigmatizing views toward LGBT communities, they also felt ill equipped and prepared to serve them (Logie, Bridge, & Bridge, 2007), given that most MSW programs did not assess student competence in relation to LGBT issues, provided few opportunities to work with LGBT seniors (e.g., 8% of schools had available field placements in elder settings), and had few faculty members with sufficient awareness of LGBT issues (Martin et al., 2009). Thus, efforts like those of Crisp, Wayland, and Gordon (2008) to instill LGBT affirming competencies across the life-course can help students reflect on heterosexist views while assisting them to acquire the skill sets that will begin to address the policies and structures within organizations and communities that diminish the visibility of LGBT seniors of color.

Limitations

Our review faced several limitations. First, the literature search focused specifically on LGBT seniors and LGBT seniors of color, and not elders of color in general. We also examined only peer-reviewed articles. These procedures limited the articles retrieved and may result in biases associated with issues of interest to the academic community versus provider-, state-, and/or local-level resources and materials regarding culturally sensitive supports and services to LGBT communities (e.g., gray literature). Hence, resources and articles located on web sites such as the National Resource Center on LGBT Aging and the American Society on Aging were not included.

It is possible that the parameters of our search did not yield all relevant articles. For example, the publication date parameters are known to have excluded an article curated as an online blog that was specifically focused on health disparities among LGBT seniors of color (Van Sluytman, 2013). This blog included articles discussing empowerment and reticence in relation to legal issues (Chin, 2013), a model of programming designed to reduce social isolation among LGBT seniors of color (Francis & Acey, 2013), improving medical access for transgender people (Kishore, 2013), and cervical cancer among Black lesbian and bisexual women (Rice, 2013)—none of which were identified due to the search parameters. Additionally, given the number of articles retrieved, we were not able to distinguish between research targeting elders and those referred to as the old-old. This is particularly important, given that, in general, the old-old are predominantly female and in poverty. Yet another limitation is our selection of databases (for example, Medline was included but not PubMed), resulting in the potential absence of articles from federally funded research projects. Last, we did not use queer as a search category. The term *queer* has potential to offend many elders in the community, given its historical usage. However, future searches for scholarship related to LGBT POC seniors may be strengthened by such an expansion in terminology in its current self-affirming incarnation and potential for creating solidarity (Morris, 2000) while questioning the hetero/homo binary (Sedgwick, 1990). These limitations highlight the need for, and difficulties of, attending to all identities and factors simultaneously and to engaging a truly intersectional and interdisciplinary lens. We hope these identified weaknesses guide future researchers forward in their efforts to address the needs of LGBTQ seniors of color.

Future research should begin to examine the overlap of themes within the literature focused on LGBT elders and those who are actively entering, or will enter, the services. Such examinations could identify significant changes in the environment (especially government recognition) that influence the disclosure and management of identity, as well as self-advocacy for LGBT specific services for elders and young adults. Furthermore, examining the experience of elder lesbian and heterosexual women could lend further support to the greater challenges of gender-based policy advocacy.

Conclusion

This study was undertaken to determine the extent to which the literature examined and addressed the needs and concerns of older LGBT POC. Content analysis of 64 articles in the international scholarly literature surfaced two articles specifically addressing the needs of LGBT older persons from racial/ethnic or indigenous populations. This finding suggests that conceptualizations of identity continue to be segmented and essentialist. Fish (2008) noted that intersectionality has not been explicitly used in LGBT health research, rendering "invisible the experiences of disabled, Black, and minority ethnic and other groups and has contributed towards the homogenisation of LGBT communities." This is true of the gerontological literature. Remaining invisible, too often POC were overlooked and few attempts at targeted recruitment were made. When researchers did endeavor to include

POC, success was limited with failures justified because they are hidden. We suggest that, rather than being invisible or hidden, LGBT seniors of color are perceived as guests in practice, policy, and research arenas who may be invited—as possible—but are generally uninvited to contribute to discussions. As a national population transforms, this failure to invite POC into such difficult dialogues demonstrates a lack of foresight.

Recently, Kropf and Adamek (2005) offered that social work is ideally situated to set the agenda and contribute to policy and practice for seniors. As it is incumbent upon the profession to advocate with, and for, those who face multiple forms of oppression (Avery & Bashir, 2003; Dalton, 1989; Wheeler, 2003), the use of an intersectional lens is critical. And, as longevity increases and marginalized communities achieve greater visibility in the United States, social workers, policymakers, and advocates must support interventions focusing on this emergent population. Over 10 years ago, McMahon and Allen-Meares (1992, p. 537) asked, "Is social work racist?" They concluded the literature that examines POC is "naïve and superficial," recommending that social work engage in transformative antiracist actions that challenge prevailing forms of structural discrimination. This is consistent with social work's professional code, which calls social workers to "strengthen relationships among people in a purposeful effort to promote, restore, maintain, and enhance the well-being of individuals, families, social groups, organizations, and communities" (National Association of Social Workers, 2000, p. 145). Our findings and these values suggest that the gerontological literature in social work must engage an antiracist stance to give voice to the experience of LGBT seniors of color and to question the structures and factors that render them invisible

REFERENCES

Administration on Aging (AoA). (2012). *A profile of older Americans: 2012*. Retrieved from http://www.aoa.gov/Aging_Statistics/Profile/2012/docs/2012profile.pdf

Administration on Aging. (2013). *Profile of older Americans: 2012*. Retrieved from http://www.aoa.gov/Aging_Statistics/Profile/2012/7.aspx

Ajrouch, K., Reisine, S., Lim, S., Sohn, W., & Ismail, A. (2010). Perceived everyday discrimination and psychological distress: does social support matter? *Ethnicity & Health*, *15*(4), 417–434.

Allen-Meares, P. (1984). Content analysis: It does have a place in social work. *Journal of Social Service Research*, 7, 51–68.

Almack, K., Seymour, J., & Bellamy, G. (2010). Exploring the impact of sexual orientation on experiences and concerns about end of life care and on bereavement for lesbian, gay and bisexual older people. *Sociology*, *44*(5), 908–924. doi:10.1177/0038038510375739

Averett, P., Yoon, I., & Jenkins, C. L. (2011). Older lesbians: Experiences of aging, discrimination and resilience. *Journal of Women & Aging*, *23*(3), 216–232. doi:10.1080/08952841.2011.587742

Avery, B., & Bashir, S. (2003). The road to advocacy-searching for the rainbow. *American Journal of Public Health, 93*(8), 1207–1210.

Babbie, E. (2004). *The practice of social research* (10th ed.). Belmont, CA: Thomson/Wadsworth.

Barker, J. C., Herdt, G., & de Vries, B. (2006). Social support in the lives of lesbians and gay men at midlife and later. *Sexuality Research & Social Policy, 3*(2), 1–23.

Barranti, C., & Cohen, H. (2001). Lesbian and gay elders: An invisible minority. In R. Schneider, N. Kropf, & A. Kisor (Eds.), *Gerontological social work: Knowledge, service settings and special populations* (pp. 343–368). Belmont, CA: Brooks/Cole.

Bass, J. K., Bolton, P. A., & Murray, L. K. (2007). Do not forget culture when studying mental health. *Lancet, 370*(9591), 918–918.

Beam, J. (1983). Racism from a Black perspective. In M. Smith (Ed.), *Black men/White men* (pp. 57–63). San Francisco, CA: Gay Sunshine Press.

Beam, J. (Ed.). (1986). *In the life: A Black gay anthology*. Boston, MA: Alyson Publications.

Behney, R. (1994). The Aging Network's response to gay and lesbian issues. *Outword: Newsletter of the Lesbian and Gay Aging Issues Network, 1*(2), 2.

Berger, R. M. (1982). The unseen minority: Older gays and lesbians. *Social Work, 27*(3), 236–242.

Boehmer, U., Miao, X., Linkletter, C., & Clark, M. A. (2012). Adult health behaviors over the life course by sexual orientation. *American Journal of Public Health, 102*(2), 292–300. doi:10.2105/AJPH.2011.300334

Bonilla, L., & Porter, J. (1990). A comparison of Latino, Black, and non-Hispanic White attitudes toward homosexuality. *Hispanic Journal of Behavioral Sciences, 12*, 437–452.

Boykin, K. (1996). *One more river to cross*. New York, NY: Anchor Books.

Brotman, S., Ryan, B., Collins, S., Chamberland, L., Cormier, R., Julien, D., & Richard, B. (2007). Coming out to care: Caregivers of gay and lesbian seniors in Canada. *Gerontologist, 47*(4), 490–503.

Brotman, S., Ryan, B., & Cormier, R. (2003). The health and social service needs of gay and lesbian elders and their families in Canada. *Gerontologist, 43*(2), 192–202.

Chin, N. (2013). *Reticence and resistance: Power of attorney and LGBT aging issues*. Retrieved from http://www.asaging.org/blog/reticence-and-necessity-power-attorney-and-lgbt-aging-issues

Cohen, S., & Wills, T. A. (1985).Stress, social support, and the buffering hypothesis. *Psychological Bulletin, 98*, 310–357.

Crisp, C., Wayland, S., & Gordon, T. (2008). Older gay, lesbian, and bisexual adults: Tools for age-competent and gay affirmative practice. *Journal of Gay & Lesbian Social Services, 20*(1–2), 5–29.

Cronin, A., Ward, R., Pugh, S., King, A., & Price, E. (2011). Categories and their consequences: Understanding and supporting the caring relationships of older lesbian, gay and bisexual people. *International Social Work, 54*(3), 421–435. doi:10.1177/0020872810396261

Dalton, H. L. (1989). AIDS in blackface. *Daedalus, 118*, 205–227.

Danforth, S., & Rhodes, W. C. (1997). Deconstructing disability: A philosophy for inclusion. *Remedial and Special Education, 18*(6), 357–366.

Davis, K. (2008). Intersectionality as buzzword: A sociology of science perspective on what makes a feminist theory successful. *Feminist Theory*, *9*(1), 67–85.

DeMuth, D. (2004). Another look at resilience: Challenging the stereotypes of aging. *Journal of Feminist Family Therapy*, *16*(4), 61–74. doi:10.1300/J086v16n04_04

de Vries, B. (2011). LGBT aging: Research and policy directions. *Policy & Aging Report*, *21*(3), 34–35.

de Vries, B., Mason, A. M., Quam, J., & Acquaviva, K. (2009). State recognition of same-sex relationships and preparations for end of life among lesbian and gay boomers. *Sexuality Research & Social Policy*, *6*(1), 90–101.

Dibble, S. L., Eliason, M. J., & Crawford, B. (2012). Correlates of wellbeing among African American lesbians. *Journal of Homosexuality*, *59*(6), 820–838. doi:10.1080/00918369.2012.694763

Dibble, S. L., & Roberts, S. A. (2002). A comparison of breast cancer diagnosis and treatment between lesbian and heterosexual women. *Journal of the Gay & Lesbian Medical Association*, *6*(1), 9–17.

Drumm, K. (2004). An examination of group work with old lesbians struggling with a lack of intimacy by using a record of service. *Journal of Gerontological Social Work*, *44*(1–2), 25–52. doi:10.1300/J083v44n01_03

Eliason, M. J., Dibble, S. L., & Robertson, P. A. (2011). Lesbian, gay, bisexual, and transgender (LGBT) physicians' experiences in the workplace. *Journal of Homosexuality*, *58*(10), 1355–1371. doi:10.1080/00918369.2011.614902

Farley, M., Golding, J. M., Young, G., Mulligan, M., & Minkoff, J. R. (2004). Trauma history and relapse probability among patients seeking substance abuse treatment. *Journal of Substance Abuse Treatment*, *27*(2), 161–167. doi:10.1016/j.jsat.2004.06.006

Fenge, L., Fannin, A., Armstrong, A., Hicks, C., & Taylor, V. (2009). Lifting the lid on sexuality and ageing: The experiences of volunteer researchers. *Qualitative Social Work: Research and Practice*, *8*(4), 509–524.

Fish, J. (2008). Navigating Queer Street: Researching the intersections of lesbian, gay, bisexual and trans (LGBTQ) identities in health research. *Sociological Research Online*, *13*(1). Retrieved from http://www.socresonline.org.uk/13/1/12.html

Francis, G. M., & Acey, K. (2013). *Reducing isolation: A community engagement service model*. Retrieved from http://www.asaging.org/blog/reducing-isolation-community-engagement-service-model

Fredriksen-Goldsen, K. I. (2011). Resilience and disparities among lesbian, gay, bisexual and transgender older adults. *Policy & Aging Report*, *21*(3), 3–7.

Fredriksen-Goldsen, K. I., & Hooyman, N. R. (2007). Caregiving research, services, and policies in historically marginalized communities: where do we go from here? *Journal of Gay & Lesbian Social Services*, *18*(3/4), 129–145. doi:10.1300/J041v18n03-08.

Fredriksen-Goldsen, K. I., Kim, H., Muraco, A., & Mincer, S. (2009). Chronically ill midlife and older lesbians, gay men, and bisexuals and their Informal caregivers: The impact of the social context. *Sexuality Research & Social Policy*, *6*(4), 52–64. doi:10.1525/srsp.2009.6.4.52

Fritsch, T. (2005). HIV/AIDS and the older adult: An exploratory study of the age-related differences in access to medical and social services. *Journal of Applied Gerontology*, *24*(1), 35–54.

Gabrielson, M. L. (2011a). "I will not be discriminated against": Older lesbians creating new communities. *Advances in Nursing Science, 34*(4), 357–373.

Gabrielson, M. L. (2011b). "We have to create family": Aging support issues and needs among older lesbians. *Journal of Gay & Lesbian Social Services, 23*(3), 322–334.

Gay and Lesbian Medical Association. (2001). *Healthy people 2010: A companion document for LGBT health*. San Francisco, CA: Author.

Goldberg, S., Sickler, J., & Dibble, S. L. (2005). Lesbians over sixty: The consistency of findings from twenty years of survey data. *Journal of Lesbian Studies, 9*(1–2), 195–213. doi:10.1300/J155v09n01_18.

Grant, J. M. (2010). *Outing age 2010: Public policy issues affecting lesbian, gay, bisexual and transgender elders*. Washington, DC: National Gay and Lesbian Task Force Policy Institute.

Hall, R. L., & Fine, M. (2005). The stories we tell: The lives and friendship of two older Black lesbians. *Psychology of Women Quarterly, 29*(2), 177–187. doi:10.1111/j.1471-6402.2005.00180.x

Hanssmann, C., Morrison, D., & Russian, E. (2008). Talking, gawking, or getting it done: Provider trainings to increase cultural and clinical competence for transgender and gender-nonconforming patients and clients. *Sexuality Research & Social Policy, 5*(1), 5–23.

Harper, P. B. (1992). Eloquence and epitaph: Black nationalism and the homophobic impulse in responses to the death of Max Robinson. In M. Warner (Ed.), *Fear of a queer planet: Queer politics and social theory* (pp. 230–263). Minneapolis: University of Minnesota Press.

Hash, K. (2006). Caregiving and post-caregiving experiences of midlife and older gay men and lesbians. *Journal of Gerontological Social Work, 47*(3/4), 121–138.

Hash, K. M., & Cramer, E. P. (2003). Empowering gay and lesbian caregivers and uncovering their unique experiences through the use of qualitative methods. *Journal of Gay & Lesbian Social Services:* Issues in Practice, Policy & Research, *15*(1–2), 47–63. doi:10.1300/J041v15n01_04

Hash, K. M., & Netting, F. (2007).Long-term planning and decision-making among midlife and older gay men. *Journal of Social Work in End-of-Life & Palliative Care, 3*(2), 59–77.doi:10.1300/J457v03n02_05

Herek, G. M., & Capitanio, J. P. (1995). Black heterosexuals' attitudes toward lesbians and gay men in the United States. *Journal of Sex Research, 32*, 95–105.

Holsti, O. E. (1969). *Content analysis for the social sciences and humanities*. Reading, MA: Addison-Wesley.

Hostetler, A. J. (2004). Old, gay, and alone? The ecology of well-being among middle-aged and older single gay men. In G. Herdt & B. de Vries (Eds.), *Gay and lesbian aging: Research and future directions* (pp. 143–176). New York, NY: Springer.

Hughes, A. K., Harold, R. D., & Boyer, J. M. (2011). Awareness of LGBT aging issues among aging services network providers. *Journal of Gerontological Social Work, 54*(7), 659–677.

Hughes, M. (2007). Older lesbians and gays accessing health and aged-care services. *Australian Social Work, 60*(2), 197–209. doi:10.1080/03124070701323824

Hughes, M. (2008). Imagined futures and communities: Older lesbian and gay people's narratives on health and aged care. *Journal of Gay & Lesbian Social Services, 20*(1/2), 167–186.

Hughes, M. (2009). Lesbian and gay people's concerns about ageing and accessing services. *Australian Social Work, 62*(2), 186–201. doi:10.1080/03124070902748878

Hughes, M. (2010). Expectations of later life support among lesbian and gay Queenslanders. *Australasian Journal on Ageing, 29*(4), 161–166. doi:10.1111/j.1741-6612.2010.00427.x

Hughes, M., & Kentlyn, S. (2011). Older LGBT people's care networks and communities of practice: A brief note. *International Social Work, 54*(3), 436–444. doi:10.1177/0020872810396254

Hyde, A., Nee, J., Howlett, E., Butler, M., & Drennan, J. (2011). The ending of menstruation: Perspectives and experiences of lesbian and heterosexual women. *Journal of Women & Aging, 23*(2), 160–176. doi:10.1080/08952841.2011.561145

Jackson, N. C., Johnson, M. J., & Roberts, R. (2008). The potential impact of discrimination fears of older gays, lesbians, bisexuals and transgender individuals living in small- to moderate-sized cities on long-term health care. *Journal of Homosexuality, 54*(3), 325–339. doi:10.1080/00918360801982298

Jacobs, R. J., & Kane, M. N. (2012). Correlates of loneliness in midlife and older gay and bisexual men. *Journal of Gay & Lesbian Social Services, 24*(1), 40–61. doi:10.1080/10538720.2012.643217

Jenkins, D., Walker, C., Cohen, H., & Curry, L. (2010). A lesbian older adult managing identity disclosure: A case study. *Journal of Gerontological Social Work, 53*(5), 402–420. doi:10.1080/01634372.2010.488280

Jessup, M. A., & Dibble S. L. (2012): Unmet mental health and substance abuse treatment needs of sexual minority elders. *Journal of Homosexuality, 59*(5), 656–674.

Jones, T. C., & Nystrom, N. M. (2002). Looking back . . . looking forward: Addressing the lives of lesbians 55 and older. *Journal of Women & Aging, 14*(3–4), 59–76. doi:10.1300/J074v14n03_05

Jönson, H., & Siverskog, A. (2012). Turning vinegar into wine: Humorous self-presentations among older GLBTQ online daters. *Journal of Aging Studies, 26*(1), 55–64. doi:10.1016/j.jaging.2011.07.003

Joyce, G. F., Goldman, D. P., Leibowitz, A. A., Alpert, A., & Bao, Y. (2005). A socioeconomic profile of older adults with HIV. *Journal of Health Care for the Poor and Underserved, 16*(1), 19–28. doi:10.1353/hpu.2005.0013

Kawachi, I., & Berkman, L. F. (2001). Social ties and mental health. *Journal of Urban Health, 78*, 458–467.

Kertzner, R. N. (1997). Entering midlife: Gay men, HIV and the future. *Journal of Gay and Lesbian Medical Association, 1*, 87–95.

Kessler, R. C., Mickelson, K. D., & Williams, D. R. (1999). The prevalence, distribution, and mental health correlates of perceived discrimination in the United States. *Journal of Health and Social Behavior, 40*(3), 208–230.

Kidd, J. D., & Witten, T. M. (2008). Understanding spirituality and religiosity in the transgender community: Implications for aging. *Journal of Religion, Spirituality & Aging, 20*(1–2), 29–62. doi:10.1080/15528030801922004

King, S. D., & Orel, N. (2012). Midlife and older gay men living with HIV/AIDS: The influence of resiliency and psychosocial stress factors on health needs, *Journal of Gay & Lesbian Social Services, 24*(4), 346–370.

Kishore, S. A. (2013). *Dying with dignity: Considerations for treating elder transgender people of color*. Retrieved from http://www.asaging.org/blog/dying-dignity-considerations-treating-elder-transgender-people-color

Knapp, G. A. (2005). Race, class, gender: Reclaiming baggage in fast travelling theories. *European Journal of Women's Studies, 12*(3), 249–265.

Knauer, N. J. (2009). LGBT elder law: Toward equity in aging. *Harvard Journal of Law and Gender, 32*, 301–358.

Knochel, K., Croghan, C. F., Moone, R. P., & Quam, J. K. (2012). Training, geography, and provision of aging services to lesbian, gay, bisexual, and transgender older adults. *Journal of Gerontological Social Work, 55*(5), 426–443. doi:10.1080/01634372.2012.665158.

Krippendorff, K. (2004). *Content analysis: An introduction to its methodology*. Thousand Oaks, CA. Sage.

Kropf, N. P., & Adamek, M. (2005). The future of social work in aging: "Everything old is new again." *Advances in Social Work, 6*(1), 121–131.

Landers, S., Mimiaga M. J., & Krinsky L. (2010): The Open Door Project Task Force: A qualitative study on LGBT aging. *Journal of Gay & Lesbian Social Services, 22*(3), 316–336.

Lanehart, S. L. (Ed.). (2009). *African American women's language: Discourse, education and identity*. Cambridge, UK: Cambridge Scholars Press.

LGBT Movement Advancement Project & Services and Advocacy for Gay, Lesbian, Bisexual and Transgender Elders. (2010) *Improving the lives of LGBT older adults*. Denver, CO: LGBT MAP.

Logie, C., Bridge, T. J., & Bridge, P. D. (2007). Evaluating the phobias, attitudes, and cultural competence of master of social work students toward the LGBT populations. *Journal of Homosexuality, 53*(4), 201–221. doi:10.1080/00918360802103472

Lovejoy, T. I., Heckman, T. G., Sikkema, K. J., Hansen, N. B., Kochman, A., Suhr, J. A., & . . . Johnson, C. J. (2008). Patterns and correlates of sexual activity and condom use behavior in persons 50-plus years of age living with HIV/AIDS. *AIDS and Behavior, 12*(6), 943–956. doi:10.1007/s10461-008-9384-2

Malebranche, D. J., Peterson, J. L., Fullilove, R. E., & Stackhouse, R. W. (2004). Race and sexual identity: Perceptions about medical culture and healthcare among black men who have sex with men. *Journal of the National Medical Association, 96*(1), 97–107.

Martin, J. I., Messinger, L., Kull, R., Holmes, J., Bermudez, F., & Sommer, S. (2009). *Council on social work education—Lambda Legal study of LGBT issues in social work*. Alexandria, VA: Council on Social Work Education.

Masini, B. E., & Barrett, H. A. (2008): Social support as a predictor of psychological and physical well-being and lifestyle in lesbian, gay, and bisexual adults aged 50 and over. *Journal of Gay & Lesbian Social Services, 20*(1–2), 91–110.

Matsuda, M. J. (1991). Beside my sister, facing the enemy of legal theory out of coalition. *Stanford Law Review, 43*(6), 1183–1192.

McFarland, P. L., & Sanders, S. (2003). A pilot study about the needs of older gays and lesbians: What social workers need to know. *Journal of Gerontological Social Work, 40*(3), 67–80. doi:10.1300/J083v40n03_06

McIntyre, L., Szewchuk, A., & Munro, J. (2010). Inclusion and exclusion in mid-life lesbians' experiences of the Pap test. *Culture, Health & Sexuality, 12*(8), 885–898. doi:10.1080/13691058.2010.508844

McMahon, A., & Allen-Meares, P. (1992). Is social work racist? A content analysis of recent literature. *Social Work, 37*(6), 533–539.

Meyer, H. (2011). Safe spaces? The need for LGBT cultural competency in aging services. *Public Policy & Aging Report, 21*(3), 24–27.

Moore, W. R. (2002). Lesbian and gay elders: Connecting care providers through a telephone support group. *Journal of Gay & Lesbian Social Services, 14*(3), 23–41. doi:10.1300/J041v14n03_02

Morris, M. (2000). Dante's left foot kicks queer theory into gear. In S. Talburt & S. R. Steinberg (Eds.), *Thinking queer: Sexuality, culture, and education* (pp. 15–32). New York, NY: Peter Lang.

Nash, J. C. (2008). Re-thinking intersectionality. *Feminist Review, 89*(1), 1–15.

National Association of Social Workers. (2000). *Code of ethics of the National Association of Social Workers*. Washington, DC: Author.

National Resource Center on LGBT Aging. (2013). *Inclusive questions for older adults: A practical guide to collecting data on sexual orientation and gender identity.* Retrieved from http://www.lgbtagingcenter.org/resources/pdfs/InclusiveQuestionsOlder%20Adults_Guidebook.pdf

Neville, S., & Henrickson, M. (2010). 'Lavender retirement': A questionnaire survey of lesbian, gay and bisexual people's accommodation plans for old age. *International Journal of Nursing Practice, 16*(6), 586–594. doi:10.1111/j.1440-172X.2010.01885.x

Orel, N. A. (2004). Gay, lesbian, and bisexual elders: Expressed needs and concerns across focus groups. *Journal of Gerontological Social Work, 43*(2–3), 57–77. doi:10.1300/J083v43n02_05

Owen, G., & Catalan, J. (2012). 'We never expected this to happen': Narratives of ageing with HIV among gay men living in London, UK. *Culture, Health & Sexuality, 14*(1), 59–72.

Persson, D. I. (2009). Unique challenges of transgender aging: Implications from the literature. *Journal of Gerontological Social Work, 52*(6), 633–646. doi:10.1080/01634370802609056

Pettinato, M. (2008). Nobody was out back then: A grounded theory study of midlife and older lesbians with alcohol problems. *Issues in Mental Health Nursing, 29*(6), 619–638. doi:10.1080/01612840802048865

Phillips, J., & Marks, G. (2008): Ageing lesbians: Marginalising discourses and social exclusion in the aged care industry. *Journal of Gay & Lesbian Social Services, 20*(1–2), 187–202.

Politi, M. C., Clark, M. A., Armstrong, G., McGarry, K. A., & Sciamanna, C. N. (2009). Patient–provider communication about sexual health among unmarried middle-aged and older women. *Journal of General Internal Medicine, 24*(4), 511–516. doi:10.1007/s11606-009-0930-z

Porter, M., Russell, C., & Sullivan, G. (2004). Gay, old, and poor: Service delivery to aging gay men in inner city Sydney, Australia. *Journal of Gay & Lesbian Social Services, 16*(2), 43–57.

Potter, W. J., & Levine-Donnerstein, D. (1999). Rethinking validity and reliability in content analysis. *Journal of Applied Communication Research, 27*, 258–284.

Quam, J. K., & Whitford, G. (1992). Adaptation and age-related expectations of older gay and lesbian adults. *Gerontologist, 32*, 367–374.

Reisner, S. L., O'Cleirigh, C., Hendriksen, E. S., McLain, J., Ebin, J., Lew, K., . . . Mimiaga, M. J. (2011). "40 & forward": Preliminary evaluation of a group intervention to improve mental health outcomes and address HIV sexual risk behaviors among older gay and bisexual men. *Journal of Gay & Lesbian Social Services, 23*(4), 523–545.

Rice, T. (2013). *Cervical cancer in elder Black lesbian and bisexual women.* Retrieved from http://www.asaging.org/blog/cervical-cancer-elder-black-lesbian-and-bisexual-women

Richard, C., & Brown, A. (2006). Configurations of informal social support among older lesbians. *Journal of Women & Aging, 18*(4), 49–65. doi:10.1300/J074v18n04_05

Riggs, M. (1991). Tongues untied. In E. Hemphill (Ed.), *Brother to brother: New writings by Black gay men* (pp. 200–205). Boston, MA: Alyson.

Robinson, W. A., Petty, M. S., Patton, C., & Kang, H. (2007). Aging with HIV: Historical and intra-community differences in experience of aging with HIV. *Journal of Gay & Lesbian Social Services, 20*(1–2), 111–128. doi:10.1080/10538720802179070

Rosenblum, D. (1994). *Queer intersectionality and the failure of recent lesbian and gay "victories"* (Paper 210). Pace Law Faculty Publications. Retrieved from http://digitalcommons.pace.edu/cgi/viewcontent.cgi?article=1209&context=lawfaculty

Scherrer, K. S. (2009). Images of sexuality and aging in gerontological literature. *Sexuality Research & Social Policy, 6*(4), 5–12. doi:10.1525/srsp.2009.6.4.5

Schope, R. D. (2005). Who's afraid of growing old? Gay and lesbian perceptions of aging. *Journal of Gerontological Social Work, 45*(4), 23–39. doi:10.1300/J083v45n04_03

Sedgwick, E. K. (1990). *Epistemology of the closet.* London, England: Penguin Books.

Sherr, L., Harding, R., Lampe, F., Johnson, M., Anderson, J., Zetler, S., & . . . Edwards, S. (2009). Clinical and behavioural aspects of aging with HIV infection. *Psychology, Health & Medicine, 14*(3), 273–279. doi:10.1080/13548500902865964

Shippy, R. (2007). We cannot go it alone: The impact of informal support and stressors in older gay, lesbian and bisexual caregivers. *Journal of Gay & Lesbian Social Services, 18*(3–4), 39–51. doi:10.1300/J041v18n03_03

Simmons, R. (1991). Tongues untied: An interview with Marlon Riggs. In E. Hemphill (Ed.), *Brother to brother: New writings by Black gay men* (pp. 50–53). Boston, MA: Alyson.

Smith, L. A., McCaslin, R., Chang, J., Martinez, P., & McGrew, P. (2010). Assessing the needs of older gay, lesbian, bisexual, and transgender people: A service-learning and agency partnership approach. *Journal of Gerontological Social Work, 53*(5), 387–401. doi:10.1080/01634372.2010.486433.

Stein, G. L., Beckerman, N. L., & Sherman, P. A. (2010). Lesbian and gay elders and long-term care: Identifying the unique psychosocial perspectives and challenges. *Journal of Gerontological Social Work*, *53*(5), 421–435. doi:10.1080/01634372.2010.496478

Tripodi, T., & Epstein, I. (1980). The use of content analysis to monitor social work performance. In T. Tripodi (Ed.), *Research techniques for clinical social workers* (pp. 103–120). New York, NY: Columbia University Press.

Van Den Bergh, N., & Crisp, C. (2004). Defining culturally competent practice with sexual minorities: Implications for social work education and practice. *Journal of Social Work Education*, *40*, 221–238.

Van Sluytman, L. G. (2013). *(Dis)parities and (in)visibility: Shifting the perception of the life course of LGBT elders LGBTQ seniors of color.* Retrieved from http://www.asaging.org/blog/disparities-and-invisibilities-shifting-perception-life-course-lgbt-elders-color

Watt, S. K. (2007). Difficult dialogues, privilege and social justice: Uses of the Privileged Identity Exploration (PIE) Model in student affairs practice. *College Student Affairs Journal*, *26*(2), 114–126.

Wheeler, D.P. (2003). Methodological issues in conducting community-based health and social services research among urban black and African-American LGBT populations. *Journal of Gay and Lesbian Social Service*, 15, 65–78.

Zaritsky, E., & Dibble, S. L. (2010). Risk factors for reproductive and breast cancers among older lesbians. *Journal of Women's Health*, *19*(1), 125–131. doi:10.1089/jwh.2008.1094

APPENDIX

TABLE A1 Comprehensive Outcomes of Literature Search

Source	Methodology	N	Men	Women	Trans	Gender Unknown	White	POC	% POC
Almack, Seymour, & Bellamy (2010)	Qualitative	15	10	15			15		
Averett, Yoon, & Jenkins (2011)	Quantitative	394		394			338	43	10.91
Averett, Yoon, & Jenkins (2012)	Mixed method	394		394			338	43	10.91
Becker et al. (2009)	Quantitative	635	635				279		
Boehmer, Miao, Linkletter, & Clark (2012)	Quantitative	164,221	69,125	95,096			81,319	72,081	43.89
Brotman, Ryan, & Cormier (2003)	Qualitative	32							
Brotman et al. (2007)	Qualitative	17	7	10					
Cronin, Ward, Pugh, King, & Price (2011)	Qualitative	36	12	24			35	1	2.78
de Vries, Mason, Quam, & Acquaviva (2009)	Quantitative	793	473	320			673	109	13.75
Dibble, Eliason, & Crawford (2012)	Quantitative	123		123			10	93	75.61
Dibble & Roberts (2002)	Quantitative	80		80			73		
Drumm (2004)	Qualitative								
Eliason, Dibble, & Robertson (2011)	Quantitative	502	350	146	6		427	70	13.94
Fenge, Fannin, Armstrong, Hicks, & Taylor (2009)	Qualitative								
Fredriksen-Goldsen & Hooyman (2007)	Literature review								
Fredriksen-Goldsen, Kim, Muraco, & Mincer (2009)	Quantitative	72	46	26			37	35	48.61
Fritsch (2005)	Qualitative	34	30	4					
Gabrielson (2011a)	Qualitative	4		4					

Gabrielson (2011b)	Qualitative	10	10	10		9	1	10
Goldberg, Sickler, & Dibble (2005)	Quantitative	100	100	100		94	6	6
Hall & Fine (2005)	Qualitative	2		2			2	100
Hash (2006)	Qualitative	19	10	9		17	2	10.53
Hash & Cramer (2003)	Qualitative	19	10	9		17	2	10.53
Hash & Netting (2007)	Qualitative	19	10	9		17	2	10.53
Hughes, A. K., Harold, & Boyer (2011)	Quantitative	86	9	77		69	14	16.28
Hughes, M. (2007)	Qualitative	14	9	5		13		
Hughes, M. (2008)	Qualitative	14	9	5		13		
Hughes, M. (2009)	Quantitative	371	243	128		299		
Hughes, M. (2010)	Quantitative	371	243	128		299		
Hughes, M., & Kentlyn (2011)	Literature review							
Hyde, Nee, Howlett, Butler, & Drennan (2011)	Qualitative	23	23	23	2	23		
Jackson, Johnson, & Roberts (2008)	Quantitative	317	107	199	9	281	26	8.2
Jacobs & Kane (2012)	Quantitative	802	802			660	134	16.71
Jenkins, Walker, Cohen, & Curry (2010)	Qualitative	1		1			1	100
Jessup & Dibble (2012)	Quantitative	15	6	9		10		
Jones & Nystrom (2002)	Qualitative	65		65		64		
Jönson & Siverskog (2012)	Qualitative	276	162	88	26			
Joyce, Goldman, Leibowitz, Alpert, & Bao (2005)	Quantitative	12,688						
King & Orel (2012)	Quantitative	316	316	316		297	16	5.06
Knochel, Croghan, Moone, & Quam (2012)	Quantitative	320						
Landers, Mimiaga, & Krinsky (2010)	Qualitative	34						
Lovejoy et al. (2008)	Quantitative	290	243	57		56	84	28.97
Masini & Barrett (2008)	Quantitative	200	137	71		180	14	7

(Continued)

TABLE A1 (Continued)

Source	Methodology	N	Men	Women	Trans	Gender Unknown	White	POC	% POC
McFarland & Sanders (2003)	Quantitative	59	37	18	3	1			
McIntyre, Szewchuk, & Munro (2010)	Qualitative	7		7			6	1	14.29
Moore (2002)	Mixed method								
Neville & Henrickson (2010)	Quantitative	2,269	1,236	1,025	13				
Orel (2004)	Qualitative	26	10	16			17	9	34.62
Owen & Catalan (2012)	Qualitative	10	10				9	1	10
Persson (2009)	Literature review								
Pettinato (2008)	Qualitative	12		12			9	3	25
Phillips & Marks (2008)	Qualitative								
Politi, Clark, Armstrong, McGarry, & Sciamanna (2009)	Qualitative	40		40			39	1	2.5
Porter, Russell, & Sullivan (2004)	Qualitative	2	2				2		
Reisner et al. (2011)	Quantitative	84	84						
Richard & Brown (2006)	Qualitative	25		25					
Robinson, Petty, Patton, & Kang (2007)	Qualitative						24	1	4
Scherrer (2009)	Qualitative								
Schope (2005)	Quantitative	183	74	109			172		
Sherr et al. (2009)	Quantitative	761	572	183			513	211	27.73
Shippy (2007)	Quantitative	155	97	57	1		103	43	27.74
Smith, McCaslin, Chang, Martinez, & McGrew (2010)	Quantitative	38	21	15	1		28	9	23.68
Stein, Beckerman, & Sherman (2010)	Qualitative	16	12	4			14	2	12.5
Zaritsky & Dibble (2010)	Quantitative	84		84			83		

Note. POC = persons of color.

Gender Transitions in Later Life: The Significance of Time in Queer Aging

VANESSA D. FABBRE

School of Social Service Administration, University of Chicago, Chicago, Illinois, USA

Concepts of time are ubiquitous in studies of aging. This article integrates an existential perspective on time with a notion of queer time based on the experiences of older transgender persons who contemplate or pursue a gender transition in later life. Interviews were conducted with male-to-female identified persons aged 50 years or older (N = 22), along with participant observation at three national transgender conferences (N = 170 hr). Interpretive analyses suggest that an awareness of "time left to live" and a feeling of "time served" play a significant role in later life development and help expand gerontological perspectives on time and queer aging.

Time, in all its conceptualizations and utilities, is an essential component of thinking about age and aging. The field of gerontology, with its varied topical domains and disciplinary traditions, offers a diverse space in which critical discussions and debates about the role of time in aging research and implications for its theorizing may be generated. This article addresses the intersection of an existential and queer perspective on time and aging across the life course. The aim is to interpret narratives about gender transitions in later life by integrating these two perspectives and generating implications for gerontological social work.

Empirical and theoretical work in gerontology has been criticized for the ways in which queer identities and experiences are marginalized (Brown, 2009). In parallel fashion, the field of queer studies has been criticized for a lack of empirical and theoretical research on aging (Sandberg, 2008). In response to these deficits in knowledge development, critical approaches to queer aging are now being explored (Hughes, 2006). Although it may be daunting to think about integrating the expansive and evolving fields of gerontology and queer studies, this article addresses one key concept rooted in the human experience—time—that is considered in both domains. I explore the experiences and reflections upon time, identity, and action in the lives of older transgender-identified persons in hopes of contributing insight into the ways in which queer identities construct meanings of aging.

TIME, GERONTOLOGY, AND QUEER THEORY

In gerontological realms, chronological time has often been the dominant conceptualization of time (Baars, 1998). Often, chronological metrics play a central role in research design and subsequent theorizing, which diminishes opportunities for examining nuanced temporalities at play in aging and identity development (Baars, 2007). In reaction to this reliance on chronological time, Baars proposed that greater attention be paid to subjective aspects of identity construction, in which personal narratives help elucidate diverse experiences and contribute to an expansion of cultural representations of aging. For example, human beings of the same chronological age can show very different aging characteristics; therefore, one cannot assume that aging processes develop in synchrony with chronological time, or that cohorts of older adults will consist of homogenous identities. In this vein, Dittmann-Kohli (2007) argued that taking an *existential time perspective*, based on the assumption that adults apprehend or perceive their own existence as situated and limited in time, is ideally suited to exploring diverse self-constructions of identity in later life. Although there is an objective reality that time to live does run out, how this fact is interpreted by transgender-identified people in later life and the influence this has on one's behavior and identity development serves as a theoretical bridge between gerontological and queer perspectives on time.

Queer theory has been used to address subjective temporal identities with respect to social structure, inequality, and the institutionalized life course as Halberstam's (2005) notion of "queer time" highlights the "the potentiality of a life *unscripted* by the convention of family, inheritance and child rearing" and claims that "queer subcultures produce *alternative* temporalities" (p. 2, italics added). Often these temporalities have been conceptualized within the context of shortened life trajectories related to marginalized status within modern Western societies. For example, the threat of severe illness and premature death experienced by many gay men during the AIDS crisis radically influenced their lifestyle choices and expectations for engaging in social life. Although many gay men were already coping with the effects of social marginalization, the added sense of diminishing future time in this community contributed to an acute existential awareness among its members that their lives and identities existed outside normative expectations of marriage, reproduction, and longevity. Halberstam's recognition of the potential for queer lives to develop with respect to unique temporal and existential concerns addresses part of the subjectivity that Baars (2007) and Dittmann-Kohli (2007) argued is needed in gerontological perspectives on identity and aging. Yet, this perspective has yet to be fully mobilized to take into account the actual experiences of aging with respect to these identities (Brown, 2009). In light of the current gay marriage movement, some scholars argue that asserting queer identities in reaction to heteronormative expectations is taking the form of "homonormativity" (Duggan, 2003), which may not constitute a queer temporality at all. The question of what queer temporalities will mean in rapidly changing political and social contexts demands more attention to longevity and queer identities over time.

Given the lack of literature on gender transitions in later life, the conceptual foundation for integrating existential and queer perspectives on late-life gender transitions in this study draws from lesbian, gay, and bisexual (LGB) research on the topic of coming out in later life. Floyd and Bakeman (2006) offered a relevant life course perspective based on their empirical work with gay, lesbian, and bisexual elders who come out later in life and argued that the process of sexual orientation identity development is driven both by maturational factors, as well as social changes. In studies of LGB grandparents, the ability to disclose sexual orientation to family members has been shown to be an important part of their identity development in later life (Orel & Fruhauf, 2013), along with acknowledgement of the years spent participating in heteronormative culture, as one of Orel's (2004) interviewees so succinctly summarized: "I just did what you were supposed to do . . . get married, have kids, and own the house with the white picket fence." (p. 69). This clear connection to heteronormative life cycles is common in narratives about coming out about one's sexuality, and I argue in this article that it is also important for transgender people contemplating a transition in later life because heteronormativity also has a constraining effect on gender expression (J. Butler, 2007). Older transgender persons who come out later in life may offer additional nuance and a longer life span perspective on Halberstam's (2005) notion of queer time, which has not been fully explored from either gerontological or queer perspectives. I argue that an integration of an existential time perspective, in which identity development is grounded in the subjective meanings derived from an awareness of having limited time to live, and the notion of queer time, in which gender variant people develop within self-constructed temporalities outside the heteronormative life course, may be integrated to contribute to knowledge development in a range of domains concerned with aging, identity and human development.

WHY EXPLORE GENDER TRANSITIONS IN LATER LIFE?

The field of gerontology has yet to explore health and wellbeing with respect to gender transitions in later life. Most writing on transgender aging has focused on critical and underexamined issues of social welfare in the lives of older transgender persons such as health, legal, financial, spiritual, trauma/abuse, and end-of-life issues (S. S. Butler, 2004; Cook-Daniels & Munson, 2010; Kidd & Witten, 2008; Minter, 2001; Persson, 2009; Porter, Ronneberg, & Witten, 2013; Williams & Freeman, 2007; Witten, 2010, Witten & Eyler, 2012). We also know that mid-life is a critical period for transgender adults as they anticipate challenges of aging (Knochel, 2011). Recently, scholars have analyzed narrative expressions of identity as a means of examining successful aging for LGBT older adults (Van Wagenen, Driskell, & Bradford, 2013), as well as narratives related to transgender embodiment and aging (Siverskog, 2012). These offer an intellectual segue within the domain of LGBT aging for exploring the significance of older transgender persons' subjective experiences of contemplating or pursuing a transition later in life.

It is well known in transgender-oriented communities that many male-to-female identified people, often the oldest of the baby boomers, have only begun to seriously contemplate gender transitions in their later years. Witten and Eyler (2012) drew attention to this reality and the potential to address normative versus nonnormative life course considerations with respect to transgender older adults, but lament the "scant" research on this topic (p. 214). From a life course perspective, the ways in which older transgender persons consider transition in later stages of life may offer insights into the ways that older adults navigate social constraints and opportunities throughout the life course. By illuminating multiple intersections between what it is to be *queer* and *aging* the participants in this study help social workers acknowledge and learn from the diversity within transgender communities so that they may both develop culturally appropriate needs assessments and services and expand their concepts and theories in aging.

METHOD

Data Collection

Sample and recruitment. Strategic sampling (Mason, 2002) was used to recruit persons, 50 years of age or older, who have seriously contemplated or have pursued a gender transition. I intentionally recruited male-to-female identified persons for interviews because they often come out/and or transition later in life than female-to-male-identified persons (Cook-Daniels, 2006). My main methods of recruitment included e-mail flyers sent to community leaders with whom I had developed relationships through activist work in Chicago, word of mouth, and snowball referrals. I was able to recruit 22 participants.

Conceptualizing the gender identities of participants is complex and multifaceted, and may best be understood from diverse theoretical and practical standpoints; addressing this complexity is beyond the scope of this article, thus my analyses explore the thoughts and use the language of older male-to-female identified persons themselves. When I speak of gender identity, I am referring to the degree to which people feel *congruent* in their body and mind, and *authentic* in their lives. In addition, gender identity, the self-conception of one's gender, is also to be distinguished from biological sex. My discussion of the ways in which people contemplate and pursue transition is intentionally nonmedical and nonlegal. For some people, a transition may mean pursuing hormone therapy or surgical modifications of their bodies; for others this means renegotiating their social and familial relationships. For others yet, it may mean the act of contemplation and discovering the power of making an informed decision about one's future. In this study, I use the word *transition* to talk about the process through which a person may decide to change from living "part time" (a term often used by participants to label expressing their preferred gender identity as female in private or only in some aspects of their lives) to "full time" (a term used to describe living in and expressing their preferred female gender 100% of the time). At the time of my interviews, 15 of the participants were living full time, three were living part time but were still not sure about transitioning, three were living part time and had decided not to transition, and one person was living part time and considered herself in preparation for transition.

Additional demographic characteristics of the 22 participants varied across race, class, and age. Eighteen participants were European American, three were African American, and one Asian American. Based on information shared during the interviews, approximately 20% expressed ongoing socio-economic challenges; 30% expressed a sense of socio-economic stability, though somewhat tenuous; and about 50% shared that their socio-economic position afforded stability and some luxury. Twelve participants were between 50 and 60 years old, seven were between 60 and 70 years old, two were between 70 and 80 years old, and one participant was 82 years old.

Interviews and participant observation. In-depth biographical interviews focused on participants' gender expression and identity over time, work and relationships, and thoughts about transitioning. They were conducted at participants' homes and, in a few cases, at public locations such as coffee shops or parks, and lasted from 1.5 to 2.5 hr. Eighteen interviews were audio-recorded and transcribed verbatim; four were recorded with hand-written notes. Participant observation (Burawoy et al., 1991; Emerson, 2001) was carried out with the permission of organizers at three national transgender conferences in the Southeast, Midwest, and Northwest of the United States. The conferences selected are unique in that they are attended by many older male-to-female identified persons, and are highly influential in this community. Participant observation at these conferences allowed me to contextualize interview data, assess similar or dissimilar cases, and sensitize myself to a social context that impacts the ways in which older transgender people think about identity and transitions. I took field notes (Emerson, Fretz, & Shaw, 2011) focused on issues of aging, late life transitions, and conference history during 170 hr in the field. This article draws from data collected through both interviews and participant observation.

Data Analysis

The findings presented in this article are based on interpretive analyses conducted as part of a larger extended case method (ECM) study (Burawoy, 1998; Burawoy et al., 1991; Samuels, 2009; Small, 2009). I used NVivo 9 qualitative data analysis software (QSR, 2012) to organize the interview and field data and develop a set of open and focused codes (Padgett, 2008). These codes identified topics, concepts and examples of the significance and function of time and time awareness in people's contemplation of a transition. I used extensive memo writing (Auerbach & Silverstein, 2003; Emerson et al., 2011) as a method of articulating early themes in the data and as my foundation for abstraction and interrogation of the data. The process of analyzing the data was an iterative one that included the use of memos, the articulation and refinement of early conceptual findings with an external observer, and presenting the data and early analyses to colleagues in a qualitative methods working group at the University of Chicago.

RESULTS

Time Left

A multitude of individual and societal factors intersect when a person comes out about their gender identity or contemplates a transition in later life, but one that stands out almost universally is an awareness of time left to live. An acute perception that there are limited days in which to embrace one's authentic self, experience the joy of feeling whole and congruent within oneself, and face death with a sense of having truly lived is central to the contemplation of transition for many people. Katherine,[1] age 62, shared one of the most poignant examples of this during our interview at a neighborhood diner:

> I don't know if you've heard these commercials on the radio about Michigan—Michigan.org.—I love the commercials . . . until—until they

---

[1]   All names in this article are pseudonyms and details have been changed to protect participants' confidentiality.

put the one on about, "An average person has 25,000 days in their life. Some of those days should be spent in Michigan." And I went, "25,000 days divided by 365—whoa, that don't give me much time left." . . . I've been obsessed with that 25,000 days ever since then. . . . I'm not afraid of dying, but I got a lot of stuff to do. And I says, "I can't die yet, not in 25,000 days!"

Barbara, age 82, a vibrant European American woman twice divorced and now happily dating, reflected on her decision to transition in her early 70s:

I was thinking, "It's time to roll the dice and go" because I was just starting to get to 70 then 71, and I knew, I figured, "I've got 20 years to go." Why shouldn't I live those 20 years as Barbara and do it right?

Similarly, Adele, an African American woman who recovered from substance abuse difficulties in her 40s, expressed to me that "at 57, I'm moving into the backside of my life, I don't have a lot of time to screw around!" Alana, also in her 50s, who has never been married and is the primary caregiver for her parents, is just starting to plan her transition on the job as a marketing analyst. She linked a sense of time and identity in this way when she said, "It's like, man, I kind of lost decades here. I gotta get going! I expect to live past 100, but still, I lost time. I could be expressing my true gender here."

For many of the people I interviewed, the realization of having only so much time left to live served as a catalyst for contemplating transition or coming out to family and friends about their gender identity. However, this was not the only narrative about time or age that played a role in their decision about a transition. One respondent, Suzanna, who at 60 years old is now enjoying life posttransition, considered her age and time left to live as possible deterrents from pursuing a transition:

There were a number of times I said I was too old. "I'm 50 some odd years old. I'm too old to make this change. I'm only going to be around another 30 years or so, why bother? Why rock the boat?" My friend Jessica, she was wonderful about this, [she said] "Of course you're not too old. You're never too old. As long as you're sucking wind, you're not too old!" So, I mean there was a little bit of that; I had to overcome my own bias in order to say that I'm going to enjoy the rest of my life.

In Suzanna's case, she was also considering whether she wanted to undergo hormone therapy and whether surgical options would be possible for her physically. Although these are concerns that people of all ages may have when contemplating a transition, the awareness of a finite time to live puts these considerations into a more overt temporal context.

For older transgender persons in this study, the knowledge of even the possibility of transitioning played an important role in their development. For example, many participants remembered hearing about Christine Jorgensen and the sensationalized news headlines about her sex change in the 1950s (Docter, 2008). As Katherine recalled:

> I heard [the news reel on Christine Jorgensen] on the radio, you know, and I forget what year it was—late '50s maybe? I think it was late '50s. I kind of thought, "That's not possible. That's got to be a mistake." And then I would listen and listen purposely to see if I could hear the story again, and I thought, "Oh, my God, *it must be possible*. They're saying it again and again and again." Really, I was just fascinated by that. I thought, "Oh, my God, there is somebody else that's like me." (italics added)

For people who have struggled with gender identity over the course of many decades, an awareness of time left takes on an existential significance that is inextricably linked with the possibilities that emerge in social context. Thus, personal narratives about identity development also take into account the ways in which social expectations and social possibilities influence people's view of themselves.

Time Served

In the context of identity development and aging, it is hard to separate looking forward from looking back. Many participants in this study who have contemplated a gender transition in their later years find themselves reflecting on their past and ways in which they have navigated the world with respect to their gender identity and expression. Through both field work and one-on-one interviews, I came across multiple ways in which people described past phases of their lives, saying they "did what they were supposed to do" or felt they "served time" conforming their gender to social expectations or demands. Having put in their time following society's expectations, many felt a sense of urgency about how they might spend the last part of their lives. Katherine expanded on her reaction to the Michigan.org commercials by evoking a prison metaphor:

> And then they came out with a second one of those [Michigan.org commercials] that said, . . . "The average person retires and they still have 3,000-some days of retirement." Wait a minute, that's only—you know, and that made it even worse . . . and now—see, I was actually thinking about writing a book. I was gonna call it *40 to Life*, and it was gonna be about, you know, for all these years you kept the secret . . . and finally you're able to be born—you know, after 40 years you were able to be

born. Most people think, "40 to life, that's a prison sentence" you know. That's why I play on words in the title.

She goes on to reflect further from the vantage point of having come out to her family recently and being able to spend more time embracing her femininity, for which she was ridiculed as a young person:

> But looking back then, it's kind of like from the aspect of, "Oh my God, all this time I could've been doing this; I could've been this; I might've even transitioned—you know, I might've made different choices," you know. . . . Well, now when I look at that, it's kind of like, "Oh, my, God, I want to do this forever." . . . Now I've only got probably, oh, 20-some years left maybe at that? That kind of drags me down when I think of it that way. . . . You know, I think back all these times where people make fun of you and, you know, all that time wasted—all that time wasted.

The notion of time wasted, or time served, was also framed with respect to feeling unsuccessful and unsatisfied with one's life. Deborah, a European American woman who runs her own business at age 55, and who recently completed her transition to living full time, reflects:

> In 2002, that started to get really hard for me. And so, I was getting close to my 50th birthday. I was like—I was what, you know, 45 at that point. Yeah, it was, like 45 or 46—and I just felt that I'd been a failure my whole life. I had my whole life—the better part of my life behind me, you know?

For several people, looking back allowed them to appreciate some aspects of their life while balancing these with the frustration of having less time to embrace their authentic gender identity. Carly, who recently retired in her early 60s, expressed no regrets about being a parent, but also recognizes that this role, which she fulfilled as a father, took away from another part of her identity:

> Yes. My daughter is—she'll be turning 40. My son is 37, now. So . . . looking at my children, oh, my God, I let them know a million times, I would not change a thing, 'cause I need them, that it's not like I was sad that I had them . . . but then that feeling [of gender conflict] stayed with me, and it progressed as you're going through your lifespan, and you're going through Erickson's different stages, I'm getting to a point in my life where I'm running out of years. I could see the light at the end of the tunnel. When you're 20 or 30, and I once smoked, I was careless about my lifestyle. You go, "Oh, I got time to recoup. I got time to regenerate my—my body cells, and all this kind of stuff." And—but then, at a certain point, you start getting a grasp that 50 isn't far away; 60 isn't

far away. And then you take a look at lifespan statistics, heart attacks, and—so you're getting closer to that, and your whole frame of reference to life starts morphing or changing. And so—so I started becoming a little bit more anxious about, "How am I gonna live?—or am I gonna die, actually pass on to the next life without experiencing being who I am?" And it gnawed at me for a long time.

One of the ways in which transgender communities have fostered this kind of reflection in social spaces, especially for those who have spent years struggling with feelings similar to those expressed by Katherine, Deborah, and Carly, has been to create special ceremonies at conferences that encourage reflection on one's growth and outlook for the future. At the start of many national conferences, first timers are often given special welcomes, and are sometimes connected with a *big sister* to help guide them through what can be an overwhelming social experience. At one such conference, I observed a private graduation ceremony in which big sisters awarded first-time attendees with a pin to signify their growth over the course of the conference. An excerpt from my field notes demonstrates the social aspect of bringing past, present, and future together in one moment:

> Nearing end of ceremony, 70-year-old first-time attendee, Summer, received butterfly pin from 'big sister' and faced the group with tears in her eyes and said, "Now I can live the rest of my life the way I want to"—I am noticing that most people have tears in their eyes at this point, myself included.

The emotionally charged dynamics that flourish in ceremonies such as this one draw attention to the role that transgender communities play in fostering queer alternatives for identity development in later life. Further, these analyses suggest that an awareness of time and the meaning given to its finitude can be a catalyst for looking back, looking forward, and pushing gender identity development into the foreground of one's later life. As Casey, age 66, so poetically summarized: "30 years alone, 30 years for other people, now 30 years for me!"

DISCUSSION

Hughes (2004) argued that queer aging is not just about "adding in" LGBT-identified people as another identity group in the gerontological sphere, just as Duggan (2003) argued that queer challenges to heteronormativity should not simply be the construction of a "homonormativity." The findings in this study suggest that the biographical narratives of older transgender persons do not simply offer additional examples of how people make decisions when perceiving a shrinking time horizon in later life. Rather, I argue that people who contemplate a gender transition in later life, especially with respect to existential time perspectives, are doing so by renegotiating the social expectations they perceive as having dominated their lives previously and thus are expanding notions of queer temporality by drawing attention to growing older in ways that do not follow heteronormative scripts. Participants in this study are conscious of social expectations for older age, most notably that they are expected to transition into their retirement years as male. Often, participants do not reject such expectations altogether; rather, they modify them to fit their developing sense of self. For example, it was common for several people I interviewed to carefully plan their final working years so that they could retire in male-mode, while also preparing for their transition to living full time as their female selves after retirement. This careful negotiation demonstrates how older transgender persons integrate an awareness of time left with the realities of time served and create a uniquely queer path through a common life phase such as retirement. Becoming aware of one's time left to live is not new to aging or human development scholarship (Carstensen, Isaacowitz, & Charles, 1999), nor to the field of gerontological social work. In fact, this existential dynamic is probably present in most work in this domain. However, this study shows that constraints on people's gender identities in earlier life heighten the significance and immediacy of these time horizons and the opportunity to experience an authentic gender identity before one dies. The narrative perspective on identity and aging emphasized by Baars (2012) and offered by participants in this study may offer a conceptual bridge between an existential and queer perspective on time and open new avenues of thought in queer aging. The notion that one's existence is meaningful with respect to its time limitation necessitates that one recognize the ways in which older people modify the nature of their existence (in this case, through gender transition) by constructing temporalities in later life that challenge heteronormative expectations (that they grow older as male).

The biographies, observations, and interpretations presented in this article demonstrate how transgender older adults acutely perceive their lives in terms of time past and time left. The ways participants in this study compared past, present, and potential future phases of life, however, show that awareness of time is also an essential component of people's sense of narrative identity. Although this may be a truism in all of human development, what is unique about people's contemplation of transition later in life is that they have achieved this narrative sense of self within a heteronormative context that has severely constrained their gender identities. Although Halberstam (2005) emphasized the analogy of a life script when discussing the ways in which queer people and culture have created space and time that is unscripted by normative social structures, I propose that the people in this study may offer more complex life course narratives that integrate experiences of having, indeed, followed a normative script, while also modifying this script to nurture identity development in later life. I further suggest that these narratives point our attention to the ways in which identity development is multifaceted and does not take place in stable and predictable ways. Halberstam (2005) argued that queer time is often marked by rapid bursts of development that do not fit neatly into normative temporal frames; the life choices made by participants in this study promote such development in later life and demonstrate how this theory is relevant in an aging context.

Gerontological social workers are poised as potential leaders in expanding research and designing interventions for working with LGBT elders. This includes leading the larger project of expanding cultural meanings of aging and expanded opportunities for identity development across the life course. In recent years, the visibility of LGBT persons has increased tremendously in the field of social work. Similarly, gerontological social work has begun to emphasize the importance of understanding aging issues with respect to LGBT persons, as clearly evidenced by this journal's special issue. However, this visibility has not yet generated the theoretical depth and breadth found in other gerontological domains. For example, Fullmer (2006) emphasized the importance of using an historical perspective and taking context into account when addressing LGBT aging, but this work could be expanded on by adding more conceptual material on transgender issues. In this regard, Burdge (2007) made a strong theoretical argument for social workers to participate in the deconstruction of the heteronormative gender binary that often oppresses transgender clients, but this argument could also be strengthened by considering the ways in which aging and growing older complicate this task.

Similarly, Davis (2008), in her thoughtful presentation of transgender issues aimed at beginning competency for social workers, did not address issues of later life, even in her section titled "Age." Social service resources, especially those developed most recently by the National Resource Center on LGBT Aging (2013) have demonstrated tremendous leadership by highlighting transgender elders as having distinct needs across the life course, but these efforts could be buoyed by the development of conceptual orientations for research and work with older transgender clients. I expand upon these efforts by suggesting that social workers challenge themselves to be cognizant of making theoretical strides along with direct service advancements in their consideration of transgender aging issues. One way to approach this is to make sure that as they gather clinical and research data, they are not only paying attention to past and present, but also exploring future opportunities for growth. Such growth fostering opportunities are often overlooked in social workers' work and research with older adults. As human beings continue to live longer lives, the understanding of the potential for development in later life will be increasingly important for expanding the knowledge base in the field of gerontological social work. From a professional perspective, social workers must also create meaningful collaborations with scholars and leaders in queer studies and gender-progressive movements. For example, issues of gender identity and sexual orientation in children and families have recently gained increasing attention, and gerontological social work has the potential to contribute insights from perspectives near the end of life that have been missing in this domain thus far. By recognizing the possibilities for identity development in later life from multiple perspectives, social workers may also discover new possibilities for their profession to more effectively and holistically support the growth and wellbeing of those with whom they work.

ACKNOWLEDGMENTS

Thank you to Linda Waite and the Center for the Economics and Demography of Aging at the University of Chicago for their support. Thank you also to the participants in this project who generously shared their experiences with me.

FUNDING

This project was supported through predoctoral student funding through the Center on Aging at the University of Chicago, National Institute on Aging T32 Training Grant.

REFERENCES

Auerbach, C. F., & Silverstein, L. B. (2003). *Qualitative data*. New York, NY: New York University Press.

Baars, J. (1998). Concepts of time and narrative temporality in the study of aging. *Journal of Aging Studies*, *11*, 283–295.

Baars, J. (2007). Chronological time and chronological age: Problems of temporal diversity. In J. Baars & H. Visser (Eds.), *Aging and time: Multidisciplinary perspectives* (pp. 1–14). Amityville, NY: Baywood.

Baars, J. (2012). *Aging and the art of living*. Baltimore, MD: Johns Hopkins University Press.

Brown, M. T. (2009). LGBT aging and rhetorical silence. *Sexuality Research and Social Policy*, *6*(4), 65–78.

Burawoy, M. (1998). The extended case method. *Sociological Theory*, *16*(1), 4–33.

Burawoy, M., Burton, A., Ferguson, A. A., Fox, K. J., Gamson, J., Gartrell, N., . . . Ui, S. (1991). *Ethnography unbound: Power and resistance in the modern metropolis*. Berkeley: University of California Press.

Burdge, B. J. (2007). Bending gender, ending gender: Theoretical foundations for social work practice with the transgender community. *Social Work*, *52*, 243–250.

Butler, J. (2007). *Gender trouble*. New York, NY: Routledge.

Butler, S. S. (2004). Gay, lesbian, bisexual, and transgender (GLBT) elders: The challenges and resilience of this marginalized group. *Journal of Human Behavior in the Social Environment, 9*(4), 25–44.

Carstensen, L. L., Isaacowitz, D. M., & Charles, S. T. (1999). Taking time seriously: A theory of socioemotional selectivity. *American Psychologist, 54*, 165–181.

Cook-Daniels, L. (2006). Trans aging. In D. Kimmel, T. Rose, & S. David (Eds.), *Lesbian, gay, bisexual, and transgender aging* (pp. 20–35). New York, NY: Columbia University Press.

Cook-Daniels, L., & Munson, M. (2010). Sexual violence, elder abuse, and sexuality of transgender adults, Age 50+: Results of three surveys. *Journal of GLBT Family Studies, 6*, 142–177.

Davis, C. (2008). Social work practice with transgender and gender noncomforming people. In G. P. Mallon (Ed.), *Social work practice with lesbian, gay, bisexual, and transgender people* (pp. 83–111). New York, NY: Routledge.

Dittmann-Kohli, F. (2007). Temporal references in the construction of self-identity: A life-span approach. In J. Baars & H. Visser (Eds.), *Aging and time: Multidisciplinary perspectives* (pp. 43–82). Amityville, NY: Baywood.

Docter, R. F. (2008). *Becoming a woman: A biography of Christine Jorgensen*. New York, NY: Haworth.

Duggan, L. (2003). *The twilight of equality: Neo-liberalism, cultural politics and the attack on democracy*. Boston, MA: Beacon Press.

Emerson, R. M. (2001). *Contemporary field research: Perspectives and formulations*. Long Grove, IL: Waveland.

Emerson, R. M., Fretz, R. I., & Shaw, L. L. (2011). *Writing ethnographic field notes*. Chicago, IL: University of Chicago Press.

Floyd, F. J., & Bakeman, R. (2006). Coming-out across the life course: Implications of age and historical context. *Archives of Sexual Behavior, 35*, 287–296.

Fullmer, E. M. (2006). Lesbian, gay, bisexual and transgender aging. In D. F. Morrow & L. Messinger (Eds.), *Sexual orientation & gender expression in social work practice* (pp. 284–303). New York, NY: Columbia University Press.

Halberstam, J. (2005). *In a queer time and place: Transgender bodies, subcultural lives*. New York, NY: New York University Press.

Hughes, M. (2004, October). *Queer ageing and social work*. Paper presented at the Reclaiming Civil Society: The 32nd Biennial Global Social Work Conference, Adelaide, Australia.

Hughes, M. (2006). Queer ageing. *Gay and Lesbian Issues and Psychology Review, 2*(2), 54–59.

Kidd, J. D., & Witten, T. M. (2008). Understanding spirituality and religiosity in the transgender community: implications for aging. *Journal of Religion, Spirituality and Aging, 20*(1/2), 29–62.

Knochel, K. A. (2011). *Are they prepared? A look at midlife transgender people and their anticipated adaptation to aging* (Doctoral dissertation). University of Minnesota, Minneapolis, MN.

Mason, J. (2002). *Qualitative researching*. London, England: Sage.

Minter, S. (2001). *Transgender elders and marriage: The importance of legal planning*. Retrieved from www.forge-forward.org/handouts/TGElders-Marriage-ShannonMinter.pdf

National Resource Center on LGBT Aging. (2013). *Improving the lives of transgender older adults*. Retrieved from http://www.lgbtagingcenter.org/resources/

Orel, N. A. (2004). Gay, lesbian, and bisexual elders. *Journal of Gerontological Social Work, 43*, 57–77.

Orel, N. A., & Fruhauf, C. A. (2013). Lesbian, gay, bisexual, and transgender grandparents. In A. E. Goldberg & K. R. Allen (Eds.), *LGBT-parent families: Innovations in research and implications* (pp. 177–192). New York, NY: Springer.

Padgett, D. K. (2008). *Qualitative methods in social work research*. Los Angeles, CA: Sage.

Persson, D. I. (2009). Unique challenges of transgender aging: Implications from the literature. *Journal of Gerontological Social Work, 52*, 633–646.

Porter, K. E., Ronneberg, C. R., & Witten, T. M. (2013). Religious affiliation and successful aging among transgender older adults: Findings from the Trans MetLife Survey. *Journal of Religion, Spirituality and Aging, 25*, 112–138.

QSR International. (2012). *NVivo 9*. Retrieved from www.qsrinternational.com

Samuels, G. M. (2009). Using the extended case method to explore identity in a multiracial context. *Ethnic and Racial Studies, 32*, 1599–1618.

Sandberg, L. (2008). The old, the ugly and the queer: Thinking old age in relation to queer theory. *Graduate Journal of Social Science, 5*, 117–139.

Siverskog, A. (2012, November). *Queer life scripts—Normativity and queerness in older LGBTQ persons' life stories*. Symposium conducted at the meeting of the Gerontological Society of America, San Diego, CA.

Small, M. L. (2009). 'How many cases do I need?' On science and the logic of case selection in field-based research. *Ethnography, 10*(1), 5–38.

Van Wagenen, A., Driskell, J., & Bradford, J. (2013). "I'm still raring to go": Successful aging among lesbian, gay, bisexual, and transgender older adults. *Journal of Aging Studies, 27*(10), 1–14.

Williams, M. E., & Freeman, P. A. (2007). Transgender health: Implications for aging and caregiving. *Journal of Gay and Lesbian Social Services, 18*, 93–108.

Witten, T. M. (2009). Graceful exits: Intersection of aging, transgender identities, and the Family/Community. *Journal of GLBT Family Studies, 5*, 35–61.

Witten, T. M., & Eyler, A. E. (2012). Transgender and aging. In T. M. Witten & A. E. Eyler (Eds.) *Gay, lesbian, bisexual & transgender aging: Challenges in research, practice & policy* (pp. 187–269). Baltimore, MD: Johns Hopkins University Press.

Resilience in Attaining and Sustaining Sobriety Among Older Lesbians With Alcoholism

NOELL L. ROWAN

School of Social Work, University of North Carolina Wilmington, Wilmington, North Carolina, USA

SANDRA S. BUTLER

School of Social Work, University of Maine, Orono, Maine, USA

This phenomenological study illuminates coping among older lesbians with alcoholism. Twenty study participants were recruited through purposive and snowball sampling; each completed 3 interviews structured to gain a deeper understanding of participants' lived experiences. This article focuses on the key situations and people that helped study participants obtain sobriety and stay sober. Five major themes emerged from the data: wake-up calls, impact of formal treatment, impact of 12-step recovery groups, consequences from other sources, and resiliency. Findings support the need for culturally sensitive approaches to practice with this subpopulation of older adults.

INTRODUCTION

Problematic use of alcohol among older adults is one of the most rapidly growing public health concerns in the United States (Axner, 2008; Blow, 2000; Center for Substance Abuse Treatment [CSAT], 1998; Farkas, 2008; Watts, 2007). Abusing alcohol creates risks for heightened medical costs, and increased morbidity and mortality particularly among older adults. An estimated 1.7 million older adults (age 50 and older) are chemically dependent, with alcohol the main drug of choice, and this group is predicted to grow to 4.4 million by 2020 (Gfroerer, Penne, Pemberton, & Folsom, 2003; Korper & Rasken, 2003; Menninger, 2002; Reardon, 2012). Yet practitioners do not routinely check for alcohol consumption when adverse health issues arise (Heuberger, 2009). As women age, metabolism and other age related changes come into play (i.e., hormonal and menopausal issues, retirement, mobility limitations, illness) and these issues place older women with alcohol problems in an important subset population with special treatment needs (Epstein, Fischer-Elber, & Al-Otaiba, 2008). One group of older adults with alcohol problems who appear to be particularly at risk are lesbians. There is growing evidence in the empirical literature that this vulnerable subset presents unique physical and mental health risks warranting attention (Gabbay &Wahler, 2002; Rowan, 2012; Satre, 2006; Shankle, Maxwell, Kutzman, & Landers, 2003).

It is difficult to estimate accurately the prevalence of alcoholism among older lesbian adults, due to a myriad of issues including stigma, the quadruple threat of marginalization (being older, female, lesbian, and having alcoholism), inadequate screening among older adults, and multiple comorbid health issues (He, Sengupta, Velkoff, & DeBarros, 2005; Hooyman & Kiyak, 2008; Rowan, 2012). Research has begun to show a substantial health risk for chemical addiction among lesbian women as they present for treatment with severe chemical abuse histories, co-occurring mental health issues, and heavy medical service utilization (Anderson, 2009; Cochran & Cauce, 2006; CSAT, 2001; Gabbay & Wahler, 2002; Mercer et al., 2007; Roberts, Tarmina, Grindel, Patsdaughter, & DeMarco, 2005; Wilsnack et al., 2008). For example, Austin and Irwin (2010) explored problem drinking among lesbians ($N = 1,141$) using a Web-based survey. Results indicated that depression and general stress were related to alcohol problems and that more research was needed to examine the relationship between specific sexual-minority stress and problem drinking. In addition, Johnson et al. (2013) examined the unique social stressors experienced by sexual-minority women. Findings suggested that hazardous drinking was associated with other mental health issues such as anxiety and depression, and that a life course perspective is vital to better understand the unique challenges of both lesbian and bisexual women.

It has also been noted that lesbian women are reluctant to disclose their sexual identity to health providers, underscoring the need for culturally sensitive assessment and intervention strategies (Mercer et al., 2007). Moreover, profound risks of hazardous drinking, depression, and history of childhood sexual abuse have been noted among lesbian and bisexual women with specific recommendations that health and mental health care providers ask about the sexual orientation of women in an effort to design more effective treatment (Wilsnack et al., 2008).

Differences between heterosexuals and sexual minorities with regard to substance use, misuse, abuse, and dependence can extend into middle age and later life (Anderson, 2009; CSAT, 2001; Jones, 2001; Satre, 2006; Valanis et al., 2000). In addition to the expected physiological, retirement, and age-related loss issues facing older adults, aging lesbians confront stressors that put them at increased risk for developing alcohol problems in later life (CSAT, 1998; Finnegan & McNally, 2002; Satre, 2006). For example, older lesbians may have experienced antigay discrimination; social or familial pressure to conceal their identity; an increased sense of isolation; and a lack of recognition in society for partner relationships and/or parental roles in their nontraditional families (Anderson, 2009; Averett, Yoon, & Jenkins, 2011; Butler, 2004; CSAT, 2001; Finnegan & McNally, 2002; Jenkins, Rowan, & Parks, 2008; McFarland & Sanders, 2003). *The Out and Aging MetLife Study of Lesbian and Gay Baby Boomers* (Metlife Mature Market, 2006) revealed that older lesbians, in particular, had no confidence that they would be treated with respect from health care providers and that they feared insensitive and unfair treatment. These additional factors illustrate the challenges contributing to stress in the older lesbian population. Furthermore, older lesbian women who are most at risk for alcohol and other drug problems appear to have low self-esteem, anxiety, depression, poorly developed social support networks or have lost social networks, and stress associated with aging (Satre, 2006).

The minimal literature about the lived experiences of older lesbian women with alcoholism and their ability to sustain recovery necessitates further research. More information is needed about older lesbians with alcoholism who have attained sobriety and their experiences with formal treatment and informal supports. Although some studies provide treatment outcomes of older adults, sexual orientation information is typically omitted (CSAT, 2001; Satre, 2006). One notable exception is a recent study ($N = 120$) comparing perceptions and outcomes of substance abuse treatment among sexual minority and heterosexual adults (Senreich, 2009). Senreich (2009) noted that sexual minority clients reported decreased satisfaction with treatment and recommended specialized and affirmative treatment for sexual minority clients. Yet only 6% of substance abuse treatment programs in the United States have specialized treatment for sexual minority clients (Substance Abuse and Mental Health Services Administration, 2010).

There is a dearth of information about what is helpful to older lesbian adults in obtaining and sustaining sobriety. Negative attitudes and heterosexism, as noted in prior research (Averett et al., 2011), can create a complex situation when older lesbian adults present for treatment for alcoholism (Eliason & Hughes, 2004). Averett and Jenkins (2012), in their review of the literature about older lesbians, clearly stated that older lesbians exhibit the ability to bounce back from adverse situations including discrimination and being marginalized in American society and that much more research is needed specifically focused on older lesbians. This study seeks to address that need by examining the lived experiences of older lesbians with alcoholism and their journey to and maintenance of sobriety.

CONCEPTUAL FRAMEWORK

The narrative gerontology perspective, which focuses on human development throughout the life course through a life review, provides a framework for this study (Kenyon & Randall, 2001). This perspective not only allows researchers the opportunity to comprehend the depth of life events and stories, but also enables study participants to interpret their experiences and life changes (Cohen, Greene, Lee, Gonzalez, & Evans, 2006; Kivnick & Murray, 2001; McInnis-Dittrich, 2005). Narratives that focus on conducting a life review can be empowering and transformative for study participants. This life review process provides a mechanism to examine life history with increased awareness of the impact of specific events as they relate to how the participants attained and sustained sobriety. This study provides information gleaned from the narrative descriptions of older lesbian women with alcoholism specific to how they have dealt with alcoholism and attained sobriety, and what they have found helpful in sustaining sobriety.

METHODS

This study was guided by a phenomenological qualitative approach, which builds on the premise that knowledge of lived experiences provides insight into the underlying meanings. This insight was achieved by being immersed in the lives of the research participants via in-depth interviews (Giorgi, 2009; Padgett, 2008; Patton, 2002; Wertz, 2005). Interest in phenomenological studies has increased due to its application and alignment with the philosophies in health research that focus on uncovering deep understandings of lived experiences (Creswell, 2007; Denzin & Lincoln, 2000; Giorgi, 1997, 2009; Padgett, 2008; Wertz, 2005; Wilding & Whiteford, 2005). Phenomenology enables a broad examination of diverse and complex situations and conditions of the participants' life experiences that would otherwise be challenging to observe or measure (Moustakas, 1994; Padgett, 2008; Wertz, 2005; Wilding & Whiteford, 2005). Phenomenology is different from other qualitative approaches in that the focus is on an in-depth understanding of people's interpretations of the world and their experiences (Padgett, 2008; Wertz, 2005). The overarching goal of this phenomenological approach is to ask the research participants to reconstruct the experiences of their lives within the context of the particular area of study (Moustakas, 1994; Seidman,

2006), which leaves the readers of the study with a much more informed and empathic understanding as if having "walked a mile in the shoes" (Padgett, 2008, p. 36) of participants.

Perhaps one of the most distinguishing characteristics of phenomenological approaches is the researcher's need to be immersed in the lives of the participants over the course of multiple interviews (Creswell, 2007; Padgett, 2008; Patton, 2002; Seidman, 2006; Wertz, 2005). In conducting this study, in-depth interviews focused on understanding the core meanings and the essence of experiencing alcoholism in the aging process of lesbian women. Moreover, allowing the phenomenon to reveal itself utilizing critical thinking and a fresh new perspective on the lived experiences is a hallmark of this approach to qualitative interviewing research (Moustakas, 1994; Padgett, 2008; Patton, 2002; Seidman, 2006; Wertz, 2005). The phenomenological approach was selected as the most effective method to fulfill the study's primary aim: to explore how older lesbian women with alcoholism make sense of their illness, obtain sobriety, transform their lived experiences into consciousness on the individual level, and create meaning out of these experiences. This article focuses on one particular research question, although the larger study included several more. The main research question explored here is "What were the key events or situations and who were the people who helped you get and stay sober?"

Sampling and Recruitment

Twenty participants meeting the inclusion criteria were included in this research, which involved a series of three in-depth interviews. To be included in the study, participants needed to be age 50 or older, self-report lesbian sexual orientation, self-report alcoholism and at minimum 1 year of continuous sobriety, and reside in a large metropolitan area in the Southeastern United States. An extra step was taken as an integrity check for the report of having alcoholism and at least one year of continuous sobriety. Each participant supplied a contact name and granted verbal permission to contact this person. The participant called the contact and introduced the person to the reason for the call and handed the phone to the first author to verify the participant's tenure of sobriety. This contact was made during the first interview and was successfully documented for each participant.

Prior to data collection, the study was approved by the Institutional Review Board of the first author's university. A combination of purposive and snowball sampling was utilized to recruit study participants. Flyers advertising the study were placed in recovery and treatment centers, Web sites, coffee shops, and volunteer participants were asked to nominate other potential participants for the study. Prior to data collection, the study was approved by the Institutional Review Board of the first author's university.

Data Collection

The main sources of data for this study were the interviews used to capture the lived experiences of older lesbian women dealing with recovery from alcoholism. The research participants were interviewed using a semistructured process and interview guide. Questions pertaining to demographics and screening of alcohol abuse versus dependence, using *DSM-IV* criteria, were included in the guide to provide specific data regarding the onset and severity of alcoholism. The first author used a semistructured phenomenologically-based interview process as described by Seidman (2006). A three-part interview structure was employed, with each interview having a specific focus on (a) life history, (b) details of experiences, and (c) reflection of the meaning given to life events and circumstances. The follow-up interviews were used to clarify issues that emerged in the prior interview(s) and for member checking. Member checking is a process of checking the content and interpreted meanings from prior interviews with the member (research participant) in an effort to improve the integrity of the research process. Open-ended questions were asked with an open-minded and nonjudgmental attitude in an effort to encourage the interviewee to share honestly and openly about her experiences with aging, being lesbian, and dealing with alcoholism. The first interview lasted approximately 90 min, and subsequent interviews (lasting about an hour each) allowed for rich and comprehensive expressions of each participant's life story. The in-depth interviews occurred at an agreed upon place (i.e., older adult's home, other community location) and each participant completed the full course of the study and received $100 for participating in the project.

Data Analysis

The audio-recorded interviews with the participants were transcribed verbatim by a research assistant. In accordance with guidelines on phenomenological research, we immersed ourselves in the data to become more fully aware of the experiences of the respondents (Padgett, 2008; Patton, 2002; Wertz, 2005) through repeatedly listening to the interview tapes and reading and rereading the transcripts (Seidman, 2006; Wertz, 2005). To foreground oblique aspects, we formed initial impressions from the data, carefully analyzed portions of the data, and then related these pieces back to the whole until the entire data set had been covered (Wilding & Whiteford, 2005). The first author had primary responsibility for conducting the data analysis, and the second author read half of the transcripts and contributed to making sense of the data. Initial themes were discussed by both authors and mutually agreed upon; final themes were fine-tuned by the first author. The computer software system *ATLASti* was used to assist in the tracking of the codes and the source material assigned to each code. Analysis began with a familiarization with the data, grouping the identified experiences and descriptions of the participants into categories, and then refining and organizing the experiences into possible themes (Giorgi, 1997, 2009). In the process of writing the findings from this project, the identified themes and categories that emerged from the data were described and examples from the actual interview transcripts were used to strengthen the description.

Enhancement of Rigor and Trustworthiness

Because qualitative research is not designed for generalization to a larger population (Padgett, 2008), elements of trustworthiness and authenticity take the place of traditional positivist elements of reliability and validity (Denzin & Lincoln, 2000). As recommended by Padgett (2008), rigor and trustworthiness were enhanced by the use of triangulation (comparing multiple data sources, e.g., interview transcripts, observations, memos) to identify congruence, peer debriefing and support, member checking, multiple interviews with each participant serving as prolonged engagement, and the use of an organized record-keeping system that produced transparency of every aspect of the study and analysis process (i.e., audit trail). In the second and third interviews, a discussion was held with the participant to review previously shared aspects of her story for accuracy and to add content that had been omitted from the prior interview(s). In addition, subsequent to each of the 60 interviews, the first author formally reflected on the interview by creating a documented memo that allowed her to debrief and make note of important points made. In this type of in-depth inquiry, it was important that the author conducting the interviews disclose her stance on the issues of alcoholism, the lesbian culture, and the aging process in an effort to join with the research participants, while simultaneously setting aside her own experiences with the phenomenon through the use of bracketing (Denzin & Lincoln, 2000; Moustakas, 1994; Padgett, 2008; Patton, 2002; Wertz, 2005), and by doing so was able to emphasize a more rigorous explanation of the data (Groenewald, 2004). We discussed our histories with the phenomena and the importance of reflexivity when examining each interview.

FINDINGS

Description of Sample

The sample consisted of 20 participants who ranged in age from 50 to 70 and had a mean age of 57.6. All participants identified as lesbian, and reported having alcoholism and continuous sobriety for a minimum of 1 year. Participants reported being sober and abstinent from alcohol for an average of 17.65 years, with a range of one year to 32 years. Table 1 further details

TABLE 1 Demographic Characteristics of the Sample

Variable	N	%
Race		
White	19	95
African American	1	5
Relationship status		
Single	6	30
Partnered (range = 1–30 yrs)	14	70
Education		
Some college	5	25
Bachelor's degree	2	10
Master's degree	12	60
Doctoral degree	1	5
Income (combined all sources)		
< $20,000	3	15
$20,000–$49,999	4	20
$50,000–$70,000	7	35
> $70,000	6	30
Employment status		
Full-time	15	75
Part-time	1	5
Retired	4	20

the race, relationship and employment statuses, education, and income of the 20 participants.

Five major themes emerged from the data relating to attaining and sustaining sobriety: *wake-up calls, impact of formal treatment, impact of 12-step recovery groups, consequences from other sources*, and *resiliency*. Each is described in the next section, using quotes from study participant interviews for illustration.

Wake-Up Calls

Participants described considerable support that aided them in attaining sobriety. This included close connections with significant others such as a partner, family members, and friends. Nearly half ($n = 8$; 40%) of study participants noted that the influence from their primary relationships (partner) assisted them in calling attention to their problem drinking. For instance, one participant noted, "My partner of the time was the contributing factor in me taking that step" to get sober as "my partner, former partner, told me that she was moving out that she couldn't live with it [my drinking] any longer and that she was going to move out." Another participant stated, "I was given the ultimatum by [my partner] . . . just, 'You either quit or I'm out of here." . . . She just had it with my behavior; I just did real screwy things."

Other participants described support in attaining sobriety through close connections with family members who played vital roles in their sobriety. More than half of the sample ($n = 11$; 55%) described important influences from members of their families of origin and families of creation (i.e., their children) as vital to attainment of sobriety. For example, one participant described waking up from a blackout:

> I forgot my [older] son had a band concert . . . and I had taken God knows what, a handful of something, and . . . the last thing I remember is sticking my legs down in a pair of black dress pants and I drove those two boys in a blackout and I thought, "Damn this ain't right; this is so not right; I got to quit; I don't know what's wrong with me but whatever it is, it's wrong."

Another participant described a death of a parent from alcoholism as instrumental in her attaining sobriety.

> Well, I had just enough clarity in my head to realize . . . my mother was an alcoholic and died of this disease when I was 12 and that's one of the things. . . . I hated alcohol growing up, ah, and I swore I'd never be like her and I was becoming like her I was pushing my family away, my kids away.

Poignant moments such as these, with intense emotions involving key family members, were repeatedly described as vital to stirring a desire to obtain sobriety or to do something radically different in their lives.

Other participants ($n = 5$; 25%) described interactions with friends or friends of family as key to attaining sobriety. This is illustrated by one participant who described how a family friend, who was also a helping professional working in an alcohol education program, assisted her to attain sobriety. She stated,

> I said to her, for the first time, I said aloud, "I think I might have a problem [with alcohol]" and so she, ah, came in and gave me one of those . . . written assessments of some sort. . . . I don't know what it was; I couldn't even tell you . . . and the result was that . . . it sort of put me in this . . . category of being . . . in the . . . early chronic stages of alcoholism.

Another participant described getting a wake-up call of sorts by noticing that several drinking friends had committed suicide and she didn't want to end up like them. She reported,

> How did I talk myself into it? What can I say? I was sick and tired of being the person I was. . . . I didn't see any future. I saw hopelessness; really I saw that I was going down the same road as my friends were that committed suicide and I heard a lot about AA [Alcoholics Anonymous] and listened to some of my friends who had been in AA.

Similar to this description, another participant traced her deep misery to the losses and ensuing behaviors caused by her excessive drinking. She stated,

> My codependency got me sober. . . . I had run out of people. I had already lost relationships, cars; . . . people were disappearing from my life one by one. And I was afraid my kids would be next. And I had a friend [who] had gotten sober and she'd been a friend for years and years, started out as my bartender, and she'd gotten sober 2 years before I did and she . . . drove me to another AA meeting. . . . And being lonely at nights sometimes I'd walk down to the corner and call her on the pay phone and . . . eventually [she] talked me into treatment. I was sick and tired of being so lonely and living like I was living.

Impact of Formal Alcoholism Treatment

Twelve participants (60% of sample) mentioned that going to formal treatment for alcoholism in myriad forms—whether as residential or inpatient treatment or intensive or traditional outpatient treatment—as helpful in their path to sobriety. One participant noted, "I see a specifically lesbian therapist. . . . I sought her out specifically because she's lesbian . . . and certified [to treat clients struggling with] drugs and alcohol." As another participant stated,

> I asked for help; one of my friends that I knew whose mom had gone into a rehab facility for alcoholism . . . and he took me over to the hospital . . . and I actually enjoyed it, . . . thought it was worthwhile; it was mostly educational; I don't remember if they brought in AA. . . . Most of the people there were not into getting sober . . . a lot of them were pretty angry about it and resentful and I was actually more like, "You know I need to stay sober;" I obviously had a problem.

Another participant described the impact that formal in-patient treatment for alcoholism had on her. She stated,

> Hearing other people's struggles helped me identify my own. The assignments helped me get in touch with feelings, thinking process, ah, that I didn't even know existed in some cases. . . . I think I started learning how to open myself up maybe so I can think back to other times when I tried psychotherapy and I always shut down any kind of anything that got too close to being like with my history with my mom, my stepmom, my first step mom and, ah, this is the first time I didn't shut down, I said, "Alright, bring it on 'cause I kind of realized it's all that crap that's down there making me hurt, making me empty."

111

Another participant discussed how intensive out-patient therapy helped her gain an understanding about her own alcoholism and the dynamics in her family. She described,

> The [out-patient] therapy group was an enormous contributor 'cause I saw in the group. . . . I got in touch with the impact of growing up in an alcoholic family for myself and my siblings and the family dysfunction and I also saw it in group members and peers. So I mean I couldn't get away from it.

Another participant spoke about the importance of her therapist being highly competent and that she was lesbian so that she could feel safe in dealing with her sexual abuse history. She stated,

> I think it [seeing my therapist] made all the difference in the world. . . . Without it I wouldn't have stayed sober . . . because I needed to address a lot of the reasons why I drank. . . . We did a lot of work primarily at the beginning with my sexual abuse from when I was a child . . . and then also at the same time . . . we did some work with keeping me sober.

Impact of 12-Step Recovery Groups

Perhaps the most pervasive impact on the participants in both getting sober and sustaining sobriety was in their involvement in 12-step recovery groups, such as AA, Alanon, and Adult Children of Alcoholics (ACOA). Seventy-five percent ($n = 15$) of participants mentioned the importance of these recovery groups in many different aspects of their ability to cope with the stressors of alcoholism. For example, one participant stated,

> I got into AA before I stopped drinking 'cause a friend had suggested that I might want to try it that it might give me more insight into my family. . . . At that point [in life] I felt something was wrong and I went to a party with a friend of mine who was in recovery [AA] and we were talking. . . . There was alcohol at the party and I was telling her about my mother and how my mother always said she had a drink every night and she never had more than two, but you know she always ended up having two drinks . . . and she talked to me about the functional alcoholic and how they can just maintain for a lengthy period of time but sooner or later it catches up and that they suffer from a slow deterioration of the soul. . . . I looked in the mirror and instead of seeing my face I saw my mom's and I realized I was turning into my mother and that slow deterioration of the soul was my deterioration.

Another participant discussed her belief that involvement in AA was vital to her during a very painful time in her life.

Well I didn't believe in God and ah just going to [AA] meetings didn't seem like it was gonna help me. . . . I felt so horrible inside, I didn't see how just going to meetings and working a step and becoming somewhat religious was going to help my insides feel better I was very much hurting inside. . . . I went to counseling for adult children of alcoholics and they talked about that it was ok to have your feelings, it was ok to cry and that I was, you know, ok and that it was ok to talk about stuff and they said to go to AA meetings and get sober and then I knew I needed to get sober. I was going to, trying to go to AA meetings which I thought were bullshit and I ran into a couple of really cool lesbians at a lesbian AA meeting and they talked about, ah, therapy and how much it helped them so that's why I did that and what I mean about cool lesbians is they had a lot of fun without drinking and they just seemed to be happy . . . and somehow . . . I saw . . . differently.

Moreover, a different participant discussed how she believed that a group of lesbians from AA helped her out when she was struggling. She stated,

They were the ones that really . . . came through for me. . . . These lesbians, I mean, I don't know what I would've done without them. I really don't. . . . They cemented me in AA, . . . These people are gonna show up and they're gonna help. . . . They walk their talk . . . That's what really got me involved with AA in a much stronger way.

Another participant described how uplifting it felt to feel a sense of belonging and connection in AA. She discussed finding a network of friends easily within the meetings and being immersed in a sense of recovery and a positive state of being and thinking. For example,

We kind of ran around together and went to tons of meetings and drank a lot of coffee and networked, . . . just hung. . . . I surrounded myself in AA; I really, really did. . . . It was like wow I mean from my first meeting I literally left there . . . and it was an astonishingly clear crisp day and I remember driving . . . and singing out loud which was something I didn't do—some little ditty . . . doo di doo di doo whatever. . . . It was just a beautiful day I'd been to an AA meeting and I felt good.

Consequences From Other Sources

Several participants ($n = 8$; 40%) mentioned other sources, such as an employer, health care provider, legal system, religious community, or school system, which provided the consequences or pertinent discussion that created the situation leading to attainment of sobriety. One participant was confronted with a need to address her alcoholism by a member of her religious community. She explained that she was mandated to attend a special alcoholism workshop and that although she went "kicking and screaming," it turned out to be a wonderful awakening experience. She stated,

> I think we were there the whole weekend because I remember leaving on a Sunday feeling so insightful . . . and was ready to go to AA. I think I went to AA the next day. . . . We, each one around the circle, . . . shared . . . about and I'm not sure that they even, well I guess they did consider themselves as alcoholic, but you know part of what we did over that whole weekend was try to come to that . . . possibly we had this disease and she did talk about the disease of alcoholism.

Another participant described how important and life changing it was when a dentist confronted her about her drinking and that overmedicating of pain pills was a problem. She described that although her partner and mother complained about how her drinking and overmedicating were caus-ing problems, it was the health care professional's words that created a desire to want to change and get sober. She said,

> Ah well, you know, that dentist . . . was really a key (laughs); the dentist said, "Oh, I see you're on valium." . . . I was very miserable by then and yes, he was the straw that broke the camel's back. . . . You know, [partner's name] had been, you know, complaining, ah, at least I'm sure for a year and my mom had really been riding me for years about how many pills I took and I just blew it off and ah, I remember. . . . my mom . . . talking about me falling asleep with a brownie, you know, falling out of my mouth just that I had started to take a bite and just passed out.

One participant identified a workplace intervention to obtain formal treatment and describes the interplay of formal and informal treatments in the personal journey to maintain that gained sobriety.

> I was having many kinds of interventions I guess and I went to the employee assistance director at my place of employment and he recom-mended that I go for an alcoholism assessment. . . . I went to in-patient treatment for 39 days . . . and I stayed there. . . . For 39 days I not only did alcoholism treatment, but I stayed an extra 8 or 9 days to do the codependent treatment . . . and then when I came home from treatment I continued . . . for another, gosh, I guess 7 or 8 years of therapy as an outpatient. . . . It was necessary for me to do a lot of outside therapy which was complemented by my involvement in Alcoholics Anonymous but I'm not so sure had I not had benefit of this therapy if I would've been able to maintain my sobriety. Ah, for me, just attending meetings and working the steps was not enough, it was complemented by the outside work, the therapy work.

Resiliency

Every participant indicated that they were at least somewhat good at bouncing back from adverse situations. Several examples illustrate how study participants saw themselves as resilient in handling life challenges, such as the coming to terms with being lesbian, aging, and dealing with having alcoholism. First, as one participant noted, "I think the fact that I can be of use to another person makes me want to recover from adversity." She went on to state, "My adversity [being lesbian, alcoholic, and older] connects me to the world and, instead of feeling rejected by it, now I feel connected." In these statements, she clearly demonstrated how she is able to make her own life stressors meaningful in her efforts to help others who may struggle with the same issues.

Another participant expressed how important her health had become as she had remained sober and gotten older. She stated,

> I just had, a year ago this month, two breast cancer surgeries so that brings health right to the forefront. . . . I was very blessed with the diagnosis [coming so early] and the outcome. . . . The first surgery they didn't get it all so they had to do a second one and with the second one they [removed it all] and they said it's completely gone. . . . The only thing I have to do is take the medication every day for 5 years . . . and get regular checkups.

Another participant described the use of prayer to cope with daily stressors and that turning her concerns over in prayer helps her to bounce back from adversity. She discussed,

> Well, I pray about it; usually that's the first thing I do. I pray about it and I try to let it go. Sometimes I pick it up again but I keep praying about it until I can just let it go and just let whatever happens happen, you know, and I never give up on me, you know, I never give up on me. As long as I am breathing, as long as I'm walking, whatever the situation is, it could change as long as I'm not stuck in being right it can change. When I think I got to be right no matter what, then I'm gonna stay stuck.

One participant described dealing with the experience of being arrested simply for being in a gay bar in the 1970s and being charged for disorderly conduct. She described this to illustrate discrimination and pervasive heterosexism in society and as an event that happened many years before attaining sobriety. She stated,

> It was like a thing that they did back then. . . . We knew that they [the police] raided gay bars and it was just part of the culture. . . . They took

everybody [from the gay bar]. . . . They used to bring the paddy wagons around and they would raid the [gay] bars and take everybody to jail. We were having a good time (laughs) [because] they took us all at the same time and we were all drunk. . . . It was a big joke. . . . There were at least 20 women and we were all in a holding cell. I worked in a bar . . . so I didn't think much about it.

Another participant discussed how coming out as a lesbian and being found out in the context of a military career was devastating to her career and her life. She described feeling as if she had to hide who she was as a lesbian.

Going under cover, . . . being quiet, not sharing who I am with people, or . . . changing the subject or, if people made fun of gays and lesbians, . . . just try to listen and go on with it, . . . being pretty nonconfrontational about it, . . . there was a lot of pressure. Well, I think somewhere you have to find, ah, meaning in it, ah, I think it's just like Viktor Frankl's book; you just have to find some meaning in whatever is going on to be able to bounce back and that's probably what's gonna help me out. . . . Probably it will be my faith and somewhere trusting that you know God still has his hand on me even if it's a difficult time.

These quotes illustrate resiliency in dealing with various adverse life situations (e.g., discrimination in a gay bar, the military) throughout their lives, including their approach to remaining sober.

DISCUSSION

The major themes that emerged from this study shed light on the distinct experiences and needs of older lesbians with alcoholism. There are distinct similarities with many groups of people, whether heterosexual or lesbian, attempting to attain and sustain sobriety. It is in the sensitivity to lesbian culture that we can accurately interpret the findings. The interviews indicate the importance of respecting the inherent dignity of older lesbians for dealing with pervasive heterosexism and the vulnerability to homophobia that they have lived with throughout their lives. Without an understanding and acknowledgement of the impact of social and individual factors at work for individuals with alcoholism, efforts to encourage recognition, treatment and ongoing support can be misguided. The participants in this research reported on feeling well cared for within their formal treatment experiences and many times sought treatment from lesbian mental health providers in an effort to gain acceptance of their identity as a lesbian and to feel safe. Other participants discussed joining informal support networks (friends or 12-step recovery meetings), which were well represented by other lesbian women as a means to feel supported in dealing with various life stressors, including the challenges associated with attaining and sustaining sobriety. As was stated earlier, alcoholism among older adults is one of the fastest growing health problems in the United States and the consequences of problem drinking to the individual, her support system, and society are tremendous. Moreover, alcoholism is often described as a chronic-relapsing condition, with only about a quarter of those treated in abstinence-based mainstream programs actually maintaining abstinence in the year following treatment (Miller, Walters, & Bennett, 2001). Therefore, this sample of 20 older lesbians with alcoholism, who have at least one year of continuous sobriety, represents one particular segment of the population of older lesbians with alcoholism, but one that well exemplifies the concept of resiliency.

The findings in this study allowed us to reveal the strengths in research participants and how their capacity to be resilient contributed to their overall health and well-being (Greene, 2002; Van Breda, 2001). According to Friend (1991), the underlying power to challenge negative stereotypes about aging and sexual orientation is the essence of successful aging specific to older lesbian and gay people. As was illustrated in several quotes from research participants, admitting to having alcoholism and with the help of treatment and 12-step recovery groups that were sensitive to their specific needs paved the way for many participants to bounce back from difficult life situations.

As described in the literature, "Resilience does not support the 'buck-up and take responsibility, because others have overcome much worse' attitude directed toward individuals and families who are experiencing difficulties" (Blundo, 2002, p. 147). Rather, resiliency involves finding a stronger and more meaningful way to deal with life difficulties and stressors (Blundo, 2002). Morrow (2001) described the importance of social workers emphasizing psychosocial strengths including resilience to assist the aging experiences among older gay and lesbian people. More specifically, social work interventions with older gays and lesbians need to take into account the historical context of homophobia, heterosexism, and the possibility that they may have survived some form of antigay violence. Such a need may be particularly heightened in an atmosphere of growing social acceptance of homosexuality to diminish or silence a person about the difficulties caused for them by attitudes and instances of homophobia. A respectful demeanor toward older lesbian and gay people is, therefore, crucial given that they may have endured much oppression and discrimination. This also can be applied to research interviews being conducted with older lesbian or gay people because qualitative interviewing requires many of the same interpersonal skillsets necessary in direct social work practice.

IMPLICATIONS FOR PRACTICE

Older lesbian adults with alcoholism have, inevitably, dealt with a complex mixture of issues related to oppression, overcoming biases, and coming to terms with their identity and recovery from alcoholism. As has been seen through the lens of the participants in this study, having supportive people who are honest enough to provide consequences such as threats to end partner relationships, employers and health care providers who call attention to problems with alcohol, and informal support networks (i.e., 12-step recovery groups), and formal treatment programs that hold individuals accountable are key to attaining and sustaining sobriety. In short, the findings from this study demonstrate that the support systems in place for older lesbians need to be attuned with the specific stressors that are common in lesbian culture (such as the history of extreme oppression, hate crimes, and the stigma of coming out as a lesbian) in addition to being savvy about the dynamics of alcoholism. Participants in this research consistently conveyed the seriousness of dealing with alcoholism within themselves; moreover, some participants discussed multiple issues within their families related to alcoholism.

These findings underscore the need to give credence to the core social work value of social justice in social work practice by respecting the unique dignity and worth of older lesbians with alcoholism. Regardless of being a largely hidden and often overlooked group of aging people in American society, this group of older lesbians presented themselves as resilient and engaged in strong social support systems. As has been supported in other research (Averett et al., 2011; Butler & Hope, 1999), study participants indicated a strong network of support and were generally functioning well in society. Even with these strengths, there remain challenges for this population, resulting from embedded heterosexism in society.

Although the purpose of this study was not to unveil participant views on oppressive practices and policies in American culture, several participants described experiencing very difficult familial and societal pressures. Hence, some implications for social work practice can be gleaned from this research. This study points to the importance of culturally sensitive treatment provisions for aging lesbians with alcoholism. As can be seen in the lived experiences of this study sample, many struggled with attaining sobriety and needed considerable aid from professional health and mental health care providers. It is vital that these professionals have at least some basic knowledge to ask respectful questions about lesbian culture, significant relationships, and be mindful of the dynamics of alcoholism. The recently established National Resource Center on LGBT (lesbian, gay, bisexual and transgender) Aging by New York's SAGE (Services & Advocacy for GLBT Elders), funded through the federal Department of Health and Human Services, is a significant step forward in preparing professionals to have the knowledge and sensitivity they need to work with older LGBT adults, including lesbians with alcoholism. The mission of the Resource Center is to provide technical assistance, training, and key resources to support LGBT older adults and can be accessed using the Web site (http://www.sageusa. org). Social work practitioners must be equipped with the cultural sensitivity to refrain from making assumptions. Instead, they need to step into the tension and ask about sexual orientation, age related issues, and significant drinking problems.

A study of 20 individuals necessarily has some limitations. The in-depth phenomenological approach requires small samples and does not have generalizability as its purpose, but rather focuses on gaining understanding of lived experiences. The lived experiences described herein come from a group of older lesbians who were largely very well educated, middle class, urban, White, and who had at least one year of sobriety. It is certainly possible that the concerns and experiences would be different for older lesbians with alcoholism who have less education; live in other parts of the country; have fewer financial resources; have different cultural, racial, or ethnic backgrounds; or less time with continuous sobriety than this particular sample. Nonetheless, this study provides a first step toward understanding the situations and events that have helped some older lesbians to attain and maintain sobriety. Future study with this particular sample of older lesbian women to attain longitudinal understanding of how they create meaning as they age would provide more in-depth understanding of sustaining sobriety while dealing with ongoing life stressors. Ultimately, future studies with more diverse samples of older lesbians with alcoholism would allow us to assess the generalizability of this study's findings.

ACKNOWLEDGMENTS

We thank the participants in this study who gave many hours of their time to tell their stories with the hope that they were being helpful to others. Special appreciation goes to Susan Buzzell for final editing of this article; Annatjie Faul, Institutional Faculty Sponsor, Kent School of Social Work, University of Louisville, who gave much support for this project; Rhonda Amer, Kent School of Social Work, who spent many hours of her time to read, transcribe and discuss the content of the participant interviews; and Kim Rogers, Administrative Associate, Kent School of Social Work, who gave much assistance with technical details of this project.

FUNDING

We thank John A. Hartford Faculty Scholars Program for the grant that supported this research project.

REFERENCES

Anderson, S. (2009). *Substance use disorders in lesbian, gay, bisexual, & transgender clients*. New York, NY: Columbia University Press.

Austin, E. L., & Irwin, J. A., (2010). Age differences in the correlates of problematic alcohol use among southern lesbians. *Journal of Studies on Alcohol & Drugs, 71*, 295–298.

Averett, P., & Jenkins, C. (2012). Review of the literature on older lesbians: Implications for education, practice, and research. *Journal of Applied Gerontology, 31*, 537–561.

Averett, P., Yoon, I., & Jenkins, C. L. (2011). Older lesbians: Experiences of aging discrimination and resilience. *Journal of Women & Aging, 23*, 216–232.

Axner, S. (2008). Substance use and abuse among older adults: Reflections from an MSW student. *Aging Times, 4*(2).

Blow, F. C. (2000). Substance abuse among older adults: An invisible epidemic. In F. C. Blow (Ed. Consensus Panel Chair), *Substance abuse among older adults* (DHHS Publication No. SMA98-3179, Treatment Improvement Protocol Series 26). Rockville, MD: Substance Abuse and Mental Health Services Administration, Office of Applied Studies.

Blundo, R. (2002). Mental health: A shift in perspective. In R. R. Greene (Ed.) *Resilience: An integrated approach to practice, policy, and research* (pp. 133–152). Washington, DC: NASW Press.

Butler, S. S. (2004). Gay, lesbian, bisexual, and transgender (GLBT) elders: The challenges and resilience of this marginalized group. *Journal of Human Behavior in the Social Environment, 9*(4), 25–44.

Butler, S. S., & Hope, B. (1999). Health and well-being for late middle-aged and old lesbians in a rural area. *Journal of Gay and Lesbian Social Services, 9*(4), 27–46.

Center for Substance Abuse Treatment. (1998). *Substance abuse among older adults* (Treatment Improvement Protocol Series, No. 26, CSAT Publication No. SMA 98-3179). Rockville, MD: US Department of Health and Human Services, Public Health Service, and Substance Abuse and Mental Health Administration.

Center for Substance Abuse Treatment. (2001). *A provider's introduction to substance abuse treatment for lesbian, gay, bisexual, and transgender individuals*. Rockville, MD: US Department of Health and Human Services. Substance Abuse and Mental Health Services Administration.

Cochran, B. N., & Cauce, A. M. (2006). Characteristics of lesbian, gay, bisexual, and transgender individuals entering substance abuse treatment. *Journal of Substance Abuse Treatment, 30*, 135–146.

Cohen, H. L., Greene, R. R., Lee, Y., Gonzalez, J., & Evans, M. (2006). Older adults who overcame depression. *Families in Society, 87*(1), 35–42.

Creswell, J. W. (2007). *Qualitative inquiry and research design* (2nd ed.) Thousand Oaks, CA: Sage.

Denzin, N. K., & Lincoln, Y. S. (Eds.). (2000). *Handbook of qualitative research* (2nd ed.). Thousand Oaks, CA: Sage.

Eliason, M. J., & Hughes, T. (2004). Treatment counselor's attitudes about lesbian, gay, bisexual, and transgendered clients: Urban and rural settings. *Substance Use & Misuse, 39*, 625–644.

Epstein, E. E., Fischer-Elber, K., & Al-Otaiba, Z. (2008). Women, aging, and alcohol use disorders. *Journal of Women & Aging, 19*, 31–48.

Farkas, K. J. (2008). Aging and substance use, misuse, and abuse. *Aging Times, 4*(2).

Finnegan, D. G., & McNally, E. B. (2002). *Counseling lesbian, gay, bisexual, and transgender substance abusers: Dual identities*. New York, NY: Haworth.

Friend, R. A. (1991). Older lesbian and gay people: A theory of successful aging. In J. A. Lee (Ed.), *Gay midlife and maturity* (pp. 99–118). New York, NY: Haworth.

Gabbay S. G., & Wahler J. J. (2002). Lesbian aging: Review of a growing literature. *Journal of Gay and Lesbian Social Services, 14*(3), 1–21.

Giorgi, A. (1997). The theory, practice, and evaluation of the phenomenological method as a qualitative research procedure. *Journal of Phenomenological Psychology, 28*(2), 235–260.

Giorgi, A. (2009). *The descriptive phenomenological method in psychology: A modified Husserlian approach*. Pittsburgh, PA: Duquesne University Press.

Gfroerer, J., Penne, M., Pemberton, M., & Folsom, R. (2003). Substance abuse treatment need among older adults in 2020: The impact of the aging baby-boom cohort. *Drug and Alcohol Dependence, 69*, 127–135.

Greene, R. R. (2002). *Resilience: An integrated approach to practice, policy, and research*. Washington, DC: NASW Press.

Groenewald, T. (2004). A phenomenological research design illustrated. *International Journal of Qualitative Methods, 3*, 1–25.

He, W., Sengupta, M., Velkoff, V. A., & DeBarros, K. A. (2005). *States* (pp. 23–209). Washington, D C: US Government Printing Office.

Heuberger, R. A. (2009). Alcohol and the older adult: A comprehensive review. *Journal of Nutrition for the Elderly, 28*, 203–235.

Hooyman, N. R., & Kiyak, H. A. (2008). *Social gerontology: A multidisciplinary perspective*. Boston, MA: Pearson.

Jenkins, D. J., Rowan, N. L., & Parks, C. (2008, November). *Recovery and resiliency in older gay addicts*. Paper presented at Gerontological Society of America Conference, National Harbour, MD.

Johnson, T. P., Hughes, T. L., Cho, Y. I., Wilsnack, S. C., Aranda, F., & Szalacha, L. A. (2013). Hazardous drinking, depression, and anxiety among sexual-minority women: Self-medication or impaired functioning? *Journal of Studies on Alcohol and Drugs, 74*, 565–575.

Jones, B. E. (2001). Is having the luck of growing old in the gay, lesbian, bisexual. transgender community good or bad luck? *Journal of Gay and Lesbian Social Services, 13*(4), 13–14.

Kenyon, G. M., & Randall, W. (2001). Narrative gerontology: An overview. In G. M. Kenyon, P. Clark, & B. de Vries (Eds.), *Narrative gerontology* (pp. 3–18). New York, NY: Springer.

Kivnick, H. Q., & Murray, S. V. (2001). Life strengths interview guide: Assessing elder clients' strengths. *Journal of Gerontological Social Work, 34*(4), 7–32.

Korper, S. P., & Raskin, I. R. (2003). The impact of substance use and abuse by the elderly: The next 20 to 30 years. In *Substance use by older adults: Estimates of future impact on the treatment system*. Substance Abuse and Mental Health Services Administration, Office of Applied Studies.

McFarland, P. L., & Sanders, S. (2003). A pilot study about the needs of older gays and lesbians: What social workers need to know. *Journal of Gerontological Social Work, 40*(3), 67–80.

McInnis-Dittrich, K. (2005). *Social work with elders: A biopsychosocial approach to assessment and intervention* (2nd ed.). Boston, MA: Allyn & Bacon.

Menninger, J. A. (2002). Assessment and treatment of alcoholism and substance-related disorders in the elderly. *Bulletin of the Menninger Clinic, 66*, 166–183.

Mercer, C. H., Bailey, J. V., Johnson, A. M., Erens, B., Wellings, K., Fenton, K. A., & Copas, A. (2007). Women who report having sex with women: British national probability data on prevalence, sexual behaviors, and health outcomes. *American Journal of Public Health, 97*, 1126–1133.

Metlife Mature Market Institute. (2006). *Out and aging: The Metlife study of gay and lesbian baby boomers*. New York: Author.

Miller, W. R., Walters, S. T. & Bennett, M. E. (2001). How effective is alcoholism treatment in the United States? *Journal of Studies on Alcohol, 62*, 211–220.

Morrow, D. F. (2001). Older gays and lesbians: Surviving a generation of hate and violence. *Journal of Gay and Lesbian Social Services, 13*, 151–169.

Moustakas, C. (1994). *Phenomenological research methods*. Thousand Oaks, CA: Sage.

Padgett, D. K. (2008). *Qualitative methods in social work research* (2nd ed.). Los Angeles, CA: Sage.

Patton, M. Q. (2002). *Qualitative research & evaluation methods* (3rd ed.). Thousand Oaks, CA: Sage.

Reardon, C. (2012). The changing face of older adult substance abuse. *Social Work Today, 12*(1), 8.

Roberts, S. J., Tarmina, M. S., Grindel, C. G., Patsdaughter, C. A. & DeMarco, R. (2005). Lesbian use and abuse of alcohol: Results of the Boston Lesbian Health Project II. *Substance Abuse, 25*, 1–9.

Rowan, N. L. (2012). Older lesbian adults with alcoholism: A case study for practitioners. *Journal of Geriatric Care Management, 22*(1), 19–24.

Satre, D. D. (2006). Use and misuse of alcohol and drugs. In D. Kimmel, T. Rose, & S. David (Eds.), *Lesbian, gay, bisexual, and transgender aging: Research and clinical perspectives* (pp. 131–151). New York, NY: Columbia University Press.

Seidman, I. E. (2006). *Interviewing as qualitative research*. New York, NY: Teachers' College Press.

Senreich, E, (2009). A comparison of perceptions, reported abstinence, and completion rates of gay, lesbian, bisexual, and heterosexual clients in substance abuse treatment. *Journal of Gay & Lesbian Mental Health, 13*, 145–169. doi:10.1080/19359700902870072

Shankle, M. D., Maxwell, C. A., Kutzman, E. S., & Landers, S. (2003). An invisible population: Older lesbians, gay, bisexual and transgender individuals. *Clinical Research and Regulatory Affairs, 20*, 159–182.

Substance Abuse and Mental Health Services Administration. (2010). *New national study shows that only six percent of substance abuse treatment facilities offer specialized services for gays and lesbians*. Retrieved from http://oas.samhsa.gov/spotlight/Spotlight004GayLesbians.pdf

Valanis, B. G., Bowen, D. J., Bassford, T., Whitlock, E., Charney, P., & Carter, R. A. (2000). Sexual orientation and health comparisons in the women's health initiative sample. *Archives of Family Medicine, 9,* 843–853.

Van Breda, A. D. (2001). *Resilience theory: A literature review.* Pretoria, South Africa: South African Military Health Service. Retrieved from http://www.vanbreda.org/adrian/resilience.htm

Watts, M. (2007). Incidences of excess alcohol consumption in the older person. *Nursing Older People, 18*(12), 27–30.

Wertz, F. J. (2005). Phenomenological research methods for counseling psychology. *Journal of Counseling Psychology, 52,* 167–177.

Wilding, C. & Whiteford, G. (2005). Phenomenological research: An exploration of conceptual, theoretical, and practical issues. *OTJR: Occupation, Participation and Health, 25*(3), 98–104.

Wilsnack, S. C., Hughes, T. L., Johnson, T., Bostwick, W. B., Szalacha, L. A., Benson, P., . . . Kinnison, K. E. (2008). Drinking and drinking-related problems among heterosexual and sexual minority women. *Journal of Studies on Alcohol & Drugs, 69,* 129–139.

Broadening Definitions of Family for Older Lesbians: Modifying the Lubben Social Network Scale

MARCENA L. GABRIELSON

Mennonite College of Nursing, Illinois State University, Normal, Illinois, USA

EZRA C. HOLSTON

College of Nursing, The University of Tennessee, Knoxville, Knoxville, Tennessee, USA

Lesbian seniors have triple vulnerability (gender, sexual orientation, and age), necessitating inquiry into their social support needs, yet research about that is scare. Investigators identify relationships between social support and senior health. The Lubben Social Network Scale, Revised (LSNS-R), has provided such evidence and has been used to study many diverse senior groups. We modified it to include a Family of Choice *category and qualitative questions to give context to responses among a sample of older lesbians. Our pilot demonstrated that the modification made a difference in accurately measuring social support among the sample, yet further investigation is warranted.*

BACKGROUND AND SIGNIFICANCE

There are one to three million lesbian, gay, and bisexual (LGB) Americans over age 65 and their numbers are expected to double by 2030 (Cahill, South, & Spade, 2000). LGB seniors are more likely to experience a disparity in social supports, compared to heterosexual seniors (National Gay and Lesbian Task Force [NGLTF], 2005), leading to an increased vulnerability to poor health outcomes. They are more likely than heterosexual seniors to age single, live alone, and have no children to provide support to them. These and other types of social disadvantages experienced by LGB seniors contribute to increased risk for health disparities as they age, compared to their heterosexual counterparts, a clear example of social disparities interacting with health over the life course (Blane, 2006). Lesbian seniors experience a triple marginalization as women, as older adults, and as a sexual minority (Kehoe, 1989), placing them at an exceptionally high risk for health disparities. Lesbians, like other women, experience career-long disparities in income, compared to men. Financial impediments can affect their access to quality and culturally competent care (Diamant, Wold, Spritzer, & Gelberg, 2000; Orel, 2004). Compared to heterosexual women, lesbians are more likely to lack health insurance and have health needs that go unmet (Heck, Sell, & Gorin, 2006; Rankow, 1995). As older adults accessing needed services (for example, supported living and long-term care) lesbians are presumed to be heterosexual and may be separated from partners, faced with bigotry and discrimination if understood to be lesbian, and may feel forced to go back into the closet to receive care (NGLTF, 2005). Further, compared to heterosexual women, lesbians are more likely to be childless, having no children to assist them with their needs as they age. Finally they are more likely to have limited support from relatives.

Care of elders is traditionally a family affair, with the implication that adult children are a natural, proper, and preferred form of social support (Gironda, Lubben, & Atchison, 1999). In fact, parenthood is considered a major contributor to social integration. Older childless adults have smaller social networks in old age than those older adults with children (Dykstra, 2006) and less financial security, poorer health outcomes, and less contact with extended family members. They often do not substitute other family members for the children they do not have to support them when they age (Dykstra, 2006). Their successful aging is significantly hindered by such barriers to adequate social support (Grossman, D'Augelli, & Hershberger, 2000).

There is a large body of research regarding associations between social support and older adult health. Social support strongly impacts the health of seniors, both mentally and physically (Berkman & Glass, 2000; Cornwell & Waite, 2009; Lubben & Gironda, 2003a; Seeman, 2001). For example, limited social support has been associated with multiple hospitalizations (Mistry, Rosansky, McQuire, McDermott, & Jarvik, 2001) and mortality (Ceria et al., 2001; Mistry et al., 2001) among older adults. Social support not only strengthens seniors' overall health experience, but also affects their perceptions of health and well-being (Cornell & Waite, 2009; Lubben & Gironda, 2003b; Lubben et. al., 2006; Rubbenstein, Lubben, & Mintzer, 1994). For instance, regardless of the actual size of the support system, seniors who perceive themselves as lacking social support, demonstrate worse mental health than those perceiving strong social support (Cornwell & Waite, 2009). Self-rated physical health reflects health status, symptoms, function, and behaviors (Fayers & Sprangers, 2002). Self-rated physical health among seniors has been associated with both actual and perceived social support. Together, limited support and perceptions of limited support are additive in their effect on self-rated poor physical health (Cornwell & Waite, 2009).

Many of the disadvantages that lesbians experience may be attributed to not having the familial social supports that research has demonstrated are vital to the well-being of heterosexual older adults. Therefore, the purpose of this cross-sectional, mixed-method pilot study with a descriptive design was to explore and describe perceived social support and associated factors among a snowball sample of older lesbians using a modified Lubben Social Network Scale, Revised (LSNS-R). The LSNS-R has been used extensively with a wide range of older adults in measuring social support received from traditionally defined family and friends. In the modified version of the instrument, *family of choice* was added to the original relative and friend categories (see Figure 1). Because of the large body of literature suggesting adult children provide substantial social support to elder parents, for analysis, we divided our sample into those with and without children.

Older lesbians often define *family* broadly so that extended family and friends are included, expanding *family* beyond simply a biological connection (Jones and Nystrom, 2002). Lesbians' "creation of family" involves the careful and conscious development of social support systems of friends over the life course (Gabrielson, 2011b). It is this constructed family from which older lesbians seek support for their physical, emotional, and spiritual health (Gabrielson, 2011a). These support systems (often comprised of other lesbians) are identified by lesbians as essential to their well-being and therefore *created families* aka *families of choice*, are basically survival systems for lesbians (Aronson, 1998; Comerford, Henson-Stroud, Sionainn, & Wheeler, 2004; Gabrielson, 2011; Grossman, D'Augelli & Hershberger, 2000; Masini & Barret, 2008; Weinstock, 2000).

Functional changes in aging reduce older adults' quantity and quality of social support from the limited ability of older adults to make social connections and the loss of friends and family (Grossman et al., 2000). Older lesbians face these same losses and may experience increased stress and conflict in addressing the losses due to their reliance on their consciously constructed social support networks (Richard & Brown, 2006). They are more likely to confront a tragic outcome: losing their family of choice due to various losses from aging at a time when it is exceptionally critical for social and personal well-being and health.

Social networks consist of social support from agencies (public and private), communities (local and regional), and individuals (Skemp Kelley, 2005). However, lesbians over 60 avoid securing support and health care

RELATIVES: Considering the people to whom you are related to by blood

1. How many relatives do you see or hear from at least once a month?
0 = none 1 = one 2 = two 3 = three or four 4 = five thru eight 5 = nine or more
2. How often do you see or hear from the relative with whom you have the most contact?
0 = less than monthly 1 = monthly 2 = few times a month 3 = weekly 4 = few times a week 5 = daily
3. How many relatives do you feel at ease with that you can talk about private matters?
0 = none 1 = one 2 = two 3 = three or four 4 = five thru eight 5 = nine or more
4. How many relatives do you feel close to such that you could call on them for help?
0 = none 1 = one 2 = two 3 = threeor four 4 = five thru eight 5 = nine or more
5. When one of your relatives has an important decision to make, how often do they talk to you about it?
0 = never 1 = seldom 2 = sometimes 3 = often 4 = very often 5 = always
6. How often is one of your relatives available for you to talk to when you have an important
decision to make? 0 = never 1 = seldom 2 = sometimes 3 = often 4 = very often 5 = always

FAMILY OF CHOICE: Considering the people to whom you are not related to by blood but you identify as
family

1. How many members of your family of choice do you see or hear from at least once a month?
0 = none 1 = one 2 = two 3 = three or four 4 = five thru eight 5 = nine or more
2. How often do you see or hear from the family of choice member with whom you have the most contact?
0 = less than monthly 1 = monthly 2 = few times a month 3 = weekly 4 = few times a week 5 =daily
3. How many members of your family of choice do you feel at ease with that you can talk about private
matters?   0 = none 1 = one 2 = two 3 = three or four 4 = five thru eight 5 = nine or more
4. How many members of your family of choice do you feel close to such that you could call on them for help?
0 = none 1= one 2 = two 3 = three or four 4 = five thru eight 5 = nine or more
5. When one of your family of choice members has an important decision to make, how often do they talk to
you about it? 0 = never 1 = seldom 2 = sometimes 3 = often 4 = very often 5 = always
6. How often is one of your family of choice members available for you to talk to when you have an important
decision to make? 0 = never 1 = seldom 2 = sometimes 3 = often 4 = very often 5 = always

FRIENDS: Considering individuals not identified as family of choice who both live in and outside
of your neighborhood

1. How many friends do you see or hear from at least once a month?
0 = none 1 = one 2 = two 3 = three or four 4 = five thru eight 5 = nine or more
2. How often do you see or hear from the friend with whom you have the most contact?
0 = less than monthly 1 = monthly 2 = few times a month 3 = weekly 4 = few times a week 5 = daily
3. How many friends do you feel at ease with that you can talk about private matters?
0 = none 1 = one 2 = two 3 = three or four 4 = five thru eight 5 = nine or more
4. How many friends do you feel close to such that you could call on them for help?
0 = none 1= one 2 = two 3 = three or four 4 = five thru eight 5 = nine or more
5. When one of your friends has an important decision to make, how often do they talk to you about it?
0 = never 1 = seldom 2 = sometimes 3 = often 4 = very often 5 = always
6. How often is one of your friends available for you to talk to when you have an important decision to make?
0 = never 1 = seldom 2 = sometimes 3 = often 4 = very often 5 = always

FIGURE 1 Modified Lubben Social Network Scale, Revised (Modified LSNS-R).

from agencies that provide conventional services because of reinforced mistrust and fear of discrimination (Goldberg, Sickler, & Dibble, 2005). Previous experiences of provider discrimination and insensitivity strengthen the propensity for care avoidance, causing a disconnection between older lesbians and potential providers of formal support services (Brotman, Ryan, & Cromier, 2003; Gabrielson, 2011a; Richard & Brown, 2006).

This care avoidance only compounds lesbians' distinct health risks. Compared to their heterosexual counterparts, older lesbians have higher rates of obesity (Cochran et al, 2001; Yancey, Cochran, Corliss, & Mays, 2003) and smoking and alcohol abuse (Burgard, Cochran, & Mays, 2005; Cochran, Keenan, Schober, & Mays, 2000; Diamant et al., 2000; Hughes & Eliason, 2002; Hughes, Wilsnack, & Richman, 2001; McCabe, Wilsnack, Bostwick, West, & Boyd, 2009). Older lesbians with nonintact informal social networks may experience greater disparities in support and health than those with intact informal networks.

Given what is known about the impact of social support on older adult well-being and health, establishing reliable tools for measuring social support and health for the lesbian population is necessary to gain a better understanding of their needs and prevent health disparities among them. It is essential to describe the impact of family of choice on social support among older lesbians to accurately measure their level of social support. Accurate assessment of social support aids in the development of interventions that strengthen social networks among older adults and are specifically tailored for diverse groups among them (Blozik et al., 2009). In this study, we tested a modified LSNS-R, including a family of choice category to determine if that modification makes a difference in accurately capturing perceived social support among older lesbians.

METHODS

Our sample was comprised of 36 lesbians age 55 and older, obtained by a snowball approach that resulted in an all-White sample. Recruitment was initiated by sending an invitation letter (including a link to the survey) to the primary investigator's professional contacts (e.g., staff, faculty, and researchers at universities across the United States). These professional contacts either met the inclusion criteria or were highly likely to have access to others meeting the criteria for participation. They were asked (a) to consider participation in the study and (b) to forward the letter and link to other individuals they knew who met the inclusion criteria.

The study was reviewed and approved by the primary investigator's university institutional review board. Complete anonymity of participation was assured. No personal information was collected. The web-based survey began with information about the study, which included the rights, risks, and benefits of participation. Participants had the choice to click either the link to not complete the survey or the link to complete it. Informed consent was conveyed by participants clicking the link to complete the study.

Instruments

Social support was measured with a modified LSNS-R. The original LSNS-R is an instrument used to identify social isolation in older adults by measuring perceived social support received by relatives and friends (see Figure 1). The modification was the inclusion of the *family of choice* category. The modified LSNS-R had a Cronbach α of .83 with a significant intraclass correlation coefficient of .83 (.73, .91). $F(30,510) = 5.86$, $p = .00$. In addition, the survey included qualitative questions to provide context to the family of choice responses.

The LSNS-R is a short instrument that usually takes only a few minutes to complete. The scale measures size, closeness, and frequency of contacts of a respondent's social network (Lubben & Gironda, 2003b). In a preliminary study by the investigators (in which the instrument was tested in its original form with lesbians 55 and older), the LSNS-R had an internal consistency of .74 (Gabrielson, Holston, & Dyck, in press). Previous internal consistency scores have been higher when the LSNS-R has been used in studies of other diverse groups of elders, ranging from .78 to .90 (Lubben & Gironda, 2003b; Wells, 2010) Over multiple studies, scores have demonstrated correlations with a variety of health indicators (Lubben & Gironda, 2003a).

LSNS-R items range from 0 (indicating responses of *never* or *none*) to 5 (indicating responses of *always* or *nine or more*). In the original 12-item LSNS-R, total score is calculated by summing each of the equally weighted items in "Relatives" and "Friends" subscales. In the modified LSNS-R, the "Family of Choice" subscale included six equally weighted items with the other two subscales. We obtained total scores by summing each of the equally weighted items in the three subscales. Total scores ranged from 0 to -90; subscale scores ranged from 0 to 30. The higher the score in a particular subscale, the higher the perceived level of social support obtained from that group. The higher the total score, the higher the level of overall perceived social support.

Demographic data were collected including age, type of housing (rent or own), employment (employed, retired, unemployed, disabled), education (level of education completed), partnered status (single, married, partnered), years in a relationship or years partnered, and income. All data were collected through a web-based survey.

Data Management

The modified LSNS-R was web based and delivered through Select Survey, a system administered through the primary investigator's home institution. This online system utilizes SSL, 128-bit encryption, and firewalls and also downloads directly into SPSS. By using Select Survey, participant responses were protected and only visible to the investigators. Following completion of the survey, the participants were directed to a debriefing page explaining the study and the primary investigator's contact information for more information or to report problems. Data files were stored electronically and are being stored indefinitely for potential secondary analysis purposes in the future.

Quantitative Data Analysis

Data were analyzed with SPSS 18.0 (Windows). Data was both continuous (age, total social support, total relative support, total friend support, and total family of choice support) and categorical (partnered status, years partnered, housing, income, number of children, employment, and education). Categories for partnered status, employment, and housing were dichotomized; total social support and its components were categorized into low support, moderate support, and high support. Descriptive analyses were used to characterize the entire sample and again when the sample was categorized into 2 groups using the variable number of children (Group 1: 0 children, $n = 15$; Group 2: 1 or more children, $n = 18$). Through dividing the sample by the variable number of children, it was possible to begin to describe correlations of having children or being childless on social support of older lesbians as measured by the modified LSNS-R. The entire sample did not have normal distribution; therefore, cross-tabulation and nonparametric statistical methods were used to analyze the data. Spearman Rho was used to determine the associations among the variables given the nonnormal distribution and sample size (Kowalski, 1972). Chi-square was computed to analyze the association of the categorical data. Mann-Whitney U was computed to determine if total social support, relative support, friend support, and family of choice support significantly differed across the 2 groups (Group 1: 0 children; Group 2: 1 or more children). Exploratory factor analysis was conducted to determine how the modified items would load given the responses of the participants. All statistics had to reach a .05 level of significance. For this observational, pilot study, a power of .66 with a moderate effect size of .39 was reached (G*Power 3.0.5 Software).

RESULTS

Descriptives—Entire Sample

The entire sample ($n = 36$) had a response rate of 94–100% for the demographics (see Table 1). Among our sample, 53% were partnered for at least 10 years ($n = 18$) with 47% less than 10 years ($n = 16$). They were young old (mean age = 62.17 ± 4.28) with 56% having at least 1 child ($n = 19$) and 44% childless ($n = 15$), 64% employed ($n = 23$), and 86% home owners ($n = 31$). In the sample, 91% had a 4-year college education ($n = 32$), with 60% having an income of at least $70K/year ($n = 21$). In regards to social support, 63% ($n = 22$) had at least moderately high total social support (48.83 ± 13.4; median = 51; range = 4–77), which was supported by moderately low relative support (REL; mean = 13.77 ± 6.8; median = 17; range = 0–28), moderate friend support (FRI; 17.18 ± 4.2; median = 17; range = 9–28), and moderate family of choice support (FOC; mean = 18.32 ± 5.8; median = 19.5; range = 0–28).

TABLE 1 Demographic Characteristics of the Sample

	Sample	
Demographic	*n*	%
Age		
56–62	22	61%
63–72	14	39%
Partnered status		
Partnered	20	59%
Single	14	41%
Years partnered		
0 months	9	25%
<12 months	1	2.8%
1–19 years	14	41%
20 or more	10	29%
Number of children		
0 (Group 1)	15	44%
1 or more (Group 2)	19	56%
Education level		
High school	1	2%
1–4 years college	6	17%
>4 years college	28	80%
Employment		
Employed	23	64%
Retired	11	31%
Unemployed	2	5%
Income		
$10,000–$29,999	1	3%
$30,000–$49,999	1	3%
$50,000–$69,999	12	34%
$70,000–$89,999	3	9%
$90,000–$109,999	5	14%
$110,000–$129,999	1	3%
$130,000–$149,999	4	11%
$150,000 or more	8	23%
Housing		
Own	31	86%
Rent	4	11%
Senior housing	1	3%

Descriptives—Two Groups

The sample was split into 2 groups using the variable *Number of children* (Group 1 = 0 children; Group 2 = 1 or more children) to see if the categorical data differed (see Table 2). Group 1 (*n* = 15) were aged pre-young old (mean age = 61.6 ± 4.1), with 57% partnered (*n* = 8), 57% in a relationship for at least 10 years (*n* = 8), 73% employed (*n* = 11), and 93% home owners (*n* = 14). Group 2 (*n* = 18) were aged pre-young old (mean age = 62.79 ± 4.4), with 47% partnered (*n* = 9), 55.6% in a relationship for at least 10 years (*n* = 10), 58% employed (*n* = 11), and 79% home owners (*n* = 15). For Group 1, 93% had a 4-year college education (*n* = 14), and 53% had an income

TABLE 2 Demographic Characteristics of the Two Groups

Demographic	Group 1 (0 Children)		Group 2 (1 or More Children)	
	n	%	*n*	%
Age				
56–62	10	67%	11	58%
63–72	5	33%	8	42%
Partnered status				
Partnered	8	57%	12	67%
Single	6	43%	6	33%
Years partnered				
0 months	3	21.5%	4	22%
< 12 months	0		1	6%
1–19 years	8	57%	6	33%
20 or more	3	21.5%	7	39%
Education level				
High school	0		1	6%
1–4 years college	4	27%	2	12%
> 4 years college	11	73%	15	82%
Employment				
Employed	11	73%	11	58%
Retired	4	27%	6	32%
Unemployed	0		2	10%
Income				
$10,000–$29,999	0		1	6%
$30,000–$49,999	0		1	6%
$50,000–$69,999	7	48%	3	17%
$70,000–$89,999	0		3	17%
$90,000–$109,999	1	6%	4	22%
$110,000–$129,999	0		1	6%
$130,000–$149,999	2	13%	2	10%
$150,000 or more	5	33%	3	17%
Housing				
Own	14	93%	15	79%
Rent	1	7%	3	16%
Senior housing	0		1	5%

of at least $90K/year ($n = 8$). Sixty percent ($n = 9$) had at least moderate total social support (mean $= 48.53 \pm 13.2$; median $= 50$; range $= 20$–77), evident by means for REL (13.53 ± 7.8; median $= 17$, range $= 0$–24), FRI (16.67 ± 5.5; median $= 16$, range $= 9$–28), and FOC (17 ± 6.6; median $= 18$, range $= 0$–25). Within Group 2, 89% had a 4-year college education ($n = 16$), and 55% had an income of at least $90K/year ($n = 10$). Fifty-six percent ($n = 10$) had at least moderate total social support (mean $= 51.33 \pm 3.3$; median $= 53$; range $= 36$–72), evident by means for REL (14.28 ± 6.0; median $= 14$; range $= 5$–28), FRI (17.67 ± 3.0; median $= 18$; range $= 11$–22), and FOC (19.39 ± 5.2; median $= 20$; range $= 10$–28). From the demographics, Group 2 had a smaller portion partnered, employed, and home owners when compared to Group 1.

Statistical Analysis

Cross-tabulation was used to analyze the association of the categorical variables across Group 1 (0 children) and Group 2 (1 or more children). There were no significant differences between the 2 groups (see Table 2).

Using Spearman Rho, there were significant correlations with p-values that ranged from .05 to .00 (see Table 3). For the entire sample, age inversely correlated with FRI item 3 (number of friends you converse with privately; $r = -.40$, $p = .02$) and FRI item 4 (number of close friends you call for help; $r = -.35$, $p = .05$). FRI item 2 (contact with friends frequently) inversely

TABLE 3 Significant Correlations ($n = 34$)

Variable$_1$	Variable$_2$	r	p	Variable1	Variable2	r	p
Age	FRI item 3	−.40	.02	REL item 6	FOC item 6	.42	.02
	FRI item 4	−.35	.05	FRI item 1	FRI item 3	.63	.00
Partner status	Years partnered	.76	.00		FRI item 4	.60	.00
Years partnered	FOC item 1	.39	.03		FOC item 3	.40	.02
Education	Employment	.44	.01		FOC item 4	.37	.04
	Housing	.47	.01	FRI item 2	FRI item 3	.36	.04
Employment	FRI item 2	−.43	.01		FRI item 4	.39	.02
Income	FRI item 2	.37	.04		FRI item 5	.48	.01
Housing	Education	.47	.01		FRI item 6	.40	.02
	FOC item 1	.39	.02	FRI item 3	FRI item 4	.80	.00
REL item 1	REL item 2	.45	.01		FRI item 5	.39	.03
	REL item 3	.50	.00	FRI item 4	FRI item 5	.46	.01
	REL item 4	.44	.01	FRI item 5	FRI item 6	.69	.00
	REL item 5	.48	.00		FOC item 2	.40	.02
	REL item 6	.70	.00		FOC item 5	.65	.00
REL item 2	REL item 4	.47	.01		FOC item 6	.48	.01
	REL item 5	.60	.00	FRI item 6	FOC item 5	.43	.01
	REL item 6	.48	.01		FOC item 6	.66	.00
REL item 3	REL item 4	.65	.00	FOC item 1	FOC item 3	.71	.00
	REL item 5	.39	.02		FOC item 4	.67	.00
	REL item 6	.45	.01	FOC item 2	FOC item 5	.58	.00
	FRI item 3	.34	.05		FOC item 6	.38	.03
REL item 4	REL item 5	.51	.00	FOC item 3	FOC item 4	.87	.00
	REL item 6	.46	.01		FOC item 6	.40	.02
REL item 5	REL item 6	.73	.00	FOC item 4	FOC item 5	.52	.00
	FRI item 2	.38	.03		FOC item 6	.57	.00
REL item 6	FRI item 6	.49	.00	FOC item 5	FOC item 6	.71	.00

Note. REL item 1 = number of relatives you see each month. REL item 2 = contact with relatives frequently. REL item 3 = number of relatives you converse with privately. REL item 4 = number of close relatives you call for help. REL item 5 = you often help relative with problem. REL item 6 = relative often helps you with problem. FRI item 1 = number of relatives you see each month. FRI item 2 = contact with friends frequently. FRI item 3 = number of friends you converse with privately. FRI item 4 = number of close friends you call for help. FRI item 5 = you often help friend with problem. FRI item 6 = friend often helps you with problem. FOC item 1 = number of family of choice members you see each month. FOC item 2 = contact with family of choice members frequently. FOC item 3 = number of family of choice members you converse with privately. FOC item 4 = number of close family of choice members you call for help. FOC item 5 = you often help family of choice member with problem. FOC item 6 = family of choice member often helps you with problem.

correlated with employed ($r = -.43$, $p = .01$) and positively correlated with income ($r = .37$, $p = .04$). FOC item 1 (number of family of choice you see each month) correlated with number of children ($r = .38$, $p = .03$) and housing ($r = .39$, $p = .02$). Certain items in FOC correlate with items in FRI. The significant correlations were between FOC item 2 (contact with family of choice members frequently) with FRI item 5 (you often help friend with problem; $r = .40$, $p = .02$), FRI item 1 (number of friends you see each month) with FOC item 3 (number of family of choice members you converse with privately; $r = .40$, $p = .02$) and FOC item 4 (number of close family of choice members you call for help; $r = .37$, $p = .04$), FOC item 5 (you often help family of choice members with problem) with FRI item 5 (you often help friend with problem; $r = .65$, $p = .00$) and FRI item 6 (friend often help you with problem; $r = .43$, $p = .01$), and FOC item 6 (family of choice members often help you with problem) with FRI item 5 (you often help friend with problem; $r = .48$, $p = .01$) and FRI item 6 (friend often help you with problem; $r = .66$, $p = .00$). Interestingly, certain items in FRI significantly correlated with those in REL. Those correlations were between FRI item 2 (contact with friend frequently) with REL item 5 (you often help relative with problem; $r = .38$, $p = .03$), FRI item 3 (number of friends you converse with privately) with REL item 3 (number of relatives you converse with privately; $r = .34$, $p = .05$), and FRI item 6 (friend often help you with problem)] with REL item 1 (number of relatives you see each month; $r = .38$, $p = .03$) and REL item 6 (relative often help you with problem; $r = .49$, $p = .00$). The items in the categories of the modified LSNS-R also correlated in each of the 2 groups (see Table 4).

Demographics for Group 1 (0 children) correlated with items in the modified LSNS-R. Age inversely correlated with FRI item 3 (number of friends you converse with privately; $r = -.56$, $p = .03$). Years partnered correlated with FOC total ($r = .68$, $p = .01$), FOC item 1 (number of family of choice members you see each month; $r = .65$, $p = .01$), FOC item 3 (number of family of choice members you converse with privately; $r = .58$, $p = .04$), and FOC item 4 (number of close family of choice members you call for help; $r = .56$, $p = .05$). Education correlated with FRI item 5 (you often help friend with problem; $r = .58$, $p = .02$) and FOC item 2 (contact with family of choice members frequently; $r = .69$, $p = .01$). Income correlated with FRI item 5 (you often help friend with problem; $r = .55$, $p = .01$).

In Group 2 (1 or more children), only one demographic correlated with one item in the modified LSNS-R. Years partnered inversely correlated with FRI total ($r = -.64$, $p = .01$).

Mann-Whitney U (MWU) test was used to determine if Group 1 (0 children) and Group 2 (1 or more children) were statistically different across the variables, especially total social support, total REL, total FRI, and total FOC. There was no statistical difference between the two groups across the variables, especially in FRI (MWU statistics $= 100.00$, $p = .22$), REL (MWU statistics $= 134.00$, $p = .99$), FOC (MWU statistics $= 107.00$, $p = .33$), and

TABLE 4 Significant Correlations by Groups

Group 1: 0 Children (n = 15)				Group 2: 1 or More Children (n = 18)			
Variable₁	Variable₂	r	p	Variable1	Variable2	r	p
Age	FRI item 3	−.56	.03	Age	Education	.51	.03
Partner status	Yrs. partnered	.61	.02	Partner status	Yrs. partnered	.52	.03
Years partnered	FOC total	.68	.01	Years partnered	FRI total	−.64	.01
	FOC item 1	.65	.01	Education	Income	.58	.01
	FOC item 3	.58	.04		Housing	.52	.03
	FOC item 4	.56	.05	REL item 1	REL item 3	.48	.05
Education	Housing	.56	.03		REL item 6	.67	.00
	FRI item 5	.58	.02	REL item 2	REL item 5	.49	.04
	FOC item 2	.69	.01		FOC item 1	−.48	.05
Income	FRI item 5	.55	.04	REL item 5	REL item 6	.58	.01
REL item 1	FRI item 6	.65	.01		FRI item 4	.55	.02
REL item 2	REL item 3	.52	.05		FOC item 1	−.50	.03
	REL item 4	.65	.01		FOC item 3	−.57	.01
	REL item 5	.68	.01	REL item 6	FRI item 4	.56	.02
	REL item 6	.57	.03		FOC item 6	.49	.05
REL item 3	REL item 4	.85	.00		FOC item 6	.69	.00
	REL item 5	.67	.01	FOC item 1	FOC item 3	.60	.01
	REL item 6	.74	.00		FOC item 4	.59	.01
REL item 4	REL item 5	.83	.00	FOC item 2	FOC item 5	−.65	.00
	REL item 6	.81	.00	FOC item 3	FOC item 4	.88	.00
REL item 5	REL item 6	.93	.00	FOC item 4	FOC item 5	.52	.03
	FRI item 6	.57	.03		FOC item 6	.65	.00
REL item 6	FRI item 6	.61	.02	FOC item 5	FOC item 6	.61	.01
FRI item 1	FRI item 3	.79	.00				
	FRI item 4	.81	.00				
	FOC item 3	.62	.02				
	FOC item 4	.63	.02				
FRI item 2	FRI item 4	.57	.03				
FRI item 3	FRI item 4	.87	.00				
	FOC item 3	.66	.01				
	FOC item 4	.62	.01				
FRI item 4	FOC item 3	.65	.01				
	FOC item 4	.70	.01				
FRI item 5	FRI item 6	.83	.00				
	FOC item 5	.60	.02				
FRI item 6	FOC item 6	.57	.03				
FOC item 1	FOC item 3	.71	.01				
	FOC item 4	.71	.01				
	FOC item 5	.82	.00				
	FOC item 6	.59	.03				
FOC item 3	FOC item 4	.78	.00				
FOC item 5	FOC item 6	.76	.00				

Note. REL item 1 = number of relatives you see each month. REL item 2 = contact with relatives frequently. REL item 3 = number of relatives you converse with privately. REL item 4 = number of close relatives you call for help. REL item 5 = you often help relative with problem. REL item 6 = relative often helps you with problem. FRI item 1 = number of relatives you see each month. FRI item 2 = contact with friends frequently. FRI item 3 = number of friends you converse with privately. FRI item 4 = number of close friends you call for help. FRI item 5 = you often help friend with problem. FRI item 6 = friend often helps you with problem. FOC item 1 = number of family of choice members you see each month. FOC item 2 = contact with family of choice members frequently. FOC item 3 = number of family of choice members you converse with privately. FOC item 4 = number of close family of choice members you call for help. FOC item 5 = you often help family of choice member with problem. FOC item 6 = family of choice member often helps you with problem.

TABLE 5 Modified LSNS-R Exploratory Factor Analysis Loading

	Factor 1	Factor 2	Factor 3	Factor 4	Factor 5
REL item 1	.695				
REL item 2	.743				
REL item 3	.710				
REL item 4	.804				
REL item 5	.795				
REL item 6	.726				
FRI item 1			.774		
FRI item 2			.543		
FRI item 3			.882		
FRI item 4			.888		
FRI item 5				.667	
FRI item 6				.920	
FOC item 1		.840			
FOC item 2					.927
FOC item 3		.897			
FOC item 4		.875			
FOC item 5					.691
FOC item 6				.694	

Note. Relative support (Factor 1; modified LSNS-R REL items 1–6), Trust in family of choice support (Factor 2; modified LSNS-R FOC items 1, 3, and 4), Trust in friend support (Factor 3; modified LSNS-R FRI items 1–4), Familiar friend's trust in reciprocity (Factor 4; modified LSNS-R FRI items 5 and 6 and FOC item 6), and Reciprocity in family of choice support (Factor 5; modified LSNS-R FOC items 2 and 5). REL item 1 = number of relatives you see each month. REL item 2 = contact with relatives frequently. REL item 3 = number of relatives you converse with privately. REL item 4 = number of close relatives you call for help. REL item 5 = you often help relative with problem. REL item 6 = relative often helps you with problem. FRI item 1 = number of relatives you see each month. FRI item 2 = contact with friends frequently. FRI item 3 = number of friends you converse with privately. FRI item 4 = number of close friends you call for help. FRI item 5 = you often help friend with problem. FRI item 6 = friend often helps you with problem. FOC item 1 = number of family of choice members you see each month. FOC item 2 = contact with family of choice members frequently. FOC item 3 = number of family of choice members you converse with privately. FOC item 4 = number of close family of choice members you call for help. FOC item 5 = you often help family of choice member with problem. FOC item 6 = family of choice member often helps you with problem.

total social support (MWU statistics = 104.00, $p = .27$). These findings for the social support suggest that the two groups do not statistically differ in total social support, total REL, total FRI, or total FOC.

Exploratory factor analysis (EFA) was used to determine how the participants' responses to the modified LSNS-R would load for the entire sample (see Table 5), especially with the high number of correlations reported earlier (see Tables 3 and 4). Five constructs were identified as follows: Relative Support (Factor 1; modified LSNS-R REL items 1–6), Trust in Family of Choice Support (Factor 2; modified LSNS-R FOC items 1, 3, and 4), Trust in Friend Support (Factor 3; modified LSNS-R FRI items 1–4), Familiar Friend's Trust in Reciprocity (Factor 4; modified LSNS-R FRI items 5 and 6 and FOC item 6), and Reciprocity in Family of Choice Support (Factor 5; modified LSNS-R FOC items 2 and 5). These five factors explained 79% of the total variance with eigenvalues greater than 1.00.

All REL items load on Factor 1, suggesting that they are measuring one construct, relative support. Three FOC items (items 1, 3, and 4) are loading on Factor 2. Four FRI items load on Factor 3, with the remaining two loading on Factor 4 with FOC item 6. FOC items 2 and 5 load on Factor 5. These results are suggesting that FRI items predominantly measure one construct, trust in friend support. Yet, FRI last two items are measuring the same construct as FOC last item, suggesting identified reciprocity in friend support overlapping with perceptions of trust in family of choice support. The remaining FOC items measure reciprocity in family of choice support. We did not run separate factor analyses for the two different groups because the sample size for each group would be too small to determine appropriate loading.

The results from the EFA suggest that for this sample, the modified LSNS-R might be identifying a type of support (FOC) that still overlaps in some ways with the FRI category but clearly differs from that of REL. In addition, this submerged support may help to understand how children contribute to the perception of social support by older lesbians. Further reliability testing of the instrument is needed with a large and diverse sample. Further modification of the items in the modified LSNS-R may be warranted if we do not see an anticipated definitive and clean three factor total (REL, FOC, and FRI) with a large and diverse sample.

Qualitative Data Analysis

Responses to the qualitative questions provide context for the findings from the quantitative and exploratory factor analyses. Four questions were asked at the end of the modified survey to supplement responses for the new family of choice (FOC) category. The number of respondents for each question is as follows:

1. Please describe here some of the relationships you have with the people you considered to be your family of choice (30 respondents/36 participants).
2. What is it about these relationships that cause you to consider these individuals your family of choice? (29 respondents/36 participants).
3. In completing the survey, how would you identify these individuals if you did not have the option of a family of choice category? What additional thoughts or comments do you have regarding that? (29 respondents/ 36 participants).
4. What additional thoughts or information would you like to add? (15 respondents/36 participants).

The analysis of the data occurred in many cycles according to the within- and across-case strategies described by Ayres, Kavanaugh, and Knafl (2003), beginning first with a process of total immersion in the data by reading each individual's responses to all four questions multiple times and then through reducing the data repeatedly to identify the overall themes of the qualitative response across each of the questions. What emerged from analysis of these data was a better contextual understanding of the nature of the relationships the respondents have with their family of choice. Family-of-choice relationships are ones that (a) replace relatives roles; (b) are characterized by longevity, safety and intimacy, and commonality; and (c) in which there is complete trust in, as well as reciprocity of, support.

Replace relatives roles. Across cases, respondents identified that family-of-choice relationships replace traditional family roles. In fact, some examples reflecting this identification include those who described these individuals as being like "sisters," a "sibling," or "son," and those who actually used terms for these roles such as "mama," "aunty," "brothers," and "sisters."

Longevity. Across cases, respondents characterized family of choice relationships as ones typified by longevity, stating that these were relationships of 25–30 years or more in some cases. They explained that family-of-choice relationships were ones with "shared history" and that were "long standing" and "time tested."

Safety and intimacy. Across cases, respondent's characterized family-of-choice relationships as ones comprised of intimacy and feelings of safety. Individuals explained that "family of choice" members "accept me as I am" and are individuals that are "nonjudgmental" and "support me no matter what." They described the relationships as ones with "a deep sense of belonging and safety" in which "anything is fair game to discuss" and even stated that "with them, I am at home."

Commonality. Across cases, respondents characterized family-of-choice relationships as ones with commonality. They stated that "family of choice" members had "common values" and "common passions" and that with them they had "shared experiences."

Trust in support, reciprocity of support. Respondents across cases identified that family-of-choice relationships were supportive and ones in which there was complete trust in that support, as well as reciprocity in the delivery of support. Relationships with "family of choice" are ones characterized by "trust" and "mutual trust." Some respondents described their complete trust in the support of family of choice with statements such as:

"They are always there for me, any time."
"They support me no matter what."

These are relationships with "complete trust" as well as "mutual trust." Some respondents described not only their trust in the support of family of choice, but also the reciprocity factor with the following statements:

"They are always available to talk with and also talk with me about decisions."

"I love and care about them, they love and care about me."

"We are there for them as well as them being there for us."

"I love and trust them and they feel the same."

"I can count on them to be there if I need them and they know I would do the same."

Respondents made many key statements that can provide some context and rationale for the significance of the family of choice and why they may replace biological family roles. One respondent explained that "I prefer their company [family of choice] more than that of my genetic (blood) family." Another individual said that, "In some ways I am closer to my family of choice than to my biological family" and another stated that describing them as friends "wouldn't begin to describe the depth of the relationships I have with my family of choice. They are not 'friends' they are my family." Further, one respondent explained her perceptions about the phenomenon with the following statement:

> The family of choice works the way a biological family OUGHT to work, but often doesn't. My biological family loves me, and I them, but they don't get what my life is about, and I have to spend a lot of energy keeping myself safe around them. My family of choice is—MY CHOICE.

Another individual may identify the crux of the phenomenon by stating, "I have friends who have had the hard experience of learning that members of their natural family weren't comfortable enough to accept their life situation and be there when needed." Finally, one participant conveyed all of the salient themes by stating,

> I have known some of these women for 30 years and they are time-tested and trusted friends. Some "hold my history," i.e., they know my secrets and my fears and my growth over the years. There is a deep sense of belonging and safety. With them I am home.

DISCUSSION

This is the first study to characterize perceived social support of older lesbians beyond the traditional categories of social support using a modified version of the LSNS-R. Results from this pilot study demonstrate that the addition of the *family of choice* category increased the accurate measurement of perceived social support by older lesbians with the modified LSNS-R. There was no overlapping of relative and friend support, as noted in a preliminary study using the original LSNS-R. With qualitative analysis, the relationships associated with *family of choice* were identified: (a) replace family roles; (b) characterized by longevity, safety and intimacy, and commonality; and (c) ones with complete trust in support, as well as reciprocity of support. Although family-of-choice support has a mean difference from relative and friend support, the family-of-choice support has elements of friend support. Family of choice may still be submerged, to some degree, in friend support with the modified LSNS-R and is submerged in both friend and relative support with the original LSNS-R. Perhaps this submergence of family of choice contributes to the lack of statistical difference between the total REL and the total FRI across the two groups. Nevertheless, the three categories of social support were not statistically different when using modified LSNS-R.

The results are supported by other studies that have reported older lesbians having broader definitions of family than just biological (Jones & Nystrom, 2002). Their families of choice are typically social support systems of friends that they have developed over the life course to support their physical, emotional, and spiritual health. They identify these support systems as essential to their well-being (Aronson, 1998; Comerford et al., 2004; Gabrielson, 2011a; Grossman et al., 2000; Masini & Barret, 2008; Weinstock, 2000). The essential nature of the family of choice was supported by our qualitative results.

Yet changes occurring as a result of the aging process (reduced mobility, losses of friends) may cause them to find this support system more difficult to keep intact at a time when it is most critical. In this study, the correlations may suggest that childless older lesbians may use support from the family of choice more than older lesbians with children.

There is, therefore, a need for targeted health and support services for this population, yet older lesbians typically avoid formal services for fears of culturally incompetent and discriminatory care (Brotman et al., 2003; Gabrielson, 2011b; Goldberg et al., 2005; Richard & Brown, 2006). It is critical that investigators work to increase providers' knowledge about older lesbians so they can provide welcoming and culturally competent and targeted care that older lesbians will access. This requires the establishment of a solid evidence base about health and social support among older lesbians.

The unfortunate reality is that lesbian elders remain one of the most invisible groups of Americans. People know little about their unique health and support needs because they have neglected to focus on them in research, and sexual orientation continues to not be identified in most aging studies (Cahill et al., 2000). Preventing older lesbian health disparities requires increasing the understanding of them through research. Healthy People 2020 recognized health disparities among the LGBT population and included a specific objective to "improve the health, safety, and well-being of lesbian, gay, bisexual, and transgender (LGBT) individuals." Healthy People

2020 calls on researchers to increase the study of health and well-being among LGBT seniors over the coming decade (US Dept. of Health & Human Services, 2010). This study contributes to moving that agenda forward.

Further reliability testing of the modified instrument is needed and further modification of its items may be warranted. The main limitations of our study were the small sample size and snowball sampling strategy, which resulted in a homogenous sample in terms of race, education, and income. Specifically, it resulted in an all-White, mostly well-educated, and middle- to upper-income sample. Further investigation using the modified instrument with a large and diverse sample is needed and is the next step in our research agenda to address health and social support disparities among the older lesbian population.

REFERENCES

Aronson, J. (1998). Lesbians giving and receiving care: Stretching conceptualizations of caring and community. *Women's Studies International Forum, 21*, 505–519.

Ayres, L., Kavanaugh, K., & Knafl, K. (2003). Within-case and across-case approaches to data analysis. *Qualitative Health Research, 13*, 871–883.

Berkman, L., & Glass, T. (2000). Social integration, social networks, social support, and health. In L. F. Berkman & I. Kawachi (Eds.), *Social epidemiology* (pp. 137–173). New York, NY: Oxford University Press.

Blane, D. (2006). The life course, the social gradient and health. In M. Marmot & R. G. Wilkinson (Eds.), *The social determinants of health* (2nd ed., pp. 54–77). New York, NY: Oxford University Press.

Blozik, E., Wagner, J. T., Gillmann, G., Iliffe, S., von Renteln-Kruse, W., Lubben, J., . . . Clough-Gorr, K. M. (2009). Social network assessment in community-dwelling older persons: Results from a study of three European populations. *Aging Clinical and Experimental Research, 21*, 150–157.

Brotman, S., Ryan, B., & Cormier, R. (2003). The health and social service needs of gay and lesbian elders and their families in Canada. *Gerontologist, 43*, 192–202.

Burgard, S., Cochran, S., & Mays, V. (2005). Alcohol and tobacco use patterns among heterosexually and homosexually experienced California women. *Drug & Alcohol Dependence, 77*, 61–70.

Cahill, S., South, K., & Spade, J. (2000). *Outing age: Public policy issues affecting gay, lesbian, bisexual and transgender elders*. New York, NY: National Gay and Lesbian Task Force Policy Institute.

Ceria, C. D., Masaki, K. H., Rodriguez, B. L., Chen, R., Yano, K., & Curb, J. D. (2001). The relationship of psychosocial factors to total mortality among older Japanese-American men: The Honolulu Heart Program. *Journal of the American Geriatrics Society, 49*, 725–731.

Cochran, S., Keenan, C., Schober, C., & Mays, V. (2000). Estimates of alcohol use and clinical treatment needs among homosexually active men and women in the U.S. population. *Journal of Consulting and Clinical Psychology, 6*, 1062–1071.

Cochran, S. D., Mays, V. M., Bowen, D., Gage, S., Bybee, D., Roberts, S. J., . . . White, J. (2001). Cancer-related risk indicators and preventive screening behaviors among lesbians and bisexual women. *American Journal of Public Health, 91*, 591–597.

Comerford, S., Henson-Stroud, M., Sionainn, C. & Wheeler, E. (2004). Crone songs: Voices of lesbian elders on aging in a rural environment. *Affilia: Journal of Women & Social Work, 19*, 418–436.

Cornwell, E., & Waite, L. (2009).Social disconnectedness, perceived isolation, and health among older adults. *Journal of Health and Social Behavior, 50*(1), 31–48.

Diamant, A. Wold, C., Spritzer, K., & Gelberg, L. (2000). Health behaviors, health status, and access to and use of health care: a population-based study of lesbian, bisexual, and heterosexual women, *Archives of Family Medicine, 9*, 1043–1051.

Dykstra, P. A. (2006). Off the beaten track: Childlessness and social integration in late life. *Research in Aging, 28*, 749–767.

Fayers, P. M., & Sprangers, M. A. G. (2002). Understanding self-rated health. *Lancet, 359*, 187–188.

Gabrielson, M. (2011a). "I will not be discriminated against": Older lesbians creating new communities. *Advances in Nursing Science, 34*, 357–373.

Gabrielson, M. (2011b). "We have to create family": Aging support issues and needs among older lesbians. *Journal of Gay and Lesbian Social Services, 23*(3), 1–13.

Gabrielson, M., Holston, E., & Dyck, M. (in press). Are they family or friends?: Social support instrument reliability in studying older lesbians. *Journal of Homosexuality.*

Gironda, M. W., Lubben, J. E., & Atchison, K. (1999). Social networks of elders without children. *Journal of Gerontological Social Work, 31*(1/2), 63–84.

Goldberg, S., Sickler, J., & Dibble, S. (2005). Lesbians over sixty: The consistency of findings from twenty years of survey data. *Journal of Lesbian Studies, 9*, 195–213.

Grossman, A. H., D'Augelli, A. R., & Hershberger, S. L. (2000). Social support networks of lesbian, gay, and bisexual adults 60 years of age and older. *Journal of Gerontology:* Psychological Sciences, *55B*, 171–179.

Heck, J., Sell, R., & Gorin, S. (2006). Health care access among individuals in same-sex relationships. *American Journal of Public Health, 96*, 1111–1118.

Hughes, T. L. & Eliason, M. J. (2002). Substance use and abuse in lesbian, gay, bisexual, and transgender populations. *Journal of Primary Prevention, 22*, 261–295.

Jones, T., & Nystrom, N. (2002). Looking back looking forward: Addressing the lives of lesbians 55 and older. *Journal of Women and Aging, 14*(3–4), 59–76.

Kehoe, M. (1989). *Lesbians over sixty speak for themselves.* New York, NY: Haworth Press.

Kowalski, C. J. (1972). On the effects of non-normality on the distribution of the sample product-moment correlation coefficient. *Journal of the Royal Statistical Society, Series C, Applied Statistics, 21*(1), 1–12.

Lubben, J., Blozik, E., Gillmann, G., Iliffe, S., von Renteln Kruse, W., Beck, J. & Stuck, A. (2006). Performance of an abbreviated version of the Lubben Social Network Scale among three European community-dwelling older adult populations. *Gerontologist, 46*, 503–513.

Lubben, J., & Gironda, M. (2003a). Centrality of social ties to the health and well-being of older adults. In B. Berkman & L. K. Harooytan (Eds.), *Social work and health care in an aging world* (pp. 319–350). New York, NY: Springer.

Lubben, J., & Gironda, M. (2003b). Measuring social networks and assessing their benefits. In C. Phillipson, G. Allan, & D. Morgan (Eds.), *Social networks and social exclusion* (pp. 20–49). Hants, England: Ashgate.

Masini, B., & Barret, H. (2008). Social support as a predictor of psychological and physical well-being and lifestyle in lesbian, gay, and bisexual adults aged 50 and over. *Journal of Gay & Lesbian Social Services, 20*(1/2), 91–110.

McCabe, S. E., Hughes, T. L., Bostwick, W. B., West, B. T., & Boyd, C. J. (2009). Sexual orientation, substance use behaviors and substance dependence in the United States. *Addiction, 104*, 1333–1345.

Mistry, R., Rosansky, J., McQuire, J., McDermott, C., & Jarvik, L. (2001). Social isolation predicts re-hospitalization in a group of older American veterans enrolled in the UPBEAT Program. *International Journal of Geriatric Psychiatry, 16*, 950–959.

National Gay and Lesbian Task Force. (2005). *Making room for all: Diversity, cultural competency and discrimination in an aging America*. Washington, DC: National Gay and Lesbian Task Force.

Orel, N. (2004). Gay, lesbian and bisexual elders: Expressed needs and concerns across focus groups. *Journal of Gerontological Social Work, 43*(2/3), 57–77.

Rankow, E. (1995). Breast and cervical cancer among lesbians. *Women's Health Issues, 5*, 123–129.

Richard, C., & Brown, A. (2006). Configurations of informal social support among older lesbians. *Journal of Women & Aging, 18*, 49–65.

Rubinstein, R., Lubben, J., & Mintzer, J. (1994). Social isolation and social support: An applied perspective. *Journal of Applied Gerontology, 13*, 58–72.

Seeman, T. (2001). How do others get under our skin? Social relationships and health. In C. D. Ryff & B. Singer (Eds.), *Emotion, social relationships, and health* (pp. 189–210). New York, NY: Oxford University Press.

Skemp Kelley, L. (2005). Minor children and adult care exchanges with community dwelling frail elders in a St. Lucian Village. *Journal of Gerontology: Social Sciences, 60B*(2), S62–S73.

United States Department of Health and Human Services. (2010). Lesbian, gay, bisexual and transgender health. In *Healthy People 2020*. Retrieved from http://www.healthypeople.gov/2020/topicsobjectives2020/overview.aspx?topicid=25

Weinstock, J. (2000). Lesbian friendships at midlife: Patterns and possibilities for the 21st century. *Journal of Gay and Lesbian Social Services, 11*(2–3), 1–32.

Wells, M. (2010). Resilience in older adults living in rural, suburban, and urban areas. *Online Journal of Rural Nursing and Health Care, 10*(2), 45–54.

Yancey, A. K., Cochran, S. D., Corliss, H. L., & Mays, V. M. (2003). Correlates of overweight and obesity among lesbian and bisexual women. *Preventative Medicine, 36*, 676–683.

GayBy Boomers' Social Support: Exploring the Connection Between Health and Emotional and Instrumental Support in Older Gay Men

JESUS RAMIREZ-VALLES and JESSICA DIRKES

School of Public Health, University of Illinois–Chicago, Chicago, Illinois, USA

HOPE A. BARRETT

Howard Brown Health Center, Chicago, Illinois, USA

We evaluate the association between emotional and instrumental support and perceived health and depression symptoms in a sample of 182 gay/bisexual men age $\geq$ 55. Perceived health was positively correlated with number of sources of emotional support and depression was negatively associated with instrumental support and health care providers' knowledge of patients' sexual orientation. Depression mediates the connection between providers' knowledge of patients' sexual orientation and perceived health. Number of sources of emotional support varied negatively with age and ethnic minority status, and positively with living with a partner. Instrumental support seemed to be dependent on living with a partner.

Social support is critical in facing the challenges of old age (White, Philogene, Fine, & Sinha, 2009). This is amplified in marginalized populations, such as gay men, who may be less socially connected (D'Augelli & Grossman, 2001; Quam & Whitford, 1992). Gay male communities, as the larger U.S society, do not value old age; thus, older gay men have limited socializing venues (Herdt, Beeler, & Rwals, 1997; Kertzner, 2001). Gay men are still often not welcome in predominantly heterosexual environments. Anecdotal data suggest that some gay men go "back to the closet" when they join assisted living facilities (Johnson, Jackson, Arnett, & Koffman, 2005, p. 96). Also, many of them (including those living with HIV/AIDS; Chesney, Chambers, Taylor, & Johnson, 2003) do not have access to traditional sources of support, such as spouses, siblings, children, and religious congregations. They are twice as likely as their heterosexual peers to live alone (Bennett, 2008b).[1] Furthermore, because the majority of older gay men do not disclose their sexual orientation to their health care providers (Funders for Lesbian and Gay Issues, 2004), these providers might not be well equipped to supply needed support and address their particular needs (Bennett, 2008a).

The current older gay male population is rapidly increasing due to the aging of what we refer to as the *gayby boomer* generation (born between 1946 and 1964; Ramirez-Valles, 2013; Rosenfeld, Bartlem, & Smith, 2012). This subcohort of gay men is different from their heterosexual baby boomer peers and the larger gay population. This was the first group of men to adopt and use the gay identity, fighting against societal stigma. This group lived through the larger sexual liberation movement. Many in this group were able to openly live with their partners or significant others and create large communities, particularly in the major US urban cities (D'Emilio, 1998). Last, this subcohort of the baby boomer generation was the hardest hit by the HIV/AIDS epidemic (Rosenfeld et al., 2012).

The purpose of this article is to explore the linkages between health and social support in older gay men. We draw on one of the premises of the stress process theory (Pearlin, Menaghan, Lieberman, & Mullan, 1981), that social support may directly, and positively, impact health regardless of the levels of stress. Social support may be expressed as emotional, instrumental, informational, and appraisal forms that may work through psychological (e.g., sense of self) and physiological (e.g., immune system) mechanisms to affect health outcomes (e.g., from onset, to management and recovery; Berkman, 1995; Cohen & Wills, 1985; House, Landis, & Umberson, 1988; Israel & Schurman, 1990). We look at two major types of support—emotional and instrumental (e.g., daily activities)—and two health outcomes—depression symptoms and perceived health. We also assess the roles of health care providers' knowledge of patients' sexual orientation and living arrangements (e.g., alone or with a partner). Furthermore, we explore how types of support are distributed across various statuses (e.g., education, race, living arrangements). Our sample comprises men of two cohorts: *gayby boomers* and the preceding silent generation (born between 1925 and 1942).

There is evidence that older gay men fare worse on health outcomes (e.g., sexual risk, mental health) and resources (e.g., social support) than

---

[1]   But see Shippy, Cantor, and Brennan (2007), who found that older gay men do have close friendships. This is based in a small sample of older gay men in New York City.

their heterosexual counterparts (de Vries & Patrick, 2006; Krehely, 2009). Gay men are at elevated risk for depression and substance and alcohol use (Lewis, 2009; Wallace, Cochran, Durazo, & Ford, 2011). In selective samples, up to one-third of older gay men report depressive symptoms (Raws, 2004; Shippy, Cantor, & Brennan, 2004), more than double the rate in the general older male population (Steffens, Fisher, Langan, Potter, & Plassman, 2009). In the National Social Life, Health, and Aging Project, a study of randomly selected noninstitutionalized older people ($N = 3,000$; 57–85 years old; Cornwell, Laumann, & Schumm, 2008; NORC, 2012), the frequency of depression symptoms among men reporting same-sex behavior was significantly higher compared the rest of the male sample (Ramirez-Valles, 2011). In a recent study of older gay, lesbian, bisexual, and transgender people (Fredriksen-Goldsen & Muraco, 2010), 41% of the sample reported lifetime suicidal ideation.

Social support has been linked to numerous positive health outcomes in older adults (White et al., 2009). In gay men, social support may buffer stigmatization (D'Augelli, Grossman, Hershberger, & O'Connell, 2001; de Vries & Blando, 2004; Ramirez-Valles, Kuhns, & Diaz, 2010). Some studies suggest that satisfaction with social support and living with a partner may be positively associated with older gay men's health (Grossman, D'Augelli, & Hershberger, 2000; Wright, LeBlanc, de Vries, & Detels, 2012) and negatively with depression (D'Augelli et al., 2001; Raws, 2004). Also, older gay men's support from friends has been found to be negatively associated with depression, anxiety, and internalized homophobia and positively associated with quality of life (Masini & Barrett, 2008). Moreover, older gay men who are out to their social networks report higher satisfaction with the support received than those whose social networks do not know their sexual orientation (Grossman et al., 2000). Overall, social support helps individuals address the challenges of aging, including the consequences of stigmatization due to sexual orientation (D'Augelli et al., 2001).

However, older gay men lose social support as they age and retire, as their partners die, and as their functional abilities decrease (Grossman et al., 2000). Older gay men are also less likely to disclose their sexuality or take on an identity as a gay man as they age (Raws, 2004), which may limit their access to social support. Research indicates that older gay men are twice as likely as their heterosexual peers to live alone (e.g., 66%; Bennett, 2008a; Grossman, et al., 2000; Shippy et al., 2004), but evidence on the levels of loneliness or isolation is inconclusive and the studies on older gay men (e.g., Grossman et al., 2000; Shippy et al., 2004) are based on samples of convenience. In a nonrandom sample of older gay men and lesbians, 27% reported no companionship and 59% stated that they have weekly contact with gay and lesbian peers (D'Augelli et al., 2001). Likewise, Shippy et al. found that 60% of gay men report lacking adequate support; Grossman et al. concluded that older gay men are satisfied with support received. In a most recent study, using a nonrandom sample of older LGBT individuals in San Francisco, 62% stated they lack companionship; 58% felt isolated, and 56% felt left out (Fredriksen-Goldsen & Muraco, 2010). Markedly, men, older participants, and ethnic minorities reported lower levels of social support.

Research on sources of social support among older gay men is more convincing. Among White older gay men, friends (or *families of choice*) are the most common source of support, followed by partners and biological families (Grossman et al., 2000; Herdt et al., 1997; Lyons, Pitts, Grierson, Thorpe, & Power, 2010; Masini & Barrett, 2008; Metlife Mature Market Institute, 2006; Shippy et al., 2004), unlike the rest of the population, in which family is the most common source of support (White et al., 2009). Partners are the most important source of emotional and instrumental, and even financial support for older gay men (Grossman et al., 2000). Having a partner, and even having a same-sex legal spouse, has been associated with fewer depressive symptoms (Wright et al., 2012). Thus, social support from friends and partners is critical to older gay men's health. Moreover, among all the possible functions that social support may furnish (e.g., emotional, instrumental), older gay men view socializing and emotional support as the most significant (Grossman et al., 2000).

As gay men age, their relationship to health care becomes critical, yet few gay men and health care providers talk about sexual orientation (Bernstein et al., 2008; Meckler, Elliott, Kanouse, Beals, & Schuster, 2006). Older gay men may be reluctant to disclose their sexual identity to health care providers because of life-long experiences of discrimination (Brotman, Ryan, & Cormier, 2003; Shankle, Maxwell, Katzman, & Landers, 2003; Stein & Bonuck, 2001; van Dam, Koh, & Dibble, 2001). This may lead to underutilization and poor care (Addis, Davies, Greene, MacBride-Stewart, & Shepherd, 2009). When health care providers are aware of the sexual identity of gay patients, health care utilization improves (Bergeron & Senn, 2003; Klitzman & Greenberg, 2002; Mayer et al., 2008; van Dam et al., 2001) and discussions of issues such as substance use, sexual behavior, and HIV are likely to take place (Klitzman & Greenberg, 2002).

This study contributes to that body of literature by looking at two specific types of support, emotional and instrumental (e.g., daily activities), and their correlation with perceived health and depression symptoms. These forms of support were chosen as they are thought of as the most important for both perceived and mental health in older (and gay male) populations (e.g., Grossman et al., 2000; Shippy et al., 2004; White et al., 2009; Wright et al., 2012). Specifically, we hypothesize (a) that perceived health is predicted by both emotional and instrumental support, living with a partner, health care providers' knowledge patients' sexual orientation, and depression symptoms; and (b) that depression is predicted by emotional and instrumental support, living with a partner, and health care providers' knowledge of patients' sexual orientation. Last, we assess what socio-demographic variables, including living with a partner, are correlated with emotional and instrumental support to elucidate subgroups of men who might be particularly vulnerable.

METHODS

Sample

Data come from a larger study (N = 307) of gay, lesbian, bisexual, and transgender people age 55 years and older collected in 2006 in Chicago. We focus on the sub-sample of men who self-identified as gay or bisexual (n = 182; 66% of total sample). Data were gathered anonymously via an internet-based protocol. The non-random sample was recruited through various means, including social and health services agencies, snowballing, and electronic lists.

The average age for the sample of gay men is 66 years (SD = 5.39; range = 56–82). About 47% of the sample is 64 years old or younger. The majority of participants (79%) are Caucasian; 11% are African American, and 5% Latino. The rest include 5% Asian American/Pacific Islander and bi- or multiracial (2% each). Complete socio-demographic information for the sample is presented in Table 1.

More than half (58%) of the men reported that they were single; 24% reported that they were partnered; 6% reported being divorced; 3% reported being married,[2] and 9% reported being widowed. In terms of living arrangements, 62% reported that they lived alone; 22% reported that they lived with their partner, and 13% reported that they lived with someone other than a partner. These percentages were similar across the three major ethnic groups.

Overall, the sample can be described as working, middle class, and highly educated. Thirty-seven percent of the sample reported an annual income between $50,000 and $100,000. Yet, 20% had an income between $20,000 and $35,000 and 18% reported less than $20,000. Caucasian men earned higher income than any other group, especially Latinos, and partnered men report higher income than those who are single. Similarly, 78% of the sample obtained a college degree or higher education. The rest did not attain a college degree. Caucasian men were more likely to have a college degree or higher than Latino and African American men.

---

[2] We cannot ascertain if participants interpreted this as being in a civil union (which is legal in Chicago) or being married. Furthermore, these respondents could have married in another state or country.

TABLE 1 Sociodemographic Variables for Study Sample ($N = 182$), Older Gay and Bisexual Men in Chicago

Variable	n	%
Ethnicity		
Caucasian	143	79%
African American	20	11%
Latino	9	5%
Asian American/Pacific Islander	4	2%
Biracial or multiracial	4	2%
Education		
Less than high school	2	1%
High school degree	15	8%
Some college	18	10%
2-year college degree	5	3%
4-year college degree	59	32%
Graduate degree	83	46%
Income		
Less than $20K	33	18%
$20K–$35K	36	20%
$35K–$50K	27	15%
$50K–$100K	68	37%
Prefer not to answer	18	10%
Relationship status		
Single	105	58%
Partnered	43	24%
Divorced	12	6%
Married	5	3%
Widowed	16	9%
Living arrangement		
Live alone	113	62%
Live with partner	41	22%
Live with others (not partner)	23	13%
Data missing	5	3%
Employment status		
Employed full-time/part-time	66	36%
Retired	96	53%
Unemployed	10	6%
Student or volunteer	4	2%

Measures

The interview protocol included the following socio-demographic information: age, employment status, education, income, relationship status, sexual identity, gender identity, race/ethnicity, and current living situation.[3] Distribution of main study variables are described next and presented in Table 2.

Perceived health. Perceived health was measured with a single item: "In general, would you say your health is." Response choices ranged from

---

[3]   Please note that no cognitive testing was done in the development of the protocol.

TABLE 2 Sample Distribution (Mean, Standard Deviation, Percentage) of Main Study Variables, $N = 182$ Older Gay and Bisexual Men in Chicago

Variable	M (SD)	Range
Perceived health	3.54 (1.02)	1 (*poor*)–5 (*excellent*)
Depression	1.51 (0.74)	1 (*not at all*)–4 (*nearly every day*)
No. of sources of emotional support	2.46 (2.96)	
No. of sources of instrumental support	1	
Primary health care providers' knowledge of patients' sexual orientation		
Primary provider knows	71%	
Primary provider does not know	16%	
Unsure if primary provider knows	9%	

$1 = poor$ to $5 = excellent$. This global measure is a national and international standard to assess overall health status and an independent predictor of mortality (Jylhä, 2009).

Depression symptoms. This variable was assessed with two items that asked about feelings over the past 2 weeks, "Over the past two weeks, how often have you been bothered by any of the following problems? a) Little interest or pleasure in doing things, and b) Feeling down, depressed, or hopeless." Response choices ranged from $1 = not at all$ to $4 = nearly every day$. Then we created an average of these two responses.

Health care providers' knowledge of sexual orientation. This item was measured with a single question, "Do you think your regular doctor, nurse or healthcare provider knows your sexual orientation/gender identity?" Response choices were, *yes, no,* or *don't know/not sure.*

Number of sources of emotional and instrumental support. These two variables were assessed by first asking participants to indicate the different kinds of support that they get from people they know. A list of persons who may provide social support was provided (e.g., partner/spouse, parent, child, coworker). For each person indicated, participants were asked to check a box that corresponded to the type of support received from that individual: financial, emotional, spiritual, healthcare, daily activities (i.e., instrumental support), and transportation. Seventy-nine percent of participants reported receiving emotional support; 53% spiritual; 49% daily activities; 38% transportation; 32% financial; and 31% reported getting health care related support. *Daily activities* is used as a proxy for instrumental support. The number of sources was added to create a count variable for each of them.

Data Analyses Plan

Bivariate analyses were first done to evaluate the association among study variables. Independent two-sample t-test, ANOVA, and correlation tests were used, depending on variable type. Next, multiple regression models were developed to assess our hypotheses. In the first model, perceived health was predicted by means of socio-demographic variables, living arrangement, number of sources of instrumental and emotional support, health care provider knowledge of respondent's sexual orientation, and depression symptoms. In the second model, we used the same independent variables to estimate their correlation to depression symptoms. The third and fourth models considered the correlates of socio-demographic variables and living arrangements with both number of sources of instrumental and emotional support.

RESULTS

As shown in Table 2, the average number of sources of emotional support was 2.46 (SD = 2.96) and the median was 2. Twenty-one percent (21%) of participants report no source of emotional support. The most frequently reported source of emotional support was friends (60%), followed by brother/sister (43%), nice/nephew (26%), and by partner and children (24%). The average number of sources of instrumental support was 1; the mean and the mode are zero. Half of the respondents reported not having a source of instrumental support. The most common source of instrumental support was friends (29%), followed by partner and child (23%, respectively).

Regarding health care providers' knowledge of patients' sexual orientation, 71% of participants expressed that their primary care providers know about their sexual orientation, and 16% indicated they do not know. Additionally, 9% stated that they do not know or are unsure whether their providers are aware of their sexual orientation.

Bivariate Analysis

Perceived health. Perceived health is positively associated with income (r = .311; p < .05) and education (r = .256; p < .05). There were differences in perceived health by education, $t(176)$ = −3.509, p < .01. Those with a college degree or higher education report better health (M = 3.68; SD =.98) than those with lower formal education (M = 3.05; SD = 1.05). There were also differences by living arrangement, $F(2, 172)$ = 4.15; p < .05. Those living with a partner reported better health (M = 3.93, SD = .88) than those living with others (M = 3.23, SD = .92). There were no differences between those living alone (M = 3.51, SD = 1.05) and those living with partners or others. Differences by relationship status indicated that partnered individuals report better perceived health (M = 3.90; SD = .88) than single individuals (M = 3.42; SD = 1.05), $t(175)$ = −2.80, p < .01. Older gay men currently employed ($M = 3.88$; $SD = .88$) reported better perceived health than retirees ($M = 3.43$; $SD = 1.07$) and those who were unemployed, volunteering, or studying ($M = 3.10$; $SD = .94$), $F(2,166) = 5.25$, $p < .01$. Caucasian men reported the highest perceived health ($M = 3.64$; $SD = 1.03$), followed by African American men ($M = 3.35$; $SD = .81$) and Latino men ($M = 2.67$; $SD = 1.00$). The only statistically significant difference was between Caucasian and Latino gay men, $F(3,172) = 2.96$, $p < .05$. Perceived health was also positively associated with instrumental support ($r = .253$; $p < .05$) and emotional support ($r = .236$; $p < .05$).

Depression symptoms. Depression was not correlated with income. Those with less than a college education experienced more frequent depression symptoms ($M = 1.76$; $SD = .86$) than those with college degrees or higher education ($M = 1.45$; $SD = .68$), $t(162) = 2.24$, $p < .05$. Older gay men living alone reported higher frequency of depression symptoms ($M = 1.58$, $SD = .81$) than those living with a partner ($M = 1.41$, $SD = .60$) and those living with others ($M = 1.35$, $SD = .54$) but the difference did not reach statistical significance. There were no differences in frequency of depression symptoms between those who were singe and partnered. Age and race were not associated with depression symptoms. Depression symptoms were associated with lower perceived health ($r = -.32$, $p < .05$).

Sources of support. Income was not correlated with number of sources of support. Those with less than college education reported fewer sources of support (of any type; $M = 2.38$; $SD = 1.80$) than those with college and higher education ($M = 3.11$; $SD = 2.20$), but this difference was not statistically significant. As anticipated, there were differences in sources support by living arrangement, $F(2, 174)=7.32$; $p < .01$. Those living alone reported fewer sources of support ($M = 2.65$; $SD = 1.89$) than those living with their partner ($M = 4.07$; $SD = 2.11$). Additionally, those who were single reported fewer sources of support ($M = 2.59$, $SD = 2.01$) than those who were partnered ($M = 3.92$, $SD = 2.18$), $t(179) = 3.84$, $p < .001$. Sources of support was negatively correlated with age ($r = -.227$, $p < .01$) and positively correlated with perceived health ($r = .192$, $p < .05$). There were no differences across ethnic groups.

In assessing sources of emotional and instrumental support separately, the number of sources of emotional support was inversely related to age ($r = -.203$; $p < .05$) and positively related to income ($r = .21$; $p < .05$) and perceived health ($r = .236$, $p < .01$) but was not associated with depression. The number of sources of instrumental support was positively associated with income ($r = .24$; $p < .05$) and perceived health ($r = .253$, $p < .01$) but was not associated with age. Those without any instrumental support have more frequent depression symptoms ($M = 1.67$, $SD = .87$) than those with at least one source of instrumental support ($M = 1.38$, $SD = .58$), $t(162) = 2.60$, $p < .05$.

Health Care Providers' Knowledge of Sexual Orientation

When comparing those whose health care providers knew about their sexual orientation against the others, we find that the former report higher perceived health ($M = 3.71$, $SD = .94$; $M = 3.05$, $SD = 1.10$, respectively), $t(170) = -3.80$, $p > .001$. Those whose health care providers knew about their sexual orientation also reported lower depression symptoms ($M = 1.46$, $SD = .67$), compared to those whose health care providers don't know ($M = 1.75$, $SD = .92$), $t(157) = 2.05$, $p < .05$.

Correlates of Perceived Health

In a multiple regression model predicting perceived health (Table 3), we found that number of sources of emotional support ($B = .229$; $p < 05$) and depression symptoms ($B = -.284$; $p < .01$) were significant. That is, having at least one source of emotional support increases the likelihood of reporting better health, and depression symptoms is inversely connected to perceived health. Notably, health care providers' knowledge of patients' sexual orientation is positively and significantly related to perceived health ($B = .203$; $p < .05$; not shown) in this model until depression symptoms is entered in the equation, suggesting mediation.

TABLE 3 Multiple Regression Models Predicting Perceived Health, Depression, and Sources of Emotional and Instrumental Support in Older Gay and Bisexual Men ($N = 182$) in Chicago

Variables	Perceived Health		Depression		Sources of Emotional Support		Sources of Instrumental Support	
	B	SE	B	SE	B	SE	B	SE
Age	.029	.016	−.103	.013	−.219**	.031	−.048	.020
Ethnic minority[a]	−.071	.208	−.175	.165	−.164*	.392	−.092	.254
Income	.112	.074	−.118	.060	.139	.145	.118	.094
Employed[b]	.130	.168	.000	.135	−.017	.337	.068	.218
Education	.149	.212	−.102	.170	−.009	.407	.039	.264
Live with other(s) (not partner)[c]	−.125	.242	−.128	.193	.059	.463	.132	.300
Live with partner[d]	.131	.220	.089	.176	.282**	.402	.352**	.261
No. sources of instrumental social support[e]	−.129	.189	−.232*	.149				
No. sources of emotional social support[e]	.229*	.095	.156	.076				
Health care provider knows sexual orientation	.144	.214	−.209*	.169				
Depression	−.284**	.113						

Note. [a]0 = Caucasian; 1 = African American, Latino, Other. [b]0 = Employed; 1 = Retired, student, other. [c]0 = Live alone; 1 = Live with other (not partner). [d]0 = Live alone; 1 = Live with partner. [e]0 = No sources of support; 1 = One or more sources of support.
*$p < .05$. **$p < .01$.

Correlates of Depression Symptoms

In the second model (Table 3), we found that only two variables were significantly associated with depression symptoms: number of sources of instrumental support ($B = -.232$; $p < .05$) and health care providers' knowledge of sexual orientation ($B = -.209$; $p < .05$). This implies that older gay men who have access to instrumental support and whose health care providers know of their sexual orientation are less likely to report depression symptoms. Furthermore, this model corroborates that depression symptoms mediate the relationship between health care providers' knowledge of patients' sexual orientation and perceived health, according to the Baron and Kenny's (1986) mediation method. Knowledge about patients' sexual orientation is associated with perceived health (as noted in the first model) and depression symptoms. Yet, as the model for predicted perceived health showed, the relationship between knowledge of patients' sexual orientation and perceived health fades when depression is included in the model.

Correlates of Source of Support

Our last models (Table 3) looked at sources of emotional and instrumental support as dependent variables and assessed their socio-demographic correlates. For number of sources of emotional support, age was inversely related ($B = -.219$; $p < .01$) as was ethnic minority status ($B = -.164$, $p < .05$). Living with partner was positively associated ($B = .282$; $p < .01$) with sources of emotional support. Yet, for number of sources of instrumental support, only living with partner was significantly associated ($B = .352$; $p < .05$).

DISCUSSION

As stated 2 decades ago, loneliness and social support are two central concerns of older gay men (Quam & Whitford, 1992). This is accentuated by the aging of the gayby boomer generation. The increasing number of older gay men poses a variety of questions ranging from the provision of human and social services, local and national policies, and health to the validity of theoretical models and the adequacy of empirical evidence. The purpose of this article has been to contribute to the nascent literature on gayby boomers' health by examining the connections between health and specific types of social support. We found that perceived health was positively correlated with number of sources of emotional support and that depression was negatively associated with instrumental support and health care providers' knowledge of patients' sexual orientation. Furthermore, the results revealed that health care providers' knowledge of patients' sexual orientation is positively associated to perceived health and that this connection is fully mediated by depression symptoms. The data also showed that the number of sources of emotional support varied negatively with age and belonging to an ethnic minority group, and positively with living with a partner; access to instrumental support seemed to be dependent on living with a partner only.

We need to consider the limitations of this study before elaborating on the implications of the findings. The nature of the cross-sectional research design prevents us from making causal inferences. Thus, the results only indicate correlations among variables. Likewise, the recruitment was biased toward Caucasian men and those with at least some level of social support. That is, ethnic minority older gay men and those in isolation were less likely to be recruited. Unfortunately, this is fairly common in the published literature. We need to improve sampling and recruitment methodologies. For example, respondent-driven sampling (RDS; Ramirez-Valles, Heckathorn, Vazquez, Diaz, & Campbell, 2005a, 2005b) might be effective in recruiting isolates and ethnic minorities. RDS, however, is expensive (this is why we did not use it in this study). Ethnographic approaches may help develop sampling and recruitment strategies (e.g., RDS), especially for ethnic and sexual minorities, by understating where and how they live, work, and socialize and how one may tap into their social networks. Moreover, our measures could have been more comprehensive—especially those about social support— and although we did not assess their validity, they are quite similar to those used in other published studies (Krause, 1999). Last, we did not collect data on HIV status because the collaborating community organizations and community members felt that such a question would have hindered response rates. This precluded us from looking at social support in what is presumed to be a vulnerable sub-group of older gay men.

The findings regarding the correlation between social support and health are consistent with the literature (Fredriksen-Goldsen & Muraco, 2010; Grossman et al., 2000; Lyons et al., 2010; Shippy et al., 2004). What our findings do is highlight the specific types of support that might be uniquely linked to health in old age. Friends and partners emerged as the most common sources of emotional and instrumental support and these two types of support seem to contribute differently to health. Emotional support appears to be more relevant for older gay men's perceptions of their own health than instrumental support, yet the opposite occurs for depression symptoms— instrumental support was the significant variable. Thus, having (and being close to) people whom older gay men trust, confide in, count on, and care for might distinctively affect health, independent of depression, living arrangements, and other socio-demographic factors. Conversely, having someone to help with daily living (e.g., cooking, grocery shopping, housekeeping) might have a singular effect on mental health. In other words, the challenges of daily life might pose a notable risk for mental health. The findings also indicate that depression symptoms are negatively associated with health care providers' knowledge of patients' sexual orientation and that depression symptoms mediate the link between providers' knowledge of patients' sexual orientation and perceived health. This could mean that older gay men who are not fully comfortable talking about their homosexuality (for fear of stigmatization or otherwise) might experience depression symptoms, which, in turn, might lead to poor perceived health. Yet, the reverse is possible, that depression symptoms lead to limited disclosure and health care providers' unawareness of patients' sexual orientation. Nonetheless, the underlying theme here is older gay men's sense of themselves as gay men, the institutional contexts that either facilitate or imped the expression of sexual orientation, and how they both shape older men's health.

The presence of a partner is another salient finding in this study. Living with a partner was not associated with perceived health or depression. This seems to contradict previous research (Grossman et al., 2000; Wright et al., 2012). However, this might be due to methodological differences across studies. For example, Grossman et al.'s (2000) analysis of the connection between health and partnership did not distinguish between gay men and lesbian women in the sample; and Wright et al.'s (2012) research found a relationship only between depression and being in a same-sex legal relationship (e.g., marriage), not living with a partner, and after controlling for emotional support (as we did). Yet, living with a partner (as opposed to living alone) was positively linked to sources of emotional and instrumental support. This, we suppose, points not at the need for gay men to partner, but rather to the risks of living alone. We were not able to discern this, but we suspect that older gay men who live with supportive peers might experience similar health benefits.

To further the understanding of gayby boomers' health, researchers next need to address questions germane to the gay (or queer and sexual minority) category (Hughes, 2006). What's the silence of gay identity? Where and how it is expressed? What are the social spaces available for older gay men, if any? How do older gay men experience and manage the stigma of old age and homosexuality? And how do ethnic and sexual minority statuses interconnect to shape social support, stress, and health? (De Vries & Patrick, 2006; Jimenez, 2003).

A clear implication from this study, taking into consideration its caveats, is that health and social services organizations and professionals may want to focus on promoting older gay men's access to emotional and instrumental support. This, we infer, requires mobilizing personal social networks, as well as service providers (e.g., home care). This effort might need to be emphasized among ethnic minorities and the older-old adults. Another repercussion is the need to promote cultural competence in health care settings so that patients and providers converse about gender identity and sexual orientation.

REFERENCES

Addis, S., Davies, M., Greene, G. MacBride-Stewart, S., & Shepherd, M. (2009). The health, social care and housing needs of lesbian, gay, bisexual and transgender older people: A review of the literature. *Health and Social Care in the Community, 17*, 647–658.

Baron, R. M., & Kenny, D. A. (1986). The moderator–mediator variable distinction in social psychological research: Conceptual, strategic, and statistical considerations. *Journal of Personality and Social Psychology, 51*, 1172–1182.

Bennett, J. (2008a, September 17). *Invisible and overlooked*. Retrieved from http://www.newsweek.com/long-invisible-gay-seniors-seek-respect-services-89161

Bennett, J. (2008b, September 17). *A lot of unknowns*. Retrieved from http://www.newsweek.com/aging-hiv-patients-face-complicated-health-issues-89175

Bergeron, S., & Senn, C. Y. (2003). Health care utilization in a sample of Canadian lesbian women: Predictors of risk and resilience. *Women & Health, 37*(3), 19–35.

Berkman, L. F. (1995) The role of social relations in health promotion. *Psychosomatic Medicine, 57*, 245–254.

Bernstein, K. T., Liu, K., Begier, E. M., Koblin, B., Karpati, A., & Murrill, C. (2008). Same-sex attraction disclosure to health care providers among New York City men who have sex with men. *Archives of Internal Medicine, 168*, 1458–1464.

Brotman, S., Ryan, B., & Cormier, R. (2003). The health and social service needs of gay and lesbian elders and their families in Canada. *Gerontologist, 43*, 192–202.

Chesney, M. A., Chambers, D. B., Taylor, J. M., & Johnson, L. M. (2003). Social support, distress, and well-being in older men living with HIV infection. *Journal of Acquired Immune Deficiency Syndromes, 33*, S185–193.

Cohen, S., & Wills, T. A. (1985). Stress, social support, and the buffering hypothesis. *Psychological Bulletin, 98*, 310–357.

Cornwell, B., Laumann, E. O., & Schumm, L. P. (2008). The social connectedness of older adults: A national profile. *American Sociological Review, 73*, 185–203.

D'Augelli, A. R., & Grossman, A. H. (2001). Disclosure of sexual orientation, victimization, and mental health among lesbian, gay, and bisexual older adults. *Journal of Interpersonal Violence, 16*, 1008–1027.

D'Augelli, A. R., Grossman, A. H., Hershberger, S. L., & O' Connell, T. S. (2001). Aspects of mental health among older lesbian, gay, and bisexual adults. *Aging & Mental Health, 5*, 149–158.

D'Emilio, J. (1998). *Sexual politics, sexual communities*. Chicago, IL: University of Chicago Press.

de Vries, B. D., & Blando, J. A. (2004). *The study of gay and lesbian aging: Lessons from social gerontology*. In H. Gilbert & B. de Vries (Eds.), *Gay and lesbian aging: Research and future directions* (pp. 3–28). New York, NY: Springer.

de Vries, B. D., & Patrick, H. (2006). The family-friends of older gay men and lesbians. In N. Teunis & H. Gilbert (Eds.), *Sexual ineqaulities and social justice* (pp. 230–249). Berkeley: University of California Press.

Fredriksen-Goldsen, K. I., & Muraco, A. (2010). Aging and sexual orientation: A 25-year review of the literature. *Research on Aging, 32*, 372–413.

Funders for Lesbian and Gay Issues. (2004). *Aging in equity: LGBT elders in America*. Retrieved from http://www.lgbtagingcenter.org/resources/pdfs/Aging%20In%20Equity.pdf.

Grossman, A. H., D'Augelli A. R., & Hershberger S. L. (2000). Social support networks of lesbian, gay, and bisexual adults 60 years of age and older. *Journal of Gerentology: Social Sciences, 55*B, 171–179.

Herdt, G., Beeler, J., & Rwals, T. W. (1997). Life course diversity among older lesbians and gay men: A study in Chicago. *Journal of Gay, Lesbian, and Bisexual Identity, 2*, 231–246.

House, J. S., Landis, K. R., & Umberson, D. (1988). Social relationships and health. *Science, 241*(4865), 540–545.

Hughes, M. (2006). Queer ageing. *Gay and Lesbian Issues and Psychology Review, 2*, 54–59.

Israel, B. A., & Schurman, S. J. (1990). Social support, control, and the stress process. In K. Glanz, F. M. Lewis, & B. K. Rimer (Eds.), *Health behavior and health education: Theory, research, and practice. The Jossey-Bass health series* (pp. 187–215). San Francisco, CA: Jossey-Bass.

Jimenez, A. D. (2003). Triple jeopardy: Targeting older men of color who have sex with men. *Journal of Acquired Immune Deficiency Syndromes, 33*, S222–S228.

Johnson, M. J., Jackson, N. C., Arnett, K., & Koffman, S. D. (2005). Gay and lesbian perceptions of discrimination in retirement care facilities. *Journal of Homosexuality, 49*(2), 83–102.

Jylhä, M. (2009). What is self-rated health and why does it predict mortality? Towards a unified conceptual model. *Social Science & Medicine, 69*, 307–316.

Kertzner, R. M. (2001). The adult life course and homosexual identity in midlife gay men. *Annual Review of Sexual Research, 12*, 75–92.

Klitzman, R. L., & Greenberg, J. D. (2002). Patterns of communication between gay and lesbian patients and their health care providers. *Journal of Homosexuality, 42*(4), 65–75.

Krehely, J. (2009). *How to close the LGBT health disparities gap*. Washington, DC: Center for American Progress.

Krause, N. (1999). Assessing change in social support during late life. *Research on Aging, 21*, 539–569.

Lewis, N. M. (2009). Mental health in sexual minorities: Recents indicators, trends, and their relationships to place in North America and Europe. *Health & Place, 15*, 1029–1045.

Lyons, A., Pitts, M., Grierson, J., Thorpe, R., & Power, J. (2010). Ageing with HIV: Health and psychosocial well-being of older gay men. *AIDS Care, 22*, 1236–1244.

Masini, B. E., & Barrett, H. A. (2008). Social support as a predictor of psychological and physical well-being and lifestyle in lesbian, gay, and bisexual adults aged 50 and over. *Gay and Lesbian Social Services, 20*, 91–110.

Mayer, K. H., Bradford, J. B., Makadon, H. J., Stall, R., Goldhammer, H., & Landers, S. (2008). Sexual and gender minority health: What we know and what needs to be done. *American Journal of Public Health, 98*, 989–995.

Meckler, G. D., Elliott, M. N., Kanouse, D. E., Beals, K. P., & Schuster, M. A. (2006). Nondisclosure of sexual orientation to a physician among a sample of gay, lesbian, and bisexual youth. *Archives of Pediatric & Adolescent Medicine, 160,* 1248–1254.

Metlife Mature Market Institute. (2006). *Out and aging: The MetLife study of lesbian and gay baby boomers.* Westport, CT: Author.

NORC. (2012). *National Social Life, Health and Aging Project.* Retrieved from http://www.norc.org/Research/Projects/Pages/national-social-life-health-and-aging-project.aspx

Pearlin, L. I., Menaghan, E. G., Lieberman, M. A., & Mullan, J. T. (1981). The stress process. *Journal of Health and Social Behavior, 22,* 337–356.

Quam, J. K., & Whitford, G. S. (1992). Adaptation and age-related expectations of older gay and lesbian adults. *Gerontologist, 32,* 367–374.

Ramirez-Valles, J. (2011). *Health and social connections of men who have sex with men in the National Social Life, Health, and Aging Project* (Unpublished report). University of Illinois at Chicago, Chicago, IL.

Ramirez-Valles, J. (2013). *Gayby boomers: The gayest generation.* Retrieved from http://gaybyboomers.blogspot.com.

Ramirez-Valles, J., Heckathorn, D. D., Vazquez, R., Diaz, R. M., & Campbell, R. T. (2005a). The fit between theory and data in respondent-driven sampling: Response to Heimer. *AIDS and Behavior, 9,* 409–414.

Ramirez-Valles, J., Heckathorn, D. D., Vazquez, R., Diaz, R. M., & Campbell, R. T. (2005b). From networks to populations: The development and application of respondent-driven sampling among IDUs and Latino gay men. *AIDS and Behavior, 9,* 387–402.

Ramirez-Valles, J., Kuhns, L. M., & Diaz, R.M. (2010). Social integration and health: Community involvement, stigmatized identities, and sexual risk in Latino sexual minorities. *Journal of Health and Social Behavior, 51,* 30–47.

Raws, T. W. (2004). Disclosure and depression among older gay and homosexual men: Findings from the urban men's health study. In H. Gilbert & B. de Vries (Eds.), *Gay and lesbian aging: Research and future directions* (pp. 117–141). New York, NY: Springer.

Rosenfeld, D., Bartlem, B., & Smith, R. D. (2012). Out of the closet and into the trenches: Gay male baby boomers, aging, and HIV/AIDS. *Gerontologist, 52,* 255–264.

Shankle, M. D., Maxwell, C. A., Katzman, E. S. & Landers, S. (2003). An invisable population: older lesbian, gay, bisexual and transgender individuals. *Clinical Research and Regulatory Affairs, 20,* 159–182.

Shippy, A. R., Cantor, M. H., & Brennan, M. (2004). Social networks of aging gay men. *Journal of Men's Studies, 13,* 107–120.

Steffens, D. C., Fisher, G. G., Langan K. M., Potter, G. G., & Plassman, B. L. (2009). Prevalence of depression among older Americans: The aging, demographics and memory study. *International Psychogeriatrics, 21,* 879–888.

Stein, G. L., & Bonuck, K. A. (2001). Original research: Physician–patient relationships among the lesbian and gay community. *Journal of the Gay and Lesbian Medical Association, 5,* 87–93.

van Dam, M. A., Koh, A. S., & Dibble, S. L. (2001). Lesbian disclosure to health care providers and delay of care. *Journal of the Gay and Lesbian Medical Association, 5,* 11–19.

Wallace, S. P., Cochran, S. D., Durazo, E. M., & Ford, C. L. (2011). *The health of aging lesbian, gay and bisexual adults in California.* Retrieved from http://escholarship.org/uc/item/9gv99494

White, A. M., Philogene, G. S., Fine, L., & Sinha, S. (2009). Social support and self-reported health status of older adults in the United States. *American Journal of Public Health*, *99*, 1872–1878.

Wright, R. A., LeBlanc, A.J., de Vries, B., & Detels, R. (2012). Stress and mental health among midlife and older gay-identified men. *American Journal of Public Health*, *102*, 503–510.

Acceptance in the Domestic Environment: The Experience of Senior Housing for Lesbian, Gay, Bisexual, and Transgender Seniors

KATHLEEN M. SULLIVAN

Seniors Services Department, L.A. Gay & Lesbian Center, Los Angeles, California, USA

The social environment impacts the ability of older adults to inter-act successfully with their community and age-in-place. This study asked, for the first time, residents of existing Lesbian, Gay, Bisexual, and Transgender (LGBT) senior living communities to explain why they chose to live in those communities and what, if any, bene-fit the community afforded them. Focus groups were conducted at 3 retirement communities. Analysis found common categories across focus groups that explain the phenomenon of LGBT senior housing. Acceptance is paramount for LGBT seniors and social networks expanded, contrary to socioemotional selectivity theory. Providers are encouraged to develop safe spaces for LGBT seniors.

Development of housing for lesbian, gay, bisexual and transgender (LGBT) seniors is new. Lucco (1987) documented that older LGBT people will move to senior housing early than their heterosexual counterparts if the staff is comprised of LGBT professionals. Additionally, LGBT seniors express fear that they would have to return to the closet, receive substandard care, and be unaccepted by other residents in long-term care facilities (Stein, Beckerman & Sherman, 2010). Community attributes of the few existing LGBT senior-housing environments have yet to be discovered. This article

is exploratory and seeks to identify the importance of the social environment for LGBT seniors in elder communities. The categories of meaning
help explain the importance of the social environment in the domestic setting for LGBT seniors. Additionally, the theory of socioemotional selectivity
theory is explored to determine relevance for the LGBT community.

By 2030, 20% of the US population will be 65 years of age or older (US
Census Bureau, 2007; US Department of Commerce, 2001). As the percentage
of people 65 years of age or older increases, the need for social and health
services, community and institutional care, and senior housing will grow;
understanding the needs is vital for the fields of social work and gerontology
(Haywood & Zhang, 2001; Hebert, Beckett, Scherr, & Evans, 2001; Knickman
& Snell, 2002; Langley, 2001). Unfortunately, minority groups are less likely to
be included in gerontological research and, as a result, the field understands
less about the aging of minority communities (Bulatao & Anderson, 2004;
Green, 2006; Kimmel, Rose, Orel, & Green, 2006). One group left out of the
literature on aging is the LGBT community. This dearth of research translates
into a lack of understanding of this group's aging process and their need
for and use of health and social services (Gabbay & Wahler, 2002; Wahler &
Gabbay, 1997).

Berger (1982), Cruikshank (1991), and Orel (2004), among others, have
noted that older lesbian and gay men were not included in studies of aging
due to ignorance, heterosexism, and purposeful marginalization. The literature on LGBT aging found that LGBT seniors had many of the same issues
adapting to aging as did their heterosexual counterparts, and they also had
issues specific to their sexual orientation and gender identity. Issues identified in the LGBT aging literature include discrimination and stigmatization,
life course diversity, social service needs, support networks, and housing
(Adelman, 1991; Beeler, Rawls, Herdt, & Cohler, 1999; Berger, 1984; Berger
& Kelly, 1986; Brotman, Ryan, & Cormier, 2003; Cahill & South, 2002; Hunter,
2005; Kimmel, 1978; Lucco, 1987; Minnigerode & Adelman, 1978; Peacock,
2000; Rosenfeld, 1999).

Social support is characterized as a coping resource by Thoits (1995),
and is a common area of LGBT aging research. The perception of social
and emotional support has a greater positive impact on mental and physical
health than does actual received support (Shippy, Cantor, & Brennan, 2004).
Research in the area of social support has reported some positive findings.
Grossman, D'Augelli, and Hershberger (2000) reported that social support
networks of lesbians, gay, and bisexual seniors were as large or larger than
the social support networks as their heterosexual counterparts. Another study
found that gay men in New York reported having larger support networks
than their heterosexual counterparts (Shippy et al., 2004).

An important aspect of social support networks of LGBT seniors is the
role of fictive kin. Fictive kin is a symbolic kinship used to describe created families (Weston, 1991). Researchers such as Krause (2001), Katz-Olson

(2001), and Williams and Dilworth-Anderson (2002) have found that African American seniors, particularly women, rely both on extended family members and fictive kin, most notably church members, for social support. In studies of the social support networks of LGBT seniors, fictive kin have been found to provide the highest level of social support after that of life partners (Grossman et al., 2000; Grossman, D'Augelli, & O'Connell, 2001; Jacobs, Rasmussen, & Hohman, 1997; Shippy et al., 2004).

The life course of LGBT seniors is diverse. The decision to reveal one's sexual orientation led to life adjustments no matter what age the decision to come out was made (Herdt, Beeler, & Rawls, 1997; Kehoe, 1989; Peacock, 2000). Indeed, Altman (1999) discussed the need for social services specific to seniors who "come out of the closet" late in life. Researchers have sought to explain how stigma, heterosexism, and internal and external homophobia produce a life course that diverged from the heterosexual life course espoused by Erikson (1975) and others (Altman, 1999; Berger, 1980; Berger & Kelly, 1986; Blando, 2001; Boxer, 1997; Cahill & South, 2002; Cass, 1979; Coleman, 1981; Dorfman et al., 1995; Herdt et al., 1997; Kimmel, 1978; Minnegerod & Adelman, 1978; Peacock, 2000; Quam, 1993; Rosenfeld, 1999; Wahler & Gabbay, 1997).

Fear of discrimination leads some to remain in, or return to, the closet. One study reported that a respondent said that she would rather commit suicide than be placed in an institution (Tully, 1989). Her fear was based upon the perception that she would be unsafe as a lesbian in an institutional setting (Tully, 1989). For some seniors, the emotional stress caused by real or perceived heterosexism and homophobia is an impetus to return to the closet, which can lead to isolation and further marginalization (Burbank & Burkholder, 2006; Friend, 1989; Herek, 2007; Rosenfeld, 1999). Indeed, two recent studies found that 65% of LGBT seniors in Los Angeles live alone, which can lead to feelings of social isolation and disconnect from society (Fredriksen-Goldsen et al., 2011; Los Angeles Department of Aging, 2011). Nationally, the rate of living alone for all persons 65 and older is 29% (Administration on Aging, 2011). Additionally, a recent study found that adults age 65 and older who have the perception of loneliness and disconnection have a 45% greater risk of death than those who felt connected to others (Perissinotto, Cenzer, & Covinsky, 2011). Isolation and marginalization, however, is not common to all LGBT seniors. Studies of older gay men and lesbians have chronicled a variety of positive coping strategies used to overcome societal stigma. Coping strategies such as the development of fictive kin, community-based social support, and fluidity in gender roles have been found to benefit older LGBT people (Adelman, 1991; Berger, 1980; Friend, 1989; Herek, Chopp, & Stohl, 2007; Kimmell, 1992; Quam, 2001; Slusher, Mayer, & Dunkle, 1996).

Housing has been a tangential and prospective issue in LGBT aging research to date (Hamburger, 1997; Kehoe, 1989; Lucco, 1987; Tully, 1989).

Lucco reported that lesbians and gay men had a strong preference to live in retirement communities staffed by lesbian and gay professionals and would move from their current dwelling to a retirement community at a younger age than their heterosexual counterparts. Several local LGBT communities have surveyed their community members about housing. One local study was done by openHouse. The study found that lesbians and gay men in San Francisco age 60 and older report higher levels of chronic disability (38% of lesbians, 36% of gay men) than did heterosexual women and men (25% of women, 16% of men), which indicates a need for support services connected to housing (Adelman, Gurevitch, De Vries, & Blando, 2006; De Vries, 2006).

The built, as well as the social, environment can greatly impact the quality of life of older adults (Scheidt & Norris-Baker, 2003; Sullivan & Neal, 2005). Life span theories study the social environment and how elders select and optimize their social environment to attain positive outcomes (Carstensen, 1992, 1998; Evans, Kantrowitz, & Eshelman, 2002; Lang, 2001; Lang, Rieckmann, & Baltes, 2002). Socioemotional selectivity theory, which explains both why and how an elder selects and optimizes his or her social environment, argues that adults reduce the total number of relationships in later life (Carstensen, 1998; Lang, 2001). Socioemotional selectivity theory posits that the context of social interaction and the goal of social interaction change with age; as people age they regulate their social contact so as to engage in social interactions that give them the highest level of emotional satisfaction (Carstensen, Mikels, & Mather, 2006). For heterosexual seniors, the relationships found most emotionally fulfilling were first those of blood relations, followed by long-term friendship (Carstensen, Fung, & Charles, 2003; Freund & Baltes, 2002; Lang et al., 2002). No research exists on the applicability of this theory for LGBT seniors. Socioemotional selectivity theory may help to explain why some LGBT seniors choose LGBT senior housing (Baltes, Wahl, & Schmid-Furstoss, 1990; Carstensen, 1992; Carstensen et al., 2006).

METHODS

The convenience sample for this study was also purposive. Only residents of three existing LGBT senior housing communities were eligible to participate. Thus, the study is limited and cannot be used to generalize to the broader LGBT senior population. Data were gathered from three LGBT senior living communities, two of which are now defunct. The sites were Rainbow Vision, Barbary Lane, and Triangle Square. In addition to participating in a focus group, participants were asked to complete a short demographic survey at the conclusion of the focus group sessions. A total of seven focus groups over a 3-month period were conducted with 38 participants. The three sites in this study were not exclusive in relation to sexual orientation or gender identity, and all were in the western United States. Participants had to meet several criteria of eligibility to be included in the study. The most basic criteria were that the participant had to identify as lesbian, gay, bisexual, or transgender and had to reside in one of the three senior housing communities. No participant in the focus groups presented with dementia or cognitive impairment. Although every effort was made to represent diverse racial and ethnic backgrounds, only one site had ethnic and racial diversity at the time of this study. The lack of racial diversity was consistent with research that found racial and ethnic minorities are more likely to live alone or with extended family, as opposed to living in long-term care or retirement communities (Orel, 2004; Taylor & Robertson, 1994).

Any resident who met the study criteria was recruited to participate in a focus group at his or her housing community. A brief description of the project was written and emailed to contact persons at each site. The project description included a brief overview of the study, a copy of the informed consent form with Human Subjects Research Review Committee approval letter, and a copy of the researcher's recruitment letter to residents. Each senior was contacted by the researcher, and if they were interested in participating were assigned to a focus group. Couples were welcome to participate, but each member was assigned to a different group. A total of three couples participated in the study.

Prior to the focus group interview, participants were asked to complete a Statement of Informed Consent, at which time the participants were told that the group would be audio recorded and transcribed verbatim by the researcher. In addition, participants were given information about the Institutional Human Subjects Review Board approval, how to contact the board, and that they could cease participation at any time. A prepared interview script was used at each focus group to ensure consistency of the inquiry. The script had five main questions and allowed for clarifying or probe questions used as needed. At the conclusion of each focus group, I asked participants to complete a simple nine-item demographic questionnaire.

Each focus group was transcribed using HyperTranscribe and analyzed using HyperResearch. Grounded theory, as found in Strauss and Corbin (1998), was used as the method of analysis. The developed codes represent the initial concepts and categories found in the text. Axial coding further defined the categories along the lines of properties and dimensions (Strauss & Corbin, 1998). For instance, acceptance is an example of a category of meaning and it included such dimensions as: not having to worry about one's neighbors, acknowledgement that being LGBT is normal, and openly grieving for a deceased partner.

The average age of the participants was 71, with the oldest being 85 and the youngest 51 years of age. Of the 38, 15 identified as women and 23 as male. There were 22 gay men, 11 lesbians, 2 bisexual and 3 transgender seniors. The average age the participants came out of the closet was 28, 16%

had been in previous heterosexual marriages and 26% had children. A large proportion (74%) was single at the time of the focus groups, and 13% were widows or widowers of a same-sex union. The majority of participants were White of European descent; two participants were African American, two were Latino/a and one identified as White of Middle Eastern descent. Four of the participants were people with disabilities. Generational differences were revealed. The older a participant was, for instance, the more likely he or she was in a previous heterosexual marriage, came out later in life, and had children, which is consistent with the literature (Herdt et al., 1997; Rosenfeld, 1999).

FINDINGS

The theme of acceptance ran throughout the data and explained why these seniors chose LGBT senior housing. Participants talked about not feeling lesser than any other person. Thus, the social context was important to participants. The social aspect of their environment produced successful behaviors, such as the desire to be inclusive of heterosexual seniors, development of new support networks, and the development of intimate (nonsexual) relationships. Acceptance provided a foundation that allowed for all other categories (or community attributes) to develop. Key categories from that data are reported in the following and quotations from participants are used to illustrate each. Please note, all names have been changed for the purposes of confidentiality.

Comfort and ease in one's domestic environment were common reasons that participants were attracted to these communities. Ease was a perception of safety, living out of the closet, and removal of negativity: "Well, I felt that this place was a place that we could live comfortably with people with like tastes and sexual orientations without fear. That was one of the major ideas that made me comfortable with this place." As Herek (2007) theorized, the lack of stigma and homophobia can lead to increased feelings of safety for sexual minorities. One participant said:

> Well, my thing being here is exactly that this is the first residence I've had as an adult where I have been comfortable with my environment, because heretofore, it has always been, you know, the back stabbers or the homophobics. So, you, you just ignore them and walk with pride. I have been more comfortable here than any other environment.

The environment provided safety and support, and this social context led some to come out of the closet for the first time in their lives. One transgender senior, closeted until age 72, described it this way: "All I am is Madeline Smith here. I never had that before. I thought this place was great. I don't have to explain that I'm transgender here, or what it is; they understand." Residents felt comfortable in their environment because they were accepted for who they were.

Community was a characteristic important to respondents. Participants felt that their community was more caring than other senior residences, and community action demonstrated the caring environment. For instance, one group member talked about residents of his community caring for a gravely ill resident. Although these kinds of actions may take place in other retirement communities, a common perception was that the level of care in the LGBT senior communities was unique.

> So, you know, you don't have to call 911 first. First you can call your friends, and if they're not home, somebody else is gonna be home and, like I said, if they couldn't physically help you or didn't know what to do they would bring somebody else over to your house. And to me that's extremely important, that sense; that is truly a sense of community.

This perceived commitment was remarkable, because residents do not have long histories with one another. The average length of residence was just 2-1/2 years at the time of the study. The community provided comfort and support to formerly isolated members.

> And I think that is what brings a lot of us here, is that we don't want to die alone. We don't have, or a lot of us don't, have children. We didn't do this back-up plan—"Oh, you're gonna take care of me in my old age [referring to children]." You get to this final stretch of life, and you don't have a back-up plan. You go, "Holy shit."

The created community at the three sites was fostered by residents' acceptance of one another. A sense of belongingness was created through shared activities, care for one another, and the shared connection of being sexual minority seniors. Freed from real or perceived societal judgments, residents had the freedom to share life experiences in a supportive, understanding, and empathetic environment.

DIVERSITY AND INCLUSIVITY

Participants desired to live in open and affirming diverse communities. What respondents appeared to mean by diversity was nonexclusivity

> I wanted to be the majority the first time in my life, and that's why I came. I didn't want to be exclusively gay, but I definitely wanted to be

the majority. And I still want to be the majority, because it ain't gonna happen anywhere else.

Participants discussed racial and ethnic diversity as a vision for all three of these communities, although it was realized in just one community. When participants discussed diversity, they primarily meant the inclusion of non-sexual minority people. One participant explained that it did not matter if a coresident was straight or gay: What was important was that each person felt comfortable there. "If I don't feel comfortable in my home, then it is not my home."

When asked if any of the group members had considered living in a tra-ditional retirement community (predominately heterosexual), the resounding answer was *no*. The attraction of their current living environment included a strong sense of community, connection with others, acceptance for who they are, safety, and a desire to live in a diverse community. Participants per-ceived that traditional retirement communities did not offer the same socially accepting living environments.

Additionally, participants gave reports of LGBT friends who lived in heterosexual retirement communities and who had gone back into the closet and isolated their true selves from their neighbors. Participants were all in agreement that they are not willing, or able, to conform or return to the closet at this stage in their lives. One participant told of a return to the closet several years ago when she was temporarily in a nursing home: "It was a very eye-opening experience, because if people who worked there would have known I was gay, I think I would have gotten worse treatment than I got."

Participants believed that LGBT seniors who decided to live openly were at a disadvantage in traditional retirement settings due to heterosex-ism. Couples expressed the desire to live together as a couple, which they perceived to be impossible in a traditional retirement community. There was a perception that there would be little or no social connection for an LGBT senior living in a heterosexual retirement community.

The ability to be open about one's life and being able to speak openly about one's life has been found to benefit LGBT seniors (Friend, 1991). Connection and normalcy of being LGBT are directly related to the feeling of acceptance and belonging, and the perception of social connection was found to be supportive of healthy aging (Perissinotto et al., 2011). Residents talked about a sense of belonging, which allowed for intimate (nonsexual) relationships. One respondent reported a complete emotional and psycho-logical breakdown after the death of her lifetime partner. This respondent required hospitalization in a mental health institution for 9 months. She felt that her life "had evaporated; it was like my entire life, the part I cared about, didn't happen. I just couldn't deal with that." It was the acceptance of others in her present senior living community that she credits with her recovery and healing. This example highlights the deep isolation some LGBT elders experienced, and evidence of a lesbian senior expanding her social network despite her age (she was 83 at the time of the interview) and despite the fact that she had moved away from her previous home of over 40 years. The acceptance and sense of belonging provided a social environment where she could heal

Acceptance was what residents sought and found at their present housing, and it was seen as both the removal of negativity and the added positive aspect of being embraced for who you are. Participants reported that they did not need to closet their lives or censor their conversations in their housing environment. These seniors desired to live an authentic life, and the acceptance found in their respective communities supported their living openly.

DISCUSSION

In contrast to the notion that as people age they contract their social networks (Carstensen, 1998), the seniors in these living communities are actually expanding their social networks. The contradiction with this life span theory for this population is one of the most significant findings of this study. The explanation for why seniors in these housing communities are, according to the data, expanding their social relationships relates to social context of place. The theory of socioemotional selectivity theory purports that people reduce the total number of their social relationships and deepen their relationships with family and long-time friends. The goals a person has for his or her relationships change from using relationships to gain knowledge from others to personal emotional satisfaction. The expansion of social networks is related to the social environment and can give social workers and aging professionals clues to how to better serve their LGBT clients.

There are perhaps two explanations for why the LGBT seniors in this study did not appear to follow the same life span trajectory that socioemotional selectivity theory hypothesizes. Peacock (2000) and others have made the argument that sexual minorities do not follow the same developmental life course as their heterosexual counterparts. An example from this study is a man in his mid-70s who, for the first time, is living in an environment that is socially accepting of his sexual orientation. As a result, this man feels that he has less stress and more freedom, and is expanding his social network. This man is not the only example of participants who were closeted for years and are now living out of the closet. One participant, a retired professor in her 80s, talked about how she had had few close friends prior to moving to her present community because, for her entire working career, she was in the closet. This highlights a possible second explanation for why socioemotional selectivity theory does not seem to apply to the seniors in this study. The theory states that as a person ages, he or she selects relationships that are both positive and emotionally meaningful (Freund & Baltes, 2002; Lang, 2001). Relationships that provide the highest level of emotional satisfaction and meet emotional goals are deepened. The combination of acceptance, inclusivity, comfort, and safety found in these communities may offer an environment that supports, for many the first time, the creation of emotionally satisfying relationships. At a time when residents should be compressing the number of relationships, many have found the first community of people with whom they can have emotionally satisfying relationships.

The expansion of social networks is healthy for seniors (Burnett, et al., 2006). Social workers and other professionals will better serve their LGBT clients if they create accepting and safe space for them in their practice. Aging professionals must first access their own comfort level with working with LGBT seniors. Understanding one's comfort level and knowledge base are key to improving care provision to this group of seniors. Next, seek out cultural competency training. Many organizations provide training to providers of care and services to seniors. Trainings, such as the L.A. Gay & Lesbian Center's *Creating Safe Spaces for LGBT Seniors*, are specifically designed to train both professionals such as long-term care administrators and frontline service workers such as certified nursing assistants. Assessment and training must then translate into practice. Intentional and conscious actions that help create safe space include: reflecting LGBT seniors in published materials, including important dates and events such as PRIDE month on agency calendars, ensuring in-take forms are inclusive, and taking the opportunity to teach others when the time and opportunity arise.

IMPLICATIONS AND FUTURE RESEARCH

Perhaps the most important contribution this study makes to the field of aging is enhancing the visibility of the participants. Few researchers have sought out this population for study, and thus there is limited information about these individuals and their experience of the aging process. This study provides a snapshot of an understudied group. In addition, the opinions of LGBT seniors who live in primarily LGBT senior housing were unknown, prior to this study. The phenomenon of LGBT senior housing is new, and this is the first effort to gain an understanding of why some seniors choose this housing and what it provides to them that previous living environments did not.

One important area of discovery was the critical importance of social relationships for this group of older adults. The seniors in this study talked about creating new family-like relationships with their neighbors. The development of new and expanded social relationships and networks in later life appears to be contrary to the tenets of socioemotional selectivity theory. An understanding of the critical importance of the social environment, and specifically an atmosphere of acceptance, to LGBT seniors is valuable for researchers and practitioners alike and highlights the great diversity in the lived experiences of seniors.

Lucco (1987) found that lesbian and gay men reported a preference for LGBT staff at retirement communities and nursing homes. Howard et al. (2002) similarly found that African American seniors preferred that nursing home staff be African American. A study focusing on whether LGBT seniors continue to have this preference, and why they have this preference, would be instructive for developers of senior living and those who provide services to seniors. Additionally, professionals who work with seniors will benefit from understanding what they can do to create open and affirming environments where all people feel safe and accepted for who they are. In particular, actions that promote acceptance over tolerance, a willingness to actively create safe spaces for sexual minority seniors, and embracing diversity will help raise the comfort level of sexual minority seniors in housing and social service arenas. As reported by Cahill and South (2002) the vast majority of the medical profession acknowledged hearing disparaging comments about LGBT patients, and more than half have knowledge of substandard care provided to LGBT seniors. A replication of the health care study cited by Cahill and Spade would help to see if the same problems persist in the same proportion. Such knowledge would aid in the development of programs that will increase the likelihood of LGBT seniors feeling accepted by medical and social service providers.

For the participants in this study, the social context of their environment was more important than the physical environment. A greater understanding of how the social context impacts the lives of sexual minority seniors will help improve interactions with this subset of the senior population.

CONCLUSION

This exploratory study seeks to provide a starting point for understanding why LGBT seniors chose to live in LGBT senior housing and what that housing provides to them. The convenience sample, as with most studies of LGBT aging, limits conclusions and does not allow for generalizability of findings. However, the triangulation of findings from three distinct communities provides some indication as to what some foundational issues may be for LGBT seniors in reference to housing. The key finding of this study was that LGBT seniors were seeking acceptance and community in their domestic environment. *Community*, for those in the LGBT community, has many meanings (Weston, 1991). Isolation continues to plague many LGBT people, and community can mean a simple seeking out of other LGBT people.

Finding community means finding others who are accepting. The knowledge that one will be treated as an equal and accepted in one's domestic environment was important to all participants. Further study of senior housing may reveal if the open and affirming qualities of the three sites studied are unique to LGBT housing or not. In particular, a study of the dominant culture found in traditional retirement communities may further highlight the need for LGBT senior housing. The quality of acceptance made the person–environment fit work in LGBT communities, and this concept would be beneficial to study in other communities in the hope of improving senior housing for all seniors.

REFERENCES

Adelman, M. (1991). Stigma, gay lifestyles and adjustment to aging: A study of later life gay men and lesbians. *Journal of Homosexuality, 20*, 7–32.

Adelman, M., Gurevitch, J., De Vries, B., & Blando, J. (2006). openHouse: Community building and research in the LGBT aging population. In D. Kimmel, T. Rose & S. David (Eds.), *Lesbian, gay, bisexual, and transgender aging research and clinical perspectives* (pp. 247–264). New York, NY: Columbia University Press.

Administration on Aging. (2011). *A profile of older Americans: 2001.* Washington, DC: US Department of Health and Human Services.

Altman, C. (1999) Gay and lesbian seniors: Unique challenges of coming out in later life. *Siecus Report, 27*(3), 14–17.

Baltes, M., Wahl, H.-W., & Schmid-Furstoss, U. (1990). The daily life of elderly Germans: Activity patterns, personal control, and functional health. *Journal of Gerontology: Psychological Sciences, 45*, 173–179.

Beeler, J. A., Rawls, T. D., Herdt, G., & Cohler, B. J. (1999). The needs of older lesbians and gay men in Chicago. *Journal of Gay and Lesbian Social Services, 9*, 31–49.

Berger, R. (1980). Psychological adaptation of the older homosexual male. *Journal of Homosexuality, 5*, 161–175.

Berger, R. (1982). The unseen minority: Older gays and lesbians. *Social Work, 27*, 236–242.

Berger, R. (1984). Realities of gay and lesbian aging. *Social Work, 29*, 57–62.

Berger, R., & Kelly, J. (1986). Working with homosexuals of the older population. *Social Casework, 67*, 203–210.

Blando, J. A., (2001). Twice hidden. *Generations, 25*(2), 87–89.

Boxer, A. M. (1997). Gay, lesbian and bisexual aging into the twenty-first century: An overview and introduction. *Journal of Gay and Lesbian Social Services, 13*, 187–197.

Brotman, S., Ryan, B., & Cormier, R. (2003). The health and social service needs of gay and lesbian elders and their families in Canada. *Gerontologist, 43*, 192–202.

Bulatao, R., & Anderson, N. (2004). *Understanding racial and ethnic differences in health in late life: A research agenda.* Washington, DC: National Academies Press.

Burbank, P., & Burkholder, G. (2006). Health issues of lesbian, gay, bisexual and transgender older adults. In P. Burkholder (Ed.), *Vulnerable older adults health care needs and interventions* (pp. 150–156). New York, NY: Springer.

Burnett, J., Regev, T., Pickens, S., Prati, L. L., Aung, K., Moore, J., & Dyer, C. B. (2006). Social networks: a profile of the elderly who self-neglect. *Journal of Elder Abuse and Neglect, 18*, 35–49.

Cahill, S., & South, K. (2002). Policy issues affecting lesbian, gay, bisexual and transgender people in retirement. *Generations, 26*(20), 49–54.

Carstensen, L. (1992). Social and emotional patterns in adulthood: Support for socioemotional selectivity theory. *Psychology and Aging, 7*, 331–338.

Carstensen, L. (1998). A life-span approach to social motivation. In J. Heckhausen & C. Dweck (Eds.), *Motivation and self-regulation across the life span* (pp. 341–364). Cambridge, UK: University Press.

Carstensen, L., Fung, H., & Charles, S. (2003). Socioemotional selectivity theory and the regulation of emotion in the second half of life. *Motivation and Emotion, 27*, 103–123.

Carstensen, L., Mikels, J., & Mather, M. (2006). Aging and the intersection of cognition, motivation, and emotion. In J. Birren & K. Schaie (Eds.), *Handbook of the psychology of aging* (6th ed., pp. 343–362). Burlington, MA: Elsevier Academic Press.

Cass, V. C. (1979). Homosexual identity formation: A theoretical model. *Journal of Homosexuality, 4*(3), 12–35.

Coleman, E. (1981). Development stages of the coming out process. *Journal of Homosexuality, 7*(2/3), 31–43.

Cruikshank, M. (1991). Lavender and gray: A brief survey of lesbian and gay aging studies. *Journal of Homosexuality, 20*(3/4), 77–88.

De Vries, B. (2006). Home at the end of the rainbow. *Generations, 29*(4), 64–69.

Dorfman, R., Walters, K., Burke, P., Hardin, L., Karanik, T., Raphael, J., & Silverstein, E. (1995). Old, sad and alone: the myth of the homosexual. *Journal of Gerontological Social Work, 24*(1–2), 29–44.

Erikson, E. (1975). *Life history and the historical moment*. New York, NY: W. W. Norton.

Evans, G., Kantrowitz, E., & Eshelman, P. (2002). Housing quality and psychological well-being among the elderly population. *Journal of Gerontology: Psychological Sciences, 57B*, P381–P383.

Fredriksen-Goldsen, K. I., Kim, H.-J., Emlet, C. A., Muraco, A., Erosheva, E. A., Hoy-Ellis, C., Goldsen, J., & Petry, H. (2011). *The aging and health report: disparities and resilience among lesbian, gay, bisexual, and transgender older adults*. Seattle, WA: Institute for Multigenerational Health.

Freund, A., & Baltes, P. (2002). The adaptiveness of selection, optimization, and compensation as strategies of life management: Evidence from a preference study on proverbs. *Journal of Gerontology: Psychological Sciences, 57B*, P426–P434.

Friend, R. A. (1991). Older lesbian and gay people: A theory of successful aging. *Journal of Homosexuality, 20*(3/4), 99–118.

Gabbay, S., & Wahler, J. (2002). Lesbian aging: Review of a growing literature. *Journal of Gay and Lesbian Social Services, 14*(3), 1–21.

Grossman, A., D'Augelli, A., & Hershberger, S. (2000). Social support networks of lesbian, gay and bisexual adults 60 years of age and older. *Journal of Gerontology*, *55B*, 171–179.

Grossman, A., D'Augelli, A., & O'Connell, T. (2001). Being lesbian, gay, bisexual, and 60 or older in North America. *Journal of Gay and Lesbian Social Services*, *13*(4), 23–40.

Hamburger, L. (1997). The wisdom of non-heterosexually based senior housing and related services. *Journal of Gay and Lesbian Social Services*, *6*, 11–25.

Haywood, M., & Zhang, Z. (2001). Demography of aging: A century of global change 1950–2050. In R. Binstock & L. George (Eds.) *Handbook of aging and social science* (Vol. 5, pp. 70–84). San Diego, CA: Academic Press.

Hebert, L. E., Beckett, L. A., Scherr, P. A., & Evans, D. A. (2001). Annual incidence of Alzheimer disease in the United States projected to the years 2000 through 2050. *Alzheimer Disease and Associated Disorders*, *15*, 169–173.

Herdt, G., Beeler, J., & Rawls, T. W. (1997). Life course diversity in older lesbians and gay men: A study in Chicago. *Journal of Gay, Lesbian, Bisexual Identity*, *2*, 231–246.

Herek, G. (2007). Beyond "homophobia": Thinking about sexual prejudice and stigma in the 21st century. *Sexuality Research and Social Policy*, *1*(2), 6–24.

Herek, G., Chopp, R., & Strohl, D. (2007). Sexual stigma: Putting sexual minority health issues in context. In I. Meyer & M. Northridge (Eds.), *The health of sexual minorities: Public health perspectives on lesbian, gay, bisexual, and transgender populations* (pp. 171–208). New York, NY: Springer.

Howard, D., Slone, P., Zimmerman, S., Eckert, K., Walsh, J., Buie, V., . . . Koch, G. (2002). Distribution of African-Americans in residential care/assisted living and nursing homes: More evidence of racial disparity. *American Journal of Public Health*, *92*, 1272–1277.

Hunter, S. (2005). *Midlife and older LGBT adults: Knowledge and affirmative practice for the social services* Binghamton, NY: Haworth.

Jacobs, R., Rasmussen, L., & Hohman, M. (1999). The social support needs of older lesbians, gay men and bisexuals. *Journal of Gay and Lesbian Social Services*, *9*, 1–30.

Katz-Olson, L. (2001). *Age through ethnic lenses*. Lanham, MD: Rowman & Littlefield.

Kehoe, M. (1989). *Lesbians over 60 speak for themselves*. New York, NY: Harrington Park Press.

Kimmel, D. (1978). Adult development and aging: A gay perspective. *Journal of Social Issues*, *43*, 113–130.

Kimmel, D. (1992). The families of older gay men and lesbians. *Generations*, *16*(3), 37–38.

Kimmel, D., Rose, T., Orel, N., & Greene, B. (2006). Historical context for research on lesbian, gay, bisexual, and transgender aging. In D. Kimmel, T. Rose, & S. David (Eds.), *Lesbian, gay, bisexual, and transgender aging research and clinical perspectives* (pp. 1–19). New York, NY: Columbia University Press.

Knickman, J., & Snell, E. (2002). The 2030 problem: Caring for aging baby boomers. *Health Services Research*, *37*, 849–884.

Krause, N. (2001). Social support. In R. Binstock & L. George (Eds.), *Handbook of aging and the social sciences* (pp. 273–294). San Diego, CA: Academic Press.

Lang, F. (2001). Regulation of social relationships in later adulthood. *Journal of Gerontology: Psychological Sciences, 56B*, P321–P326.

Lang, F., Rieckmann, N., & Baltes, M. (2002). Adapting to aging losses: Do resources facilitate strategies of selection, compensation, and optimization in everyday functioning? *Journal of Gerontology: Psychological Sciences, 57B*, P501–P509.

Langley, J. (2001). Developing anti-oppressive empowering social work practice with older lesbian women and gay men. *British Journal of Social Work, 31*, 917–932.

Los Angeles Department of Aging. (2011). *Needs assessment survey* [Unpublished raw data].

Lucco, A. J. (1987). Planned housing preferences of elder homosexuals. *Journal of Homosexuality, 14*(3/4), 35–55.

Minnigerode, F. A., & Adelman, M. (1978). Elderly homosexual women and men: A report on a pilot study. *Family Coordinator, 27*, 451–456.

Orel, N. (2004). Gay, lesbian, and bisexual elders: Expressed needs and concerns across focus groups. *Journal of Gerontological Social Work, 43*(2–3), 57–77.

Orel, N. (2006). Lesbian and bisexual women as grandparents: The centrality of sexual orientation in the grandparent-grandchild relationship. In D. Kimmel, T. Rose, & S. David (Eds.), *Lesbian, gay, bisexual, and transgender aging research and clinical perspectives* (pp. 175–194). New York, NY: Columbia University Press.

Peacock, J. R. (2000). Gay male adult development: Some stage issues of an older cohort. *Journal of Homosexuality, 40*(2), 13–29.

Perissinotto, C., Cenzer, I., & Covinsky, K. (2011). Loneliness in older persons a predictor of functional decline and death. *Archives of Internal Medicine, 172*, 1078–1084.

Quam, J. (1993). Gay and lesbian aging. *Siecus Report, 21*(5), 10–12.

Quam, J. (2001). Adaptation and age related expectations of older gay and lesbian adults. *Gerontologist, 32*, 367–374.

Rosenfeld, D. (1999). Identity work among lesbians and gay elderly. *Journal of Aging Studies, 13*, 121–140.

Scheidt, R., & Norris-Baker, C. (2003). Many meanings of community: Contributions of M. Powell Lawton. *Journal of Housing for the Elderly, 17*, 55–66.

Shippy, A., Cantor, M., & Brennan, M. (2004). Social networks of gay men. *Journal of Men's Studies, 13*, 107–120.

Slusher, M. P., Mayer, C. J., & Dunkle, R. E. (1996). Gays and lesbians: Older and wiser (GLOW): A support group for older gay people. *Gerontologist, 36*, 118–123.

Stein, G., Beckerman, N., & Sherman, P. (2010). Lesbian and gay elders and long-term care: identifying the unique psychosocial perspectives and challenges. *Journal of Gerontological Social Work, 53*, 421–435.

Strauss, A., & Corbin, J. (1998). *Basics of qualitative research: Techniques and procedures for developing grounded theory* (2nd ed.). Thousand Oaks, CA: Sage.

Sullivan, K., & Neal, M. (2005, November). *Queer aging: Aging literature of lesbian, gay, bisexual and transgender people*. Presentation at the Gerontological Society of America Annual Conference, Orlando, FL.

Taylor, I., & Robertson, A. (1994). The health needs of gay men: a discussion of the literature and implications for nursing. *Journal of Advanced Nursing, 20,* 560–566.

Thoits, P. (1995). Stress, coping, and social support processes: Where are we? What's next? *Journal of Health and Social Behavior, 35*(Extra Issue), 53–79.

Tully, C. T. (1989). Caregiving: What do midlife lesbians view as important? *Journal of Gay and Lesbian Psychotherapy, 1,* 87–103.

US Census Bureau. (2007). *U.S. census state and city quick facts.* Retrieved October 15, 2010 from http://quickfacts.census.gov/qfd/states/35/3570500.html

US Department of Commerce. (2001). *US census: Profile of general demographic characteristics.* Washington, DC: US Census Bureau.

Wahler, J., & Gabbay, S. G. (1997). Gay male aging: A review of the literature. *Journal of Gay and Lesbian Social Services, 6*(3), 1–20.

Weston, K. (1991). *Families we choose: Lesbians, gays kinship.* New York, NY: Columbia University Press.

Williams, S. W., & Dilworth-Anderson, P. (2002). Systems of social support in families who care for dependent African-American elders. *Gerontologist, 42,* 224–233.

The Highs and Lows of Caregiving for Chronically Ill Lesbian, Gay, and Bisexual Elders

ANNA MURACO

Department of Sociology, Loyola Marymount University, Los Angeles, California, USA

KAREN I. FREDRIKSEN-GOLDSEN

School of Social Work, University of Washington, Seattle, Washington, USA

This study examines informal caregivers' and LGB care recipients' best and worst experiences of care within their relationship. Communal relationship theory guides the research. The work uses qualitative interview data from a sample of 36 care pairs (N = 72), divided between committed partners and friends, to understand the similarities and differences in the care norms employed in varied relationship contexts. Findings from the study show that relationship context influences the experiences that caregivers and care recipients identify as best and worst, but often focus on the relationship and needs met at bests, and conflict and fear of worsening health as worsts.

Caregiving, which includes hands-on personal care, instrumental assistance with household needs, and emotional support (Wrubel & Folkman, 1997), has been the focus of many academic studies. Typically, studies that address the significance of the relational contexts of care focus on spousal dyads, adult child–parent relationships, and neighbors (Barker, 2002). Little of the existing research, however, has addressed the relational context in caregiving for lesbian, gay, and bisexual (LGB) adults age 50 and older, an understudied population that differs from other populations due to its invisibility, marginalization, unique types of support systems, and lack of legal protections. Both sexual orientation and the context of the caregiving relationship (i.e., relationships between committed partners and friends, straight and LGB) are expected to have an influence on the perception, experiences, and quality of care.

This study focuses on the care experiences indicated to be the best and worst informal care experiences according to both care recipients and caregivers, and contextualizes these experiences within the theory of communal relationships. The evaluation of best and worst instances in the contexts of caregiving by the study participants in both committed partnerships and friendships serves as a vehicle for attaining a deeper understanding of the ways that individuals experience care within the relational context. Asking the participants, both caregivers and care recipients, to identify and describe the best and worst experiences of care revealed a wealth of thematic material that serves as a basis of this study. Our work uses interview data from a sample of 36 pairs of older LGB care recipients and their informal (unpaid) caregivers, who consist of either a committed partner or a friend ($N = 72$) to understand how the care recipients and caregivers differently perceive and experience noteworthy moments in the caregiving process. Theoretically, we engage theories of reciprocity and social exchange and conclude that Clark's (1981) theory of communal relationships provides the optimal framework for understanding the dynamics that occur in these informal care relationships. The article concludes with a discussion of implications for practice, given our findings.

There are more than 62 million caregivers providing unpaid care in the United States, at an estimated economic value of more than $450 billion (Feinberg, Reinhard, Houser, & Choula, 2011). There are likely more than 2 million US older adults that self-identify as LGB (Cahill, South, & Spade, 2000; Fredriksen-Goldsen et al., 2011). The exponential growth of the 50 and older population in the next 2 decades suggests the number of LGB older adults may more than double by 2030 (Fredriksen-Goldsen, et al., 2011), yet, the informal caregiving of sexual minority adults 50 and older has received limited attention.

The existing research on LGB caregiving illustrates that formal services are less often utilized than in other populations; additionally, the duration of the care provided by friends or extended kin relationships may be shorter (Coon, Thompson, Steffen, Soccoro, & Gallagher-Thompson, 2003; Family Caregiver Alliance, 2002). The relational aspect of informal caregiving, which is the relational context in which the care occurs, affects the perceived quality and challenges inherent in the care context. Informal caregiving, for the purposes of this study, is defined as hands-on personal care (e.g., assistance with dressing or bathing), instrumental assistance with household needs (e.g., housekeeping, transportation, and coordination of care), and emotional support (e.g., emotional reassurance) provided by a committed partner or spouse, friend, or community member who is neither paid nor a volunteer affiliated with a service organization.

REVIEW OF LITERATURE

Much research on caregiving has been built on the theoretical foundations of stress and coping theories or on sociological theories of work. When studies focus on the relational contexts in which care takes place, they typically address heterosexual spouses and adult child–parent relationships (Adams, McClendon, & Smyth, 2008; Guada, Hoe, Floyd, Barbour, & Brekke, 2012) and tend to focus on either caregiver or care recipient perceptions, not both. When care recipient characteristics and outcomes have been examined, the care recipient and caregiver outcomes and burdens tend to be viewed as separate from their relational interactions (Coeling, Biordi, & Theis, 2003; Cox & Dooley, 1996; Lyons, Zarit, Sayer, & Whitlatch, 2002; Pruchno, Burant, & Peters, 1997). Often, studies fail to consider the recipient of care as an active participant in the dyadic care process (Lyons, et al., 2002; Sauter, 1996), which ignores a primary player in the care relationship and limits our understanding of the relational context of caregiving.

For heterosexuals, marital spouses are most commonly selected to provide care when needed due to norms of intimacy (Allen, Goldscheider, & Ciambrone, 1999), care, and commitment (Cancian, 1987) within marital relationships. LGB adults' ability to marry a same-sex partner has been legally limited (or prohibited), although relationship norms consistent with marital relationships appear to govern same-sex partnerships in that when asked to whom they would turn to for caregiving needs, older LGB adults would first turn to partners, then to friends and other family members (Cahill et al., 2000).

Perceived reciprocity or mutuality in the relationship as a pattern of exchange characterized by the giving and receiving of assistance affects relationship quality. In a dyadic relationship the caregiver and care recipient agree, over time, upon a mutually, generally unspoken, defined set of rules or norms that govern their interactions (Coeling et al., 2003; LeBlanc & Wight, 2000). Mutuality can exist even if both dyad members do not contribute equally, because caregiving conditions change over time. Norms of obligation and generalized rules of reciprocity are more salient in spousal and parent–child relationships than among extended kin or friends (Call, Finch, Huck, & Kane, 1999; Coeling, et al., 2003). On the other hand, level of perceived support, rather than actual support, may be salient among the extended friendship network of LGB older adults (LeBlanc & Wight, 2000).

Communal Relationships

Some studies about caregiving for older adults have framed the discussion using exchange theories of relationships (Ingersoll-Dayton & Antonucci, 1988; Walker, Pratt, & Oppy, 1992), which focus on the importance of power and reciprocity in dyadic relationships. With respect to caregiving relationships, the receipt of help perpetuates a power dynamic where the caregiver has more power vis-à-vis the care recipient, even when the care relationship occurs among committed relationship partners. Such power relations may extend to decision-making about the provision of care in covert ways (Pyke, 1999) and affect the everyday interactions within the care dyad (Beel-Bates, Ingersoll-Dayton, & Nelson, 2007).

A theoretical framework related to exchange theory that elucidates the dynamics in caregiver–care recipient relationships, especially in the case of LGB older adults, is the communal relationships theory. According to Clark (1981), communal relationships constitute an implicit agreement to take care of one another to the best of their ability, with less significance placed on how much any one person expects reciprocation from the relationship. In the case of committed partners, care recipients may use the expression of vulnerable emotion (i.e., anxiety, fear, sadness) to communicate their needs, rather than to defer power, to the caregivers. Expressing gratitude to a partner enhances perception of the relationship's communal strength (Lambert, Clark, Durtschi, Fincham, & Graham, 2010). Prior findings show that in communal relationships, expressions of vulnerability may signal: (a) a need and desire for care, (b) a lack of need or the success of care, (c) appreciation of care, or (d) love and care for the partner (Clark, Fitness, & Brisette, 2001; Graham, Huang, Clark, & Helgeson, 2008). Among married couples expressing vulnerable emotions, reports of less caregiving stress and greater sensitivity to the care recipient's needs by caregiving spouses led to greater feelings of being mutually cared for by both spouses (Clark et al., 2001; Graham et al., 2008; Monin, Martire, Schulz, & Clark, 2009).

In the case of LGB older adults who need care, communal relationship theory explains why friends, neighbors, and community members step up to provide care for others with seemingly little to gain from the interaction. Clark explained the dynamics of communal relationships:

> Since at any given time, the needs and preferences of members of a communal relationship are unlikely to be exactly the same, members should be unlikely to give and receive exactly comparable benefits within a short period. Indeed, members may actively avoid giving benefits directly comparable to benefits they may have recently received since

doing so might imply a preference for a different and less valued type of relationship. (Clark, 1981, p. 375)

In LGB older adult populations, committed partners are cited as the most common caregivers, followed by friends as the second more common relational type (Cahill et al., 2000; Cantor, Brennan & Shippy, 2004), yet the balance of exchanges may vary when chronic illness and caregiving are involved.

Based on the literature, we decided to explore the relational aspects of the caregiving relationships for older LGB adults and elucidate the norms, both formal and informal, that regulate these relationships. We asked our sample a range of questions about their caregiving experiences, which ranged from the challenges they faced to the day-to-day actions that comprise caregiving. Here, we focus on the events that participants identified as best and worst in their interviews because these questions address some of the challenges and rewards that both caregivers and care recipients experience in the contexts of care. Moreover, these questions illuminate the often unspoken norms employed by caregivers and care recipients in navigating informal care relationships.

METHOD

Participants

The interview data that guide this research were collected in 2005–06 in an urban area of Washington state. Trained researchers interviewed a sample of 36 pairs of older LGB care recipients and their caregivers ($N = 72$). For the purposes of this research, *care recipient* was defined as a self-identified LGB adult, age 50 or older, who requires assistance with daily needs. *Caregiver* was defined as the person designated by the LGB older adult as the informal helper who assists most with daily needs, and is neither paid nor a volunteer affiliated with a service organization and could include committed partners or friends. The caregiver was required to be age 18 or older, but did not need to be of sexual minority status. Only the primary informal caregiver to the older adult participated in the study.

Participants were recruited through an extensive search of community and health services that cater to older adults or LGB individuals. Specifically, we recruited participants by sending e-mails, posting flyers, and making presentations in locations where the targeted populations were expected to frequent (e.g., health clinics, support groups, buddy programs, community-based churches, and social groups). Recruiting from various sites minimized biases compared to relying on a sample drawn solely from one site, such as a support group or health clinic. The recruitment materials stated that participants would be paid $25 each for their time and participation in the study.

Procedures

Prior to the onset of the study, the Institutional Review Boards of our respective institutions approved all procedures. Face-to-face interviews were conducted with chronically ill LGB older adults and their caregivers at a time and location of their choice where privacy could be insured. The older adults and their caregivers were interviewed in separate rooms, but simultaneously, to insure that dyad members did not influence each other's responses. The interviews lasted between 75 and 90 min and were audio recorded with the permission of the participants. Interviewers were trained in the social and behavioral sciences and experienced working with lesbian, gay male, and bisexual populations. Interviewers also were trained in methods and techniques for effective interviewing of adults with functional disabilities and their caregivers.

The interviews were conducted face-to-face in the location of the participants' choosing. As such, we conducted interviews in public spaces (such as libraries and cafes), in private homes, and in the university research offices. Prior to beginning the interview, the caregiver and care recipient reviewed and signed an informed consent form. At the end of the interview, each participant was paid $25 as a token of appreciation for her or his time and participation in the study.

Open-ended qualitative questions were asked at the termination of a series of quantitative questions, about an hour into the interview period. The interview began with the interviewer asking the participant a series of quantitative survey questions, which are not being addressed in this study, but have been published elsewhere (see Fredriksen-Goldsen, Kim, Muraco, & Mincer, 2009). The quantitative questions included standard measures of physical and mental health, the types of illnesses and disabilities that required care, and measures of dyadic relationship quality. By the point in the interview when the interviewer asked open-ended questions, the interviewer and the participant had developed a degree of rapport. The open-ended questions addressed a range of topics about the nature of care and the ways that care affected the relationship. The questions for the caregiver that provided the most fruitful data for this study were: "Please describe the best experience you've had providing care for [care recipient]" and "Please describe the worst experience you've had providing care for [care recipient]." The questions for the care recipient that provided the majority of data for this study were: "Please describe your best experience of receiving care from [caregiver]" and "Please describe your worst experience of receiving care from [caregiver]."

The qualitative interview data were transcribed verbatim and then coded by examining responses to a series of questions. The data are exploratory in that they address experiences of LGB care recipients, age 50 and older, and their caregivers, who are either committed partners or friends. Given the difficulty in recruiting this largely invisible population, we established the greatest possible sample that was available at the time of recruitment; therefore, the standard qualitative benchmark of saturation was not the sampling goal. The experiences of this sample are not intended to be representative of all LGB adults age 50 and over, nor are they generalizable to other populations; rather the findings from this study can help one to better understand the norms that guide the caregiving context of the sample.

The data were coded through the process of open coding (LaRossa, 2005), where the material was reviewed repeatedly to identify common themes or concepts that emerged from the interviews. In particular, we carefully examined the interview data and then created subcodes for the most common themes related to the relationships between partners and friends who provide and receive care. We conducted the initial phase of open coding; subsequently, an undergraduate research assistant performed a second round of coding according to the themes we had identified. In the final phase of coding, we reviewed the research assistant's coding to reach the final analysis of the data. To provide structure to the coding process, we used NVivo 8, a qualitative data analysis program.

RESULTS

The self-identified relationship context of the caregiving pairs ($N = 36$) was 50% committed partners, 47% friends, and 3% other, including neighbors and others. The sample characteristics by age for care recipients was 74% age 50–59, 17% age 60–69, and 9% age 70 and older; for caregivers 69% was under age 50, 17% age 50–59, 8% age 60–69, and 6% age 70 and older. In terms of ethnicity, approximately 50% of both the care recipients and caregivers were Caucasian, 20% of the care recipients and 31% of the caregivers were African American, 17% of care recipients and 13% of caregivers were multiethnic, 9% of care recipients were Latino, 3% of caregivers were Asian, and 3% of both care recipients and caregivers were Native American. The sexual orientation of the care recipients was 67% lesbian or gay and 33% bisexual; the caregivers were 63% lesbian or gay, 17% bisexual, and 20% heterosexual.

The relationship characteristics of the committed partnership portion of the sample by relationship type and gender ($n = 18$) are as follows: 50% of the committed partnerships were male/male, 33% of were female/female, and 16% were male/female (one transgender individual and two bisexual individuals were members of these partnerships). Of the dyads characterized as friends or other ($n = 18$), 50% were male/male, 44% were female/female, and 22% were male/female. Of the male/female friendship dyads ($n = 4$), 25% were comprised of a male care recipient and a female caregiver, and 75% were comprised of a female care recipient and a male caregiver.

Care recipient participants suffer from one or more of the following conditions: mental condition including bipolar, schizophrenia, and depression (66.6%); HIV/AIDS (62.5%); arthritis (44%); high blood pressure (37.5%); diabetes (31.5%); and Alzheimer's disease (18.5%). Most of the sample of care recipients had three or four of the aforementioned conditions. In a typical week, 17% of caregivers provided care for 4 hr or less, 14% provided 5-9 hr, 31% provided 10-19 hr, and 38% provided 20 or more hr.

The themes that emerged from the qualitative data are presented here according to the dyads comprised of committed partners and friends. We make this analytical distinction because there are relational differences between partnerships and friendships, which affect the contexts in which caregiving is performed. In particular, given prior research findings, caregiving in the context of a partnership is an implicit relationship expectation, although caregiving in friendship embodies the norm of caring for each other, but may have limits to the care friends are willing to give over the long term, especially when decision-making is required (Muraco & Fredriksen-Goldsen, 2011).

Partners: Care Recipients' Best and Worst Experiences

One of the most common themes present in the qualitative data was that the care recipients perceived the best experiences of caregiving in terms of the relationship context. In particular, many of the best caregiving experiences were identified as expressions of love and commitment to the relationship. One care recipient noted that the best experience of receiving care is found in the caregiving partner's "love ... the willingness to do anything that's needed." Other care recipients found it difficult to identify one particular best experience:

> On the one hand, the whole thing's been a good experience; he's seen me through a hell of a lot and he's not walked away. He works to understand. And I guess you do see deeper and deeper [commitment] as time goes on, and I want to be able to return it, too. I can certainly see his commitment to me, you know, that he's stayed with me through some of the stresses that he's had to go through. It helps me understand the depth of the commitment that's there, and I would certainly do the same for him.

Here, we see that to the care recipient, the caregiver's ongoing assistance comprises the best experience because it signifies strength and commitment in the relationship.

Another common experience identified as the best by care recipients was the caregiving partners' recognition and fulfillment of needs, both day-to-day and in crises. One lesbian care recipient said that the best experience of receiving care is that her partner cooks her meals. Another gay male care recipient noted that his partner is "very conscious of my likes and dislikes. . . . He's very considerate and has an eye out for things for me that he thinks I would like. So it's more an ongoing thing than just a single example." Some of the care recipients' best experiences of care were more notable instances when caregivers saw a developing health crisis and responded immediately. One gay male care recipient remembered his best experience:

> Probably last month when I had rapid heart beat, because I woke up in the morning and I knew something was wrong but I wasn't sure what it was, but he immediately, when he woke up, just called 911 and that was it. So he just took care of it there on the spot.

In part, the care recipients acknowledge the categorization of optimum caregiving is related to fear of managing the difficult circumstances of their illnesses. One lesbian care recipient explained,

> I would say there would be times that I was absolutely terrified and she would still be there, and that could be as simple as trying to take a bath when I had parts of me that couldn't have water on them. And she always managed to pull it off.

The most common response to the question of the worst caregiving experience by care recipient partners was that there was "no worst experience." When care recipient partners were able to identify a worst experience, it tended to either be a pointedly embarrassing situation they had endured (especially those dealing with incontinence) or a feeling of being a burden to the caregiver. One lesbian care recipient explained that the worst experience was, "When I lost control of myself and wet the bed and everything, and that was so embarrassing. And of course she had to take care of me." A gay male care recipient similarly explained,

> Well, it's only been bad when the experience is bad. You know, like when you're incontinent and things are a mess and he'll help me into the shower and then help clean up the bed and everything. That's the—I mean, he doesn't mind doing it, it's very seldom it's happened, but that's like the worst.

Others acknowledge that they worry about being a burden to their partner. One lesbian care recipient explained, "I just feel like sometimes [my partner] wants to give up—and I wouldn't blame her." Another noted that the most frustrating experiences are when she has to ask her partner for assistance, "Knowing she's going to be irritated, but having to ask."

Partners: Caregivers' Best and Worst Experiences

Like care recipients, caregiving partners also focus on the best experiences of caregiving in terms of the relationship context. In particular, many of the best caregiving experiences were identified as those that represent the love and commitment they have for their partner. One gay male caregiver said, "I hope it doesn't sound trite, but every day that I wake up with him is the best experience. . . . It's the fact that he's still here." Other caregivers identify the best experiences as being able to provide enjoyment by going on trips or outings that the care recipient would not be able to attend otherwise. A lesbian caregiver noted that the best experience was when she was able to help her partner attend a local music festival that she greatly enjoyed by figuring out how to navigate the grounds, setting up transportation, and bringing her food. Other caregiving partners considered the best experiences to be their ability to provide financial and emotional support to their partner. As one lesbian caregiver explained,

> OK, the best thing I think that I've done is that I'm in a position where she does not have to work. And so that was the main thing, because she got fired after so many years because of the headaches and not being able to function. So that just caused her a lot of fear—How am I going to support myself? So I stepped in and I was helping her along.

Another lesbian caregiver reiterated that the best experiences occur in the day-to-day actions of caregiving and being a partner, rather than in more grandiose activities:

> I think it's just the support that I provide her, overall. I mean, you're talking about the best kind of caregiving and that kind of thing, but it's just every day. I think it's the overall support that I can provide her and do provide her.

One of the ways in which the caregiving partners most differed from other respondents was in identifying difficult and conflict-filled moments in caregiving as best experiences. Some caregiving partners reported their awareness that their relationship was different because of the illness, yet the couple would survive the challenge. One gay male caregiver explained:

> It was one of those cathartic moments; he had come home from the hospital after about a 4-day stay, and was on a whole lot of medication which was making him absolutely stupid as well as nauseous and incontinent. And besides holding down a fulltime job . . . and I was just getting so angry and frustrated and we were both that way. And I started to lose it; I just started to scream. He started to cry, and I just realized then that it was OK for another human being to depend on someone, particularly me, and that I could do this and that if given all the choices in the world,

he would not ever want to be a 3-year-old again and how hard it was for him to have to ask for help. It was one of those great moments of inner growth, and growth on both parts, where we both let go our expectations that were no longer reasonable in the situation that existed, and became OK with it.

A similar type of best experience identified by caregiving partners was when they experienced physical vulnerability, which caused them to better understand themselves and empathize with their partners' limitations. One gay male caregiver explained that he had broken his ankle and was on crutches at the same time his partner was in a wheelchair for his chronic condition. He noted,

> I think that's one of the most memorable [experiences], because for the first time I could really understand where he was, I could understand that—OK, you had the mobility really jacked up—I broke my ankle and my mobility was really jacked up, I realized how bad this feels, when something like that's taken away. But I then felt guilt about that, too, because I knew mine was going to correct itself and his wasn't.

The worst experiences acknowledged by the caregiving partners related to their own limitations. Some caregivers focused on fear of being unable to take care of their partner or that their partner's health would worsen. Some of the worst experiences were based on actual events that had occurred; for example, one caregiving partner recalled not being able to lift his partner out of the bathtub, which made him realize that his partner had needs that he could not meet. A lesbian caregiving partner admitted that, sometimes, pushing her partner's wheelchair is physically exhausting, especially when going up and down hills. Other caregivers' fears centered on worries about their partners' declining health. One lesbian caregiving partner said, "I don't like it that her health is going downhill and I'm afraid for her health, I'm just totally worried." One gay male caregiving partner recalled that it was difficult to see his partner in so much pain during a particularly bad spell.

Partners less frequently, but still commonly, reported worst experiences of conflict and feelings of frustration. One gay male caregiver noted that an argument occurred when his partner was feeling like he was not able to fully contribute to the relationship, "And I don't remember how things were worded exactly, but I had said something that made him feel like I had called him stupid. . . . We slept in separate beds that night. That was the worst." Other caregiving partners described overwhelming caregiving circumstances as being their worst experiences. For example, one lesbian caregiver recalled an instance where her partner fell out of bed and broke both of her feet:

> When it gets very bad is when in a period of a week she's got so many conditions that there will be a crisis with this condition, a crisis with that condition, like three different urgent things and I'm trying to be there

with her in some way with all of them and it's just absolutely exhausting. That's very hard for me.

Friends: Care Recipients' Best and Worst Experiences

Similar to the partners, those who receive care from friends identify best experiences of care to be related to their relationship, as well as the recognition and fulfillment of needs. One care recipient commented that the best experiences of care by his caregiver occurs when they attend concerts together

> and we're both sort of connected to the event in the same way, she has a way of nudging me that is like a very loving nudge, and a happy nudge, too, that I translate into her openness of being able to do such an act, and also we're not making anything out of it as being a sexual thing it's just—I enjoy your company and I'm very happy that I'm here to have this wonderful time right now.

Care recipients also identified the best experiences as those in which they felt taken care of by their caregiving friend. One gay male care recipient explained that when he was hospitalized, none of his family members came to visit and, "all the things that they should have done, could have done, ought to have done – [my friend] did that." Another gay male care recipient reported that his caregiving friend is, "Always there if I call him. He calls me every morning. . . . And if I don't answer, he'll get in the car and just drive here." The consistent care and connection with the caregiving friend seems to be important in classifying an event as the best. Other care recipients remembered the best experience of caregiving as special efforts taken by the friend. One gay male care recipient identified the best experience of caregiving happened when his friend baked chicken at home and brought it to him while he was in the hospital. Others noted their best experiences occurred when their friends fill prescriptions for them and go to the store and buy groceries for them.

Similar to the care recipient partners, the care recipient friends' most common response to the question about the worst care experience was "none." The few care recipient friends who identified a worst care experience indicated that there have been conflicts with the caregiver; for example, one care recipient said, "Overall she's been a very positive influence, but on a couple of occasions we've had some blowups. I guess that's the closest thing I can [identify as] a problem."

Friends: Caregivers' Best and Worst Experiences

Many of the caregiving friends characterized the best experiences of caregiving as related to relatively ordinary interactions within the friendship, such as spending time together or providing emotional support. One caregiver said that the best caregiving experiences happen when they are simply "hanging out" together,

> When we're just sitting around and laughing and talking about what's going on. But the laughing part, I think it far outweighs any grocery-shopping trip. I mean, when we go to the store, we hop a bus and it's just the company, our company.

Another caregiver noted, "Just some normal friendship things that friends do."

A second theme to emerge from caregiving friends' best experiences was instances of help from the caregiver, both in day-to-day and in serious situations. The caregiver's assistance ranged from keeping them company in hospital waiting rooms to taking action that ultimately saved their lives. One caregiving gay male friend noted that he reminds the care recipient to take his medication and helps him to understand his doctors' orders. Another caregiver, a lesbian friend, recalled a very frightening scene with her friend:

> I went to see her and she was really cold. . . . For the most part she doesn't go out or she's confined to her bed, but this time she's in the bed and under the covers with a sweater on just freezing and I called 911 and had her taken to the hospital. . . . She was in real danger and she could have had kidney failure; they probably could have shut down. She just thought she was cold and she couldn't get warm and I felt good that I could just come and [take care of her]—I thought, "This is not natural," and she said, "Oh, I'll be all right," and I'm like, "No, you won't; I'm calling 911."

In these instances, caregiving friends felt good about the assistance they were able to provide to friends in times of real need.

Personal benefit was one final best experience identified by caregiving friends. In particular, friends responded that caregiving makes them feel good about themselves. One lesbian caregiver noted that when her friend came out of surgery, she was waiting for her: "When she came out, she looked up smiling with no teeth; that was my best experience because I felt, I don't know, I felt needed." Another way that caregivers articulated the best experiences was by explaining how providing assistance to their friend improved their self-esteem. One male caregiver noted, "Now, this is going to sound greedy, but . . . it raises my self esteem that I'm helping somebody."

Some of the worst experiences voiced by the caregiving friends were conflicts brought about by misunderstandings and short tempers. Others' comments reflected concerns about acute or worsening illnesses. One of the caregivers recalled the worst experience as being one where her friend was far sicker than she'd understood,

189

[The neighbor] called 911 and took her to the hospital and she'd had a heart attack. . . . She is ill so much of the time that I sort of play it off in my head that it's not quite as bad as she says it is. But when I saw her in that bed with all the tubes and a ventilator on and all the tubes going into her arms and her nose—it was very scary, pretty scary for me.

Fear about the care recipient friends' actions also were designated as some of the worst experiences by caregivers. In particular, one caregiver noted that his hospitalized friend called him to tell him that he was going to pull out all of his tubes and leave the hospital. The friend recalled, "I was trying to talk to him, tell him 'Please don't leave the hospital. If you take the tubes out, you could die.'" Serious past situations also had arisen where the care recipient indicated that they wanted to end their own life. One caregiver said, without hesitation, that the worst situation arose when the care recipient tried to kill herself. She explained, "I didn't know if I should call 911 or not," which reflects her concern about whether or not she should honor her friend's wishes. Another caregiver encountered a related situation, where her friend told her that she wanted to end her life because no one cared. The friend responded: "I'm here. I care. That's selfish to think that when you at least have one friend. Most people don't even have a friend in life."

In summary, there were many similarities, but also differences between the experiences that caregivers and care recipients, both partners and friends, identified as the best and worst. The most common best experiences to be identified by all dyad types, that is partners and friends, and by both caregivers and care recipients were related to the relationship itself, rather than any specific act or circumstance. For care recipients, having needs met by either a partner or friend were also commonly expressed as best experiences. Care recipients also most commonly noted that there were no worst experiences in caregiving by partners or friends. Some differences between partner and friend care dyads were expressed. Conflict was uniformly identified in terms of worst experiences for friend dyads, whereas partners sometimes indicated that conflict was a worst experience, but other times noted that conflict or challenges were best experiences because they drew the partners together or raised the caregiver's level of empathy. Finally, caregiving friends were the only group of participants that identified personal benefit as a component of a best care experience.

DISCUSSION

Approaching the care relationship as a communal relationship, rather than an exchange relationship, allows for a greater understanding of the expectations of caregiving experiences for both the caregiver and care recipient. Although the participants in this study did not address how they define caregiving and the inherent expectations in their own words, we can glean from their evaluations of the most and least optimum care experiences what they view as central or normative to caregiving. As such, this study is exploratory in that we examine what caregivers and care recipients identify as the best and worst experiences of care that they have encountered in their particular care relationship.

Differences by Relationship Context

Within the partnership dyad, the description of best and worst experiences differs for the caregiver and the care recipient, which is to be expected given the findings of prior studies that address issues such as caregiver stress (Pearlin, Mullan, Semple, & Skaff, 1990), as well as care recipients' emotional strain and deferential actions (Beel-Bates et al., 2007; Newsom & Schulz, 1998). Interestingly, rather than focusing on experiences of care, which was the basis of the interview prompt, a majority of care recipients and caregivers who were partners instead focused on the best experiences of caregiving as representative of relationship commitment. In contrast, when discussing worst experiences of caregiving, caregiving partners were more likely to address their own fears and shortcomings in ably dealing with the needs of their partner. Care recipients typically downplayed the worst experiences of receiving care saying that they had "no bad experiences." Those who did identify worst experiences of caregiving identified feeling burdensome and embarrassment at the root of the events.

In this study, caregivers in both partner and friend dyads were able or willing to articulate various best and worst experiences with more frequency than the care recipients. In partnership dyads and friendship dyads alike, the care recipients were most likely to respond that there were "no worst experiences" in their caregiving relationship. Viewing the care recipient's inability or unwillingness to name a worst experience through the lens of the communal relationship theory, the assistance they receive fits within their expectations of care from a partner or friend. Because they do not expect any more than the caregiver provides, they do not view any experiences as particularly negative.

Differences and Similarities in Norms and Experiences

Different norms govern the partnership and friendship dyads; this finding is reasonable, given the greater level of commitment between the caregiver and care recipient to their relationship. In particular, caregiving partners tend to identify conflict, and the growth that emerges from the negotiation of conflict, as best, rather than worst experiences. Such an evaluation relates to prior studies' (Clark et al., 2001; Graham et al., 2008) identification of vulnerable expressions as barometers of the communal relationship, such that a care recipient's voicing of a need for care or the lack of need for a particular type of care can affect the caregiving dynamic. The conflicts described by the caregivers typically were related to uncertainty that they could effectively meet the needs of their care recipient partner. For instance, one caregiver explained that because of a particularly pointed conflict, he and his care recipient partner both let go of their expectations that were no longer reasonable, given the condition of the care recipient's health. In so doing, both the caregiver and care recipient expressed vulnerability, which improved their ability to navigate the new challenges that arose in the care relationship and thus, strengthened their relationship.

Another common theme to emerge from the data is that both the caregivers and care recipients in partnership dyads identify best experiences as connected to the relationship and commitment they share, rather than any singular high point in giving or receiving care. When partner caregivers do identify a best experience, they often refer to a circumstance where they were able to provide a pleasurable event for the care recipient or a time when they felt satisfaction that they could meet a care recipient's needs. The care recipients, on the other hand, point to the day-to-day ways that the caregivers meet their needs and are willing and able to help in a crisis.

Breaches in Relationship Norms

The worst experiences, according to partnered caregivers and care recipients, were those in which the relationship expectations or the care aspects of the relationships were breached. In particular, the caregivers identified the worst experiences as those where they felt that they could not meet the needs of the care recipient and conversely, the care recipients noted the worst experiences as ones filled with embarrassment or where they felt bothersome. The norms of the communal relationship suggest that when a person takes a caregiving role, they make an implicit agreement to provide care to the best of their abilities (Clark, 1981). If a caregiver feels that she was unable to meet the needs of the care recipient, for example, then she may feel as if she has not upheld the agreement, regardless of whether the demands she experienced were too great to accomplish. The communal relationship theory also helps to understand that a care recipient's embarrassment related to her incontinence is a physical, rather than emotional, form of vulnerability that is not accounted for in the normative relationship expectations of care undertaken by adult peers. Were the needs voiced in a vulnerable emotional manner, they would be considered a care recipient's expression of appreciation for the caregiver's actions (Clark et al., 2001; Graham et al., 2008). Because the circumstance (incontinence) emerged from an inability to manage one's physical self, it represents a breach of relationship norms and, thus, is viewed as a particularly negative experience of care based on the care recipient's, rather than caregiver's failing.

Benefits to Care Recipients and Caregivers

Similar to the findings of the partnership dyads, both caregivers and care recipients in friendship dyads identify the best care experiences as relational, related to everyday support and valued time spent together. In contrast to the partnership dyads, caregiving friends are more likely to articulate their own feelings of increased self-esteem as a benefit gained from providing help to a friend. Perhaps the self-focus has to do with validation of membership in a communal relationship; by participating in a process that signals a communal tie, the caregiver's own status in a communal system is reinforced. A second way that caregiving friends focus on their own benefit from providing care is in framing the best experiences of caregiving as being able to meet real needs of their friends, which also corresponds with the communal norm of providing care to the best of one's ability.

The care recipient friends most commonly note the best experiences as related to the ability to rely upon the friend as a safety net that stands between them and an unmet need for care. Others point to feeling cared for as a best experience provided by their caregiving friend. Both of these findings illustrate the care recipient reliance upon communal relationship norms, which suggests that when in need, they will find willing community members who will provide care. Unfortunately, there also exists the possibility that the care recipients may have to rely upon different community members to provide care over time, as research shows that there are limits to some friends' willingness or ability to provide unlimited care (Muraco & Fredriksen-Goldsen, 2011).

Conflict

One of the most notable differences between partnership and friendship dyads in the study is in the focus on the outcomes for the partnership versus the outcomes for individuals, which is illustrated in the way that the dyads view conflict. In caregiving and care recipient friend dyads, both groups identify conflicts and misunderstandings as being worst care experiences, a finding that differs from partnership dyads. Whereas in partnership dyads, conflict led to growth, which ultimately strengthened the relationship, none of the friendship dyads viewed conflict as beneficial to their relationship. It is possible that conflict negates the beneficial feelings that caregiving friends feel they gain from providing care, although no existing research about communal relationships addresses the effect of interpersonal conflict. The focus of this interpersonal conflict, however, appears to lie in the individual versus dyadic outcomes. Moreover, because the communal relationship does not depend on how any care recipient expects reciprocation from any particular caregiver, in times of conflict, caregivers may desire to reallocate their care to another communal member. Lacking the firm commitment toward the care recipient that is present in partnership relationships, conflict may threaten the duration of the dyadic relationship between friends.

One final finding that deserves attention is the caregiving friends' reactions to a care recipient's suicide attempt. Although different religious and ethical arguments could shape an individual's response to a suicide attempt, the communal relationship framework interprets such an action as severing a communal tie. An attempt to end one's life signals a failure of both the caregiver and the care recipient to abide by the norms of the communal relationship, which places community membership and engagement as the center of informal care.

This study contributes to the relationships, older LGB adults, and caregiving literatures by connecting the experiences that caregivers and care recipients identify as best and worst to the broader theoretical framework of communal relationship theory. In so doing, this work illustrates the differential norms at work in informal caregiving arrangements by partners and friends and helps us to better understand why partners and friends engage in informal caregiving.

The communal relationship framework illustrates the pivotal role of relationship commitment and day-to-day care within LGB caregiving relationships, yet most caregiving services and public policies were not designed to support these diverse caregiving relationships. Most services and policies were developed to assist legally married spouses and other biological family members providing care and often are not accessible to same-sex caregiving partners or to friends, those that typically provide caregiving in LGB communities.

In contrast to most employers, and federal and state leave policies, the National Family Caregiver Support Program (NGCSP), established in 2000 through the US Administration on Aging, broadly defines informal or family caregivers as adult family members, friends, or neighbors who provide care without pay. LGB caregivers and care recipients are able to access NFCSP services such as service information and access, counseling and support, and respite care (Administration on Aging, 2012). The NFCSP provides an example of the significance of defining caregiving broadly. Yet, most existing policies intended to help older adults and their caregivers exclude or limit LGB same-sex partners or friends further increasing the risk for emotional stress and conflict.

Professionals need ongoing training and consultation to increase their understanding of how best to provide services for LGB older adults and their caregivers. Social workers and other service providers need to better understand how the relational context may impact these caregivers and care recipients, and that training needs to be responsive to conflict and changing care situations, especially among caregiving friends when caregiving demands exceed their expectations or abilities to provide on-going care. Such training programs need to address the critical importance of care planning and the use of care teams and other caregiving advocates if needed (Fredriksen-Goldsen et al., 2011).

Although this research makes strong contributions, it also has limitations. One limitation is that we did not ask the caregiving participants why they engage in informal caregiving; thus, our application of the communal relationship theory is based on our interpretations of interview data, rather than on specific questions that directly connect the theory to the data. A second limitation lies in methodological procedure we used for this research. At the outset of the study, we opted to interview participants separately, but simultaneously, to allow the participants to speak more candidly than they may have were their dyad mates present. Although our methodological choice provided rich data, it also limited the degree to which we can understand the interpersonal dynamics that occurred within the care dyads, because we did not observe the way the participants interacted when together.

The findings of this study point to several avenues that would be fruitful for future research. One area that deserves to be the focus of additional research is a longitudinal study that follows care dyads over time, to better understand the duration, character, and quality of the relationships that occurs as the health statuses of these individuals change. Given that our study was cross-sectional, it can only tell us about the dynamics between the care dyads at one point in time. Another study worthy of research attention would place more focus on the existing norms for caregiving and receiving care. Although some of these norms emerged from the interview data in our study, making norms of optimal caregiving and care receiving a more central focus of research may help us to better understand existing, but often unstated, expectations.

CONCLUSION

This work serves as a step toward understanding not only the relational contexts in which caring occurs, but also the expectations that both the caregiver and care recipient have for the care activities. As the older adult population in the United States becomes increasingly older and more diverse, it is imperative that people consider experiences of caregiving and care receiving across divergent groups, including within LGB communities. Given their histories of marginalization and invisibility, LGB older adults likely rely heavily on informal care supports, including care provided by partners and friends. By utilizing communal relationships theory to examine the best and worst experiences of caregiving, similarities as well as differences in communal norms by both role and type of caregiving relationship emerge. Communal expectations and engagement have important implications for both caregiving and care receiving in later life.

ACKNOWLEDGMENTS

We acknowledge Mark Williams, Hyun-Jun Kim, Nerissa Irizarry, and Charles Hoy-Ellis for their assistance in the completion of this work.

FUNDING

The work presented in this article was supported by a grant received from the National Institutes of Health and the National Institute on Aging (R01 AG026526; PI: Fredriksen-Goldsen) and a grant from the Hartford Foundation (PI: Fredriksen-Goldsen). A Summer Research Grant from Loyola Marymount University to Anna Muraco provided additional support.

REFERENCES

Adams, K. B., McClendon, M. J., & Smyth, K. A. (2008) Personal losses and relationship quality in dementia caregiving. *Dementia: International Journal of Practice and Research, 7*, 301–309.

Administration on Aging. (2012). *National Family Caregiver Support Program.* Retrieved from http://www.aoa.gov/aoa_programs/hcltc/caregiver/index.aspx#purpose

Allen, S. M., Goldscheider, F., & Ciambrone, D. A. (1999) Gender roles, marital intimacy, and nomination of spouse as primary caregiver. *Gerontologist, 39*, 150–158.

Barker, J. C. (2002) Neighbors, friends, and other non-kin caregivers of community living dependent elders. *Journal of Gerontology: Social Sciences, 57*, 158–167.

Beel-Bates, C. A., Ingersoll-Dayton, B., & Nelson, E. (2007) Deference as a form of reciprocity among residents in assisted living. *Research on Aging, 29*, 626–643.

Cahill S., South K., & Spade J. (2000) *Outing age: Public policy issues affecting gay, lesbian, bisexual and transgender elders.* Washington, DC: National Gay and Lesbian Task Force.

Call, K. T., Finch, M. A., Huck, S. M., & Kane, R. A. (1999) Caregiver burden from a social exchange perspective: Caring for older people after a hospital discharge. *Journal of Marriage and Family, 61*, 688–699.

Cancian, F. M. (1987) *Love in America: Gender and self development.* New York, NY: Cambridge University Press.

Cantor, M. H., Brennan, M., & Shippy, A. (2004) *Caregiving among older lesbian, gay, bisexual, and transgender New Yorkers.* New York, NY: National Gay and Lesbian Taskforce Policy Institute.

Clark, M. S. (1981) Noncomparability of benefits given and received: A cue to the existence of friendship. *Social Psychology Quarterly, 44*, 375–381.

Clark, M. S., Fitness, J., & Brisette, I. (2001) Understanding people's perceptions of relationships is crucial to understanding their emotional lives. In G. Fletcher

& M. S. Clark (Vol. Eds.), *Blackwell handbook of social psychology: Vol. 3. Interpersonal processes* (pp. 253–278). Oxford, UK: Blackwell.

Coeling, H. V., Biordi, D. L., & Theis, S. L. (2003) Negotiating dyadic identity between caregivers and care receivers. *Journal of Nursing Scholarship, 35*, 21–25.

Coon, D. W., Thompson, L., Steffen, A., Soccoro, K., & Gallagher-Thompson, D. (2003) Anger and depression management: Psychoeducational skill training interventions for women caregivers of a relative with dementia. *Gerontologist, 43*, 678–689.

Cox, E. O., & Dooley, A. C. (1996) Care-receivers' perception of their role in the care process. *Journal of Gerontological Social Work, 26*, 133–152.

Family Caregiver Alliance. (2002). *Fact sheet: LGBTI caregiving: Frequently asked questions*. San Francisco, CA: Author.

Feinberg, L., Reinhard, S. C., Houser, A., & Choula, R. (2011). *Valuing the invaluable: 2011 update—The growing contributions and costs of family caregiving.* AARP Public Policy Institute. Retrieved from http://assets.aarp.org/rgcenter/ppi/ltc/i51-caregiving.pdf

Fredriksen-Goldsen, K. I., Kim, H. J., Emlet, C. A., Muraco, A., Erosheva, E. A., Hoy-Ellis, C. P., . . . Petry, H. (2011). *The aging and health report: Disparities and resilience among lesbian, gay, bisexual, and transgender older adults.* Seattle, WA: Institute for Multigenerational Health.

Fredriksen-Goldsen, K., Kim, H. J., Muraco, A., & Mincer, S. (2009) Chronically ill midlife and older lesbians, gay men, and bisexuals and their informal caregivers. *Sexuality Research and Social Policy, 6*, 52–64.

Goldsen, K. I. (2003, November). *Resiliency and AIDS caregiving.* Paper presented at the 56th Annual Scientific Meeting of the Gerontological Society of America, San Diego, CA.

Graham, S. M., Huang, J. Y., Clark, M. S., & Helgeson, V. S. (2008) The positives of negative emotions: Willingness to express negative emotions promotes relationships. *Personality and Social Psychology Bulletin, 34*, 394–406.

Guada, J., Hoe, M., Floyd, R., Barbour, J., & Brekke, J. S. (2012) How family factors impact psychosocial functioning for African American consumers with schizophrenia. *Community Mental Health Journal, 48*, 45–55.

Ingersoll-Dayton, B., & Antonucci, T. (1988) Reciprocal and nonreciprocal social support: Contrasting sides of intimate relationships. *Journal of Gerontology, 43*, 565–573.

Lambert, N. M., Clark, M. S., Durtschi, J., Fincham, F. D., & Graham, S. M. (2010) Benefits of expressing gratitude to a partner changes one's view of the relationship. *Psychological Science, 21*, 574–580.

LaRossa, R. (2005) Grounded theory methods and qualitative family research. *Journal of Marriage and Family, 67*, 837–857.

LeBlanc, A. J., & Wight, R. G. (2000) Reciprocity and depression in AIDS caregiving. *Sociological Perspectives, 43*, 631–649.

Lyons, K. S., Zarit, S. H., Sayer, A. G., & Whitlatch, C. J. (2002) Caregiving as a dyadic process: Perspectives from caregiver and receiver. *Journals of Gerontology: Series B, 57B*, P195–P204.

Monin, J. K., Martire, L. M., Schulz, R., & Clark, M. S. (2009) Willingness to express emotions to caregiving spouses. *Emotion, 9*, 101–106.

Muraco, A., & Fredriksen-Goldsen, K. I. (2011) "That's what friends do": Informal caregiving for chronically ill LGBT elders. *"Journal of Social and Personal Relationships, 28*, 1073–1092.

Newsom, J. T., & Schulz, R. (1998) Caregiving from the recipient's perspective: Negative reactions to being helped. *Health Psychology, 17*, 172–181.

Pearlin, L. I., Mullan, J. T., Semple, S. J., & Skaff, M. M., (1990) Caregiving and the stress process: An overview of concepts and their measures. *Gerontologist, 30*, 583–594.

Pruchno, R. A., Burant, C. J., & Peters, N. D. (1997) Understanding the well-being of care receivers. *Gerontologist, 37*, 102–109.

Pyke, K. (1999) The micropolitics of care in relationships between aging parents and adults children: Individualism, collectivism, and power. *Journal of Marriage and the Family, 61*, 661–672.

Walker, A. J., Pratt, C. C., & Oppy, N. C. (1992) Perceived reciprocity in family caregiving. *Family Relations, 41*, 82–85.

Wrubel, J., & Folkman, S. (1997) What informal caregivers actually do: The caregiving skills of partners of men with HIV. *AIDS Care, 9*, 691–706.

Older Lesbians and Bereavement: Experiencing the Loss of a Partner

CAROL L. JENKINS

School of Social Work, East Carolina University, Greenville, North Carolina, USA

AMANDA EDMUNDSON

Department of Occupational Therapy, East Carolina University, Greenville, North Carolina, USA

PAIGE AVERETT and INTAE YOON

School of Social Work, East Carolina University, Greenville, North Carolina, USA

There is very little research focused on older bereaved lesbians. This study is a response to the lack of knowledge about the issues for older lesbians who lose a partner. We examined bereavement issues for 55 older lesbians. The study asked participants to describe their concerns and experiences after losing a partner. Qualitative analysis identified several themes that ran throughout, including disenfranchised grief, the loneliness of isolation, and the frustration of relentless battles. These findings indicate the need for social workers to educate themselves and others about the particular needs facing this vulnerable group of older women.

INTRODUCTION

Experiencing the death of a person with whom one has shared a close relationship is often difficult for the surviving partner. Some bereaved individuals have their grief further laden with battles against prejudice and discrimination. A majority of the research conducted on bereavement analyzes the experience of heterosexual couples grieving the loss of a partner, but the occurrence among homosexual couples has received little attention. The small amount of existing literature primarily focuses on the experience of gay men losing their partners due to AIDS. Considered an invisible population, older lesbians are at risk of being overlooked due to a combination of factors including their age, gender, and sexual orientation (Averett, Yoon, & Jenkins, 2011). This tendency results in a lack of information about older lesbians' experiences in general, and even less information related to the experience of bereavement.

This article adds to the current literature to create a better understanding of the unique issues that older, bereaved lesbians face while dealing with the loss of a partner. It first provides an overview of the few studies related to bereavement among lesbian women. It then describes results of a qualitative study of experiences surrounding the loss of a partner for a sample of older lesbian women. The authors discuss the implications of their analysis and offer suggestions for practice. It is important that healthcare and service providers—particularly social workers—be aware of the unique circumstances facing older lesbians who have lost a partner. Given this information, providers can improve their understanding of these clients' singular struggles and experiences and be better able to enhance the quality of services they provide.

BACKGROUND

Research surrounding the loss of a partner in an LGBT relationship is relatively recent. As a result, there are few articles available and very few of those are focused on lesbians or are based on empirical studies. An early article by Doka (1987) introduced the concept of disenfranchised grief that is experienced by a person in a nontraditional relationship whose partner dies. This happens when society does not recognize the relationship and an equal level of importance is not given to the loss of the partner.

When a spouse dies in a heterosexual relationship, the bereaved partner receives emotional support from family and friends that can help alleviate the negative consequences associated with the loss, such as psychological distress, depression, and increased morbidity (Burton, Haley, & Small, 2006; Fry, 2001; Holm & Severinsson, 2012; O'Connor, 2010). The bereaved partner of a same-sex couple often does not receive such support and may be refused rituals and rights that would typically be granted to spousal partners (Bent & Magilvy, 2006).

In one article related to this issue, Broderick, Birbilis, and Steger (2008) pointed out that the lack of research has resulted in an absence of current knowledge about lesbians and their relationships for professionals such as social workers and grief counselors. They discuss what the literature has reported about lesbian relationships in general, and use this knowledge to offer recommendations for practice when working with women who have lost a partner.

The few empirical studies that have been published are focused primarily on gay men and the loss of a partner, especially to AIDS (e.g., Glackin & Higgins, 2008; Oerlemans-Bunn, 1988). Two exceptions are studies published by Jones and Nystrom (2002) and Bent and Magilvy (2006). Jones and Nystrom reported on a study in which semistructured interviews were conducted with 62 lesbians, 55 years and older. They identified worries about the impacts of losing a partner as one of their major concerns related to aging, and were particularly concerned about the loss of support.

Bent and Magilvy (2006) provided results of in-depth interviews with a small sample ($n = 6$) of women who self-identified as lesbians and who had lost a life partner. They found that positive support following the death led to relationships with the partner's family, to an ability to handle business matters satisfactorily, and to a strengthened ability to cope with the loss. Negative support (e.g., ongoing legal battles, being shut out of the hospital room, friends not recognizing the relationship) led to a longer period of bereavement and to less resolution of the grief.

Given this near absence of published research, we really know very little about the bereavement experiences of lesbians and the issues surrounding the loss. This study addresses the lack of knowledge about this important topic.

METHODOLOGY

Procedure

This article focuses on presenting and discussing the results of a qualitative study of responses to an open-ended survey question about the experience of losing a partner. The participants are a subsample (14%) of a larger national sample of older lesbian women ($n = 394$) who responded to an online survey consisting of 115 questions. The study protocol was approved by a university-based Institutional Review Board. Convenience sampling methods were used to gather data. A full description of the methods for the larger study, conducted in 2010-2011, can be seen in Averett et al. (2011).

Sample

The sample for this study consisted of 55 lesbian women who responded to an open-ended question asking them to describe their personal concerns and experiences surrounding the loss of their partners. Demographic information can be seen in Table 1.

TABLE 1 Demographic Characteristics

Variable	Score
Age	
Mean	64.6 years
Range	55–82 years
Education	
High school	3.6% ($n = 2$)
Associate degree	9.1% ($n = 5$)
Bachelor degree	23.6% ($n = 13$)
Master's degree	32.7% ($n = 18$)
Doctoral degree	30.0% ($n = 11$)
Income	
$\leq$\$10,000	.02% ($n = 1$)
\$10,000–\$20,000	9.0% ($n = 5$)
\$20,000–\$30,000	14.5% ($n = 8$)
\$30,000–\$40,000	16.3% ($n = 9$)
\$40,000–\$50,000	16.3% ($n = 9$)
$\geq$\$50,000	34.5% ($n = 19$)
Race/ethnicity	
Caucasian	81.8% ($n = 45$)
Latino	3.6% ($n = 2$)
Native American	1.8% ($n = 1$)
Multiracial	1.8% ($n = 1$)
Other/unknown	11.0% ($n = 6$)

Three questions were targeted at older lesbians who had experienced the death of a partner while they were together. The first was simply an identifier, inquiring about whether the participant had experienced the loss of a partner while they were together. Those responding in the affirmative were provided with two additional questions. The first of these asked the participants to identify which of four obstacles were encountered in dealing with the death of their partner: legal, financial, social, and emotional. Respondents were allowed to indicate multiple responses to this question.

Finally, participants were asked to describe their personal concerns and experiences surrounding the loss of their partners. An unlimited text box was available for participants to respond to the third question, and many wrote at length about their experiences. Fifty-seven women provided responses to this question but two of the responses were not actually related to the loss of a partner, leaving 55 respondents who addressed the issue. Eight of the responses indicated that the women had not yet faced the death of a partner, but one or the other was currently experiencing serious health problems. Some of these women described their experiences within the health care setting, while others discussed what they anticipated would happen when their partner died. Two of the women described how their partners were no longer part of their life because they had been admitted to full-time care within a skilled nursing facility. The remaining 45 responses were from women who had actually experienced the loss of a partner to death; two of these women had lost two partners and described both of those losses. Thus, the qualitative analysis that follows was based on responses from these last 45 women. It should be noted, however, that the responses from the remaining 10 participants were similar in nature to those of the larger subsample as they described discriminatory actions from health care providers and/or the sense of loss they either felt with a partner who was absent physically from them or that they had begun to anticipate.

Responses to the second question provided categorical results that offer a snapshot of the proportion of the 55 respondents who had experienced difficulty with any of the obstacles identified. Information from the final question provided rich, in-depth qualitative data that were analyzed via emergent themes (Patton, 2002). The responses were read through to get a sense of the whole. Then the responses were categorized based upon similarities within responses. The emergent themes that had a large set of participant responses were prioritized as a finding, and the smaller themes were reexamined to see if they then could be combined to create a more robust theme. Two of the authors assumed primary responsibility for this part of the analysis. They first worked individually, reading and rereading the responses to identify issues, feelings, and incidents that seemed essential to the respondents' experience. They then compared results to identify the emerging themes and subthemes, discussing their findings while continuing to reread the responses. Notes related to the discussions and decisions were maintained. The remaining authors reviewed the results of the analysis for accuracy. The resulting themes are presented in the following.

RESULTS

Obstacles

Participants who identified themselves in the first question as having lost a partner were requested to indicate whether they had experienced any of four categories of obstacles in dealing with the death, including emotional, social, legal, and financial obstacles. They were able to select all that were applicable to their experience, and many participants identified obstacles in more than one category. The category identified most often was emotional obstacles: About 76% of participants had faced some type of obstacle related to emotional issues at the loss of their partner. Over 40% of respondents reported they had encountered obstacles related to social and legal issues, and over a third encountered some sort of financial obstacle. This information provides only a broad overview of the issues facing participants; the last question was intended to gather detailed information that would elaborate on impacts of the obstacles and on the personal experience of each woman.

Themes

Two of the respondents reported positive experiences: One woman "had the support of her [partner's] family" and the other stated, "Friends, neighbors, children, coworkers were supportive." The remaining respondents discussed negative experiences, with four broad themes emerging from the qualitative analysis: disenfranchised grief, discriminatory actions, the loneliness of isolation, and the frustration of relentless battles. Patterns of experience were identified within some of the broader themes and are indicated by subheadings in the discussion of themes that follows. It was evident during the analysis that some of the themes were intertwined due to the relationship among the issues discussed by the respondents.

DISENFRANCHISED GRIEF

Discussion of experiences related to this theme was evident throughout the participants' responses. The concept of disenfranchised grief covers the personal attitudes and responses that are a result of not giving equal value to a loss in this kind of relationship.

Respondents were clear that they believed their experiences were very different from those of women who lost a spouse in a traditional relationship, particularly in the attitudes that others had toward them and their loss. The importance and depth of their loss was devalued by many of the people with whom they came in contact, including family and friends and the broader public. Many respondents described the disrespect they believed was shown by members of the community and the way in which the death was often ignored completely by the people with whom they associated. One respondent noted: "Many people did not acknowledge or generally take my loss to be as significant as it was—they basically ignored her death." Another wrote about her experience: "Our relationship was under the radar due to her high profile in the community. My feelings at her death were not able to be acknowledged."

As difficult as it was to receive this type of treatment from individuals outside their immediate support network, it was often devastating to find that family members (of both partners) were also likely to discount the importance of the experience. This was particularly true for members of the partner's family. As one respondent reported, "Once she died, her family did not consider me at all. We have known each other for over 25 years. Her family knew." Another reported that she was not even allowed the solace of keeping any of her partner's belongings: "My partner's family took her personal possessions."

This discounting of the validity of the relationship and of the loss negatively impacted the ability to adequately grieve the loss. As one respondent wrote, "Nobody was willing to honor my 30-year relationship with her in that I was not considered to be a 'widow' by them." Another described her experience when seeking grief counseling: "I am a widow. Went to a grief support group and the facilitator didn't relate to me as a widow."

DISCRIMINATORY ACTIONS

Respondents provided a great deal of discussion related to discriminatory actions that resulted from a refusal of rights—both legal and social—that would typically be granted to spousal partners in a heterosexual relationship. These actions were experienced from an array of sources including the legal and health care systems, the workplace, and the community.

Legal/financial issues. Legal issues remain an area of great concern for same-sex partners because they have limited or no legal recourse in most states. Several respondents discussed being faced with legal battles, usually with their partner's family members. This proved to be an added strain for respondents during a time when they were dealing with the emotional loss of their partner. The fact that it often resulted in financial loss for the women added to the stress they were experiencing.

Most of these conflicts were around maintaining access to their partner's resources and most resulted in negative financial consequences for the respondent. One respondent described it this way: "Because the law wouldn't recognize our relationship, everything in her estate, little that it was, went to her daughter." Even when the partners had attempted to take legal precautions, families still disputed them, as described by this response: "It was especially difficult dealing with her biological family in spite of all of the legal papers and arrangements we made in advance."

Another area of concern was related to financial responsibilities facing the respondents at a time when their income was reduced due to the loss of the partner's financial resources. Responses detailed the older women's experiences adjusting to the loss of income, as well as to facing tax penalties for the few who discussed actually inheriting the partner's estate. Examples of this are seen in the following statements: "When my partner died, I had to pay a huge inheritance tax on 'her half of our house' in order to sell the house we shared." "Half of my home went into her 'estate' so I had to pay inheritance taxes." Other respondents were denied access to benefits to which they felt legally entitled: "I applied for her income tax return and the IRS would not give it to me even though I was the beneficiary of her estate."

There were instances in which the relationship was selectively recognized. This often led to negative consequences for the couple, as can be seen in the following response:

> Ironically, while she was terminally ill, without insurance, and applying for public assistance, the state counted my income in determining her eligibility for assistance as if we were married, and decreased her benefit amount accordingly; yet I wasn't able to put her on my health insurance as a spouse or dependent, because it would have violated state law.

One respondent was held responsible for her partner's health care expenses: "I was stuck with $150,000 of my deceased partner's medical bills."

Other benefits that a surviving spouse is entitled to but that were denied our respondents included pensions and Social Security benefits, as seen in the following statements: "Because we had not formed a legal partnership by the time she died I was not entitled to any of her pension, etc." "I was not able to get her Social Security nor the death benefit I would have had if I was with a man." In certain cases, the benefits withheld were a significant amount: "I would have three times the Social Security I get now if our relationship was honored."

Health care system issues. Respondents were often in contact with the health care system during the time period preceding the death. Their experiences tended to be negative because their relationship was at best tolerated, but more often disrespected or ignored. Without being legally considered as a family member, partners lost their ability to help, or sometimes even to be present with, their partners in a health care facility. As one participant pointed out, she was "not given access in the hospital." Thus, this woman was denied the small comfort of being able to be with the person she loved at a time when it was vitally important for both of them to be able to be together.

One respondent's experience was especially poignant as she described the moment she and her partner were separated at the hospital, and the events that followed: "I was not allowed to be with my partner when she died in the hospital." Thus, their last opportunity to be together—and the chance to say a final good-bye—was denied to them.

Some respondents reported that they had anticipated difficulties and had taken legal precautions they hoped would help them avoid problems. Despite their attempts to be prepared, they still faced obstacles. For example: "I was on all the paperwork having her power of attorney (to make medical and financial decisions) but they [hospital staff] put up a fuss anyhow."

Workplace issues. Workplace issues were related to the lack of legal recognition for the partnerships. There are few protections for same-sex couples in the workplace, as they are denied most benefits offered to heterosexual couples, such as health care insurance and leaves of absence to provide care. One respondent, referring to health care benefits, stated, "I have excellent health insurance. I would like for my partner to be able to participate in it. That is not possible, because I am a US government retiree." Even requesting a leave of absence to care for their loved one is difficult to justify when there is no legal recognition of the relationship: "We have no legal rights or understanding at our jobs. If one of us gets sick, we can't take time off legally."

Community issues. Community issues were related to a lack of social recognition of the relationship. Some respondents reported having difficulty when dealing with community organizations that provide services at the time of a death. For example, one respondent described her experience with a local newspaper as follows:

> Our 22-year relationship was greatly devalued and disrespected. Even the newspaper refused to refer to me as her partner and instead listed me as one of many "friends," even though I had been the breadwinner for several years and was the primary caregiver and hospice caregiver the last 3 years of her life.

Another respondent reported her experience with personnel at the funeral home: "[They] refused to talk to me, they talked to her son."

THE LONELINESS OF ISOLATION

From the lost partner. Respondents reported that a major challenge after the loss was the task of learning to live alone after having shared a home with the person they loved. In one respondent's words: "Emotionally, I just had trouble functioning for over a year; I would walk into a room and expect her to be there, and sometimes just not believe she was gone."

From the partner's family. Many of the respondents indicated that isolation from their partner's family was a major issue with which they were challenged. This isolation presented them with an additional and unexpected loss. They described how they had developed social relationships with partners' families over the years of the relationship and considered them as a part of their support network. It was devastating to discover after the death that some of these family members did not return those feelings. One respondent noted, "The worst emotional toll was that her family pulled away and I don't get to see the grandkids I helped raise." A similar report was made by another of the respondents when she disclosed, "[Her] family was not happy that she was a lesbian. After she died, they pulled away from me. I was very involved with a set of grandkids who live only an hour away and I lost them after she died."

From the support system. Descriptions of being isolated were not limited to the perception of being cut off from family support systems. Respondents also identified themselves as experiencing feelings of isolation from others who either were or who might have been perceived as part of their support network. For example, one respondent wrote that she was "Socially not sure where one fits. Most of my friends are coupled," while another described the difficulty of staying ". . . connected to the women who were really her [i.e., the partner's] friends." Respondents also found themselves with fewer friendships, as evidenced by one who wrote: "Because most of us become invisible as we become older, it becomes harder to find other lesbians to interact with. This is so isolating that it is the most difficult thing to overcome."

The task of finding others who could identify with their experiences and empathize with them proved to be even more formidable. As one wrote,

207

"I had no support system, and as I met women, as soon as they heard I had lost my partner they evaporated."

THE FRUSTRATION OF RELENTLESS BATTLES

Losing a person one loves is a trying experience for any person, but for the survivor of a same-sex couple, the emotional stress of the loss can be amplified by a relatively constant stream of battles—with one's own emotions, with family and the partner's family, and with other individuals in the broader social system (e.g., health care and legal professionals). Our respondents described how they experienced anger and sadness at not having the relationship recognized, at not being allowed to spend time with the loved one in her final hours, at being denied access to financial resources they had shared, and at not finding the support they had hoped for from family and friends. Respondents discussed the frustration and weariness they felt with the constant struggle to get through this difficult time in their lives.

Many of the respondents disclosed their feelings of disappointment and frustration that they were unable to find persons in whom they could confide. Although this is related, in part, to the theme of being isolated, it is focused more on the feelings that were evoked by respondents' experiences with isolation. In the words of one participant it was "hard to find someone to express emotions to." Even when granted the opportunity, sharing their experiences proved difficult in groups where they were the only lesbian. As one respondent put it, "I was offered help through hospice, but as the only lesbian, I was not able to have anyone who could—or would—validate my experience at losing a life partner."

Participants described the vexation generated through social encounters after the death of their partners, reporting a great deal of resistance from their families, as well as the families of their partners. One respondent noted:

> Her family tried to stop me from making all health care decisions when she was terminally ill, despite our legal documents that we had in place. I had to fight, fight, fight all the time with my late partner's family to leave us alone.

Another respondent indicated the lack of support from her own family:

> Only a few people attended the service because my partner was not "out" prior to her passing and I outed her in her obituary. . . . None of my family attended the funeral. . . . I have loads of anger about how I was treated by others over her passing.

Respondents also described the frustration they experienced when dealing with the community in general, and the various organizations they

encountered at the time of the death. This is best summarized by the statement of one respondent, "There isn't even a word to describe the situation—
you had to use 'widowed,' which is legally incorrect." This quote illustrates
a recurring experience described by respondents, which is that their wid-
owhood was not recognized or acknowledged. This provides a theme that
is interwoven throughout all of the others, leading to disenfranchised grief,
discriminatory actions, feelings of isolation, and relentless battles.

IMPLICATIONS AND FUTURE DIRECTIONS FOR SOCIAL WORK PRACTICE

This research has provided important information regarding an issue about
which little is known, i.e., the impacts on the survivor of a lesbian couple
when one partner dies. We have learned that the emotional distress accom-
panying the loss of a loved one for any person, as well as legal and financial
issues that can arise, can be magnified for older lesbians in many ways. Their
grief may not be legitimized by recognition of their relationship in the way it
is for heterosexual couples. They are often denied the legal rights available to
heterosexual couples: health care coverage for the partner, leaves of absence
to provide care, decision-making authority in health care settings, and access
to financial resources such as pensions. They can experience reduced, or no,
access to the one they love at the most trying time when they are separated
in a health care facility. They may find their economic well-being jeopar-
dized by the loss of their partner's financial resources and are often denied
access even to personal possessions that could provide comfort in their time
of loss. They may not find the support they hoped to have from family and
friends and are left feeling isolated and alone.

Many of these issues would be resolved if same-sex partners were
allowed to marry legally. Two landmark rulings by the Supreme Court in June
2013 will dramatically improve the status of couples who are married in states
that legally permit same-sex unions. At the time of the rulings, this was only
possible in 12 states—Connecticut, Delaware, Iowa, Massachusetts, Maine,
Maryland, Minnesota, New Hampshire, New York, Rhode Island, Vermont,
and Washington—and the District of Columbia ("Did you know?", 2013).
Same-sex couples in these states can receive benefits at the state level as
married couples.

In one ruling, the Court declined to rule on a challenge to Proposition 8,
passed by California voters in 2008, which banned gay marriage. In effect,
this decision will allow same-sex marriage to resume there as soon as a
federal appeals court lifts a stay on marriage licenses for same-sex couples
issued by a lower judge (Williams & McClam, 2013). California had temporarily allowed same-sex marriages between June 16 and November 4, 2008, and
still recognizes the marriages performed during that time frame.

In the second ruling, the Court struck down the Defense of Marriage Act (DOMA), passed by the US Congress and signed by President Clinton in 1996. DOMA prohibited federal recognition of same-sex marriages and allowed states to refuse to recognize such marriages performed in other states. Because DOMA was a federal law, couples married under the provisions of a state law were not entitled to federal protections. Nor were they entitled to benefits such as Social Security survivor benefits or retirement benefits extended to spouses ("Same-sex couples' legal rights," 2013). In the wake of this decision, legal analysts indicate that couples in a legally-recognized marriage will have access to over 1,000 "federal privileges and programs that use marital status as a criteria for eligibility" (Arkin, 2013, p. 1). Government agencies do not always adhere to the same statues and regulations, however, which means that couples living in the 38 states that don't allow same-sex marriages may not have full access to all benefits (Arkin, 2013).

Another potential means of ensuring legal rights to same-sex couples is through domestic partnership laws. This type of law results in a same-sex couple being granted nearly the same rights and benefits as a married heterosexual couple, including some tax benefits and employment benefits (e.g., family or medical leave). Domestic partnership laws vary widely by state, however, and can even vary within states, which results in a confusing system of guarantees ("Domestic partnership laws," 2013). More important, however, is the fact that they do not guarantee same-sex couples the same protections as heterosexual couples and they effectively perpetuate the premise that same-sex couples should be treated differently under the law.

Until the legal status of same-sex marriage is widespread, it is vitally important to develop alternative means of helping lesbian women deal with the issues surrounding the loss of a partner. This is particularly important for social workers who are often the front-line service providers with whom these women come into contact.

The primary focus for social workers should be on education—for themselves, for co-workers, for policymakers, and for students preparing to enter the field of social work. First, social workers need to learn about the issues themselves. They need to understand the implications of disenfranchised grief for clients: Delegitimization of their loss by others, denial of their need to grieve, lack of access to shared resources, loss of social and emotional support, and feelings of isolation. They should consider recommending grief assessment and counseling, preferably to a counselor who is culturally competent and understands the special needs of bereaved lesbian women. Bent and Magilvy (2006) suggested that social workers might be advocates with the deceased partner's family in an effort to reduce the tensions that can exist. A referral to legal services may be appropriate when there is an issue with settling the estate or in accessing other benefits that might be available.

Social workers should be informed about the domestic partnership laws in their state and locality (i.e., county, city) so they will be able to help identify any legal rights a bereaved lesbian client might have. They also need to encourage their clients who are in a same-sex relationship to take proper measures to plan for future events. The creation of wills and living wills are a means by which same-sex couples can legally protect their rights and wishes (Riggle, Rostosky, & Prather, 2006). It is important to encourage clients to name their health care proxies as well.

Social workers should do all they can to educate other professionals about the issues, including those within their own agency and others who might be involved in providing services to bereaved lesbians (e.g., nurses, physicians, funeral home directors). The importance of educating others needs to be recognized, particularly those who work with the older population, as well as those suffering from serious or chronic medical conditions (Stein & Bonuck, 2001). Neustifter (2008) noted that it is important for providers to be knowledgeable about the influence of societal prejudices on older lesbians' quality of life. This may be especially important for health care providers because research shows that older lesbians have concerns about how they are treated in the health care system (Stein, Beckerman, & Sherman, 2010). It is possible that some professionals are not aware of the significant impact their behavior has on the bereaved because they do not understand the multiple and singular issues facing these women (e.g., loss of social and emotional support, loss of access to family members such as grandchildren from the partner's side of the family).

One of the core values of social work is advocacy. An important part of advocating for clients is to educate policymakers. It is particularly important to help policymakers understand the issues facing the survivors of same-sex relationships to help them see the importance of improving the legal status of such relationships. It may also aide them in developing workplace policies that are fairer and more beneficial for same-sex couples.

Another important group to educate about these issues is students in social work programs. They are the future of the profession and may be able to be the *change agents* that are needed to bring about the transformation in thinking of so many members of society that will be necessary to improve the lives of all individuals in same-sex relationships.

It should be noted that there are limitations associated with this study. One is the use of an online survey. This data collection method impacted the composition of our sample because Internet users are more likely to be middle- and upper-middle class individuals (Matsuo, McIntyre, Tomazic, & Katz, 2004). It is likely that this partially explains the high levels of both education and income reported by our participants. It should be noted, however, that past research has demonstrated that gays and lesbians generally have higher educational levels than heterosexuals and that lesbian women typically earn more income than heterosexual women (Black, Gates, Sanders, & Taylor, 2000).

Our study also shares limitations related to the lack of diversity in our sample that has been acknowledged by many previous researchers, due to the difficulty in accessing the old-old and racial minorities (Averett & Jenkins, 2012; Jacobsen, 1995). Our sample was predominately middle-aged and young-old, as well as predominately Caucasian. Despite our attempts to specifically reach these difficult-to-access populations, we were relatively unsuccessful, which limits the generalizability of our findings.

Attention to lesbian women, in general, and their issues has increased in recent years. Despite this recent interest, social workers still know little about their lives as they get older and they are especially sadly lacking in knowledge about how they cope when a partner dies. This study augments the understanding of what is known about grieving among lesbian women and offers practical recommendations for addressing some of the issues they face.

REFERENCES

Arkin, D. (2013). *Gay couples stand to receive thousands of benefits in wake of DOMA decision*. Retrieved from http://usnews.nbcnews.com/_news/2013/06/26/19100907-gay-couples-stand-to-receive-thousands-of-benefits-in-wake-of-doma-decision

Averett, P., & Jenkins, C. L. (2012). Review of the literature on older lesbians: Implications for education, practice and research. *Journal of Applied Gerontology, 31*, 537–561.

Averett, P., Yoon, I., & Jenkins, C. L. (2011). Older lesbians: Experiences of aging, discrimination and resilience. *Journal of Women & Aging, 23*, 216–232.

Bent, K. N., & Magilvy, J. (2006). When a partner dies: Lesbian widows. *Issues in Mental Health Nursing, 27*, 447–459.

Black, D., Gates, G., Sanders, S., & Taylor, L. (2000). Demographics of the gay and lesbian populations in the United States: Evidence from available systematic data sources. *Demography, 37*, 139–154.

Broderick, D. J., Birbilis, J. M., & Steger, M. F. (2008). Lesbians grieving the death of a partner: Recommendations for practice. *Journal of Lesbian Studies, 12*, 225–235.

Burton, A. M., Haley, W. E., & Small, B. J. (2006). Bereavement after caregiving or unexpected death: Effects on elderly spouses. *Journal of Mental Health, 10*, 319–326.

"Did you know?" (2013). Retrieved on July 5, 2013 from http://gaymarriage.procon.org/

Doka, K. J. (1987). Silent sorrow: Grief and the loss of significant others. *Death Studies, 11*, 455–469.

"Domestic partnership laws." (2013). Retrieved on March 8, 2013 from http://www.legalmatch.com/law-library/article/domestic-partnership-rights-by-state.html

Fry, P. S. (2001). Predictors of quality of life perspectives, self-esteem, and life satisfactions of older adults following spousal loss: An 18-month follow-up study of widows and widowers. *Gerontologist, 4*, 787–798.

Glackin, M., & Higgins, A. (2008). The grief experience of same-sex couples within an Irish context: Tacit acknowledgement. *International Journal of Palliative Nursing, 14,* 297–302.

Holm, A. L., & Severinsson, E. (2012). Systematic review of the emotional state and self-management of widows. *Nursing and Health Sciences, 14,* 109–120.

Jacobsen, S. (1995). Methodological issues in research on older lesbians. *Journal of Gay and Lesbian Social Services, 3,* 43–56.

Jones, T., & Nystrom, N. (2002). "Looking back . . . Looking forward: Addressing the lives of lesbians 55 and older." *Journal of Women & Aging, 14*(3/4), 59–76.

Matsuo, H., McIntyre, K., Tomazic, T. & Katz, B. (2004). The online survey: Its contributions and potential problems. In *Proceedings of the Survey Research Methods section of the American Statistical Association.* Retrieved from http://www.amstat.org/sections/srms/Proceedings/y2004/Files/Jsm2004-000440.pdf

Neustifter, R. (2008). Common concerns faced by lesbian elders: An essential context for couple's therapy. *Journal of Feminist Family Therapy: An International Forum, 20,* 251–267.

O'Connor, M. (2010). PTSD in the older bereaved people. *Aging & Mental Health, 14,* 310–318.

Oerlemans-Bunn, M. (1988). On being gay, single, and bereaved. *American Journal of Nursing, 88,* 472–476.

Patton, M. (2002). *Qualitative research and evaluation methods* (3rd ed.). Thousand Oaks, CA: Sage.

Riggle, E. B., Rostosky, S. S., & Prather, R. A. (2006). Advance planning by same-sex couples. *Journal of Family Issues, 27,* 758–776.

"Same-sex couples' legal rights." (2013). Retrieved on March 8, 2013 from http://www.legalmatch.com/law-library/article/faq-same-sex-couples-legal-rights.html

Stein, G. L., Beckerman, N. L., & Sherman, P. A. (2010). Lesbian and gay elders and long-term care: Identifying the unique psychosocial perspectives and challenges. *Journal of Gerontological Social Work, 53,* 421–435.

Stein, G. L., & Bonuck, K. A. (2001). Attitudes on End-of-Life Care and Advance Care Planning in the Lesbian and Gay Community. *Journal of Palliative Medicine, 4,* 173–190.

Williams, P., & McClam, E. (2013). *Supreme Court strikes down defense of marriage act, paves way for gay marriage to resume in California.* Retrieved from http://nbcpolitics.nbcnews.com/_news/2013/06/26/19151971-supreme-court-strikes-down-defense-of-marriage-act-paves-way-for-gay-marriage-to-resume-in-california

Developing Understanding of Same-Sex Partner Bereavement for Older Lesbian and Gay People: Implications for Social Work Practice

LEE-ANN FENGE

National Centre for Post-Qualifying Social Work, Bournemouth University, Bournemouth, UK

There is little research and literature exploring same-sex partner bereavement in later life or end-of-life experiences of lesbian and gay elders in the United Kingdom. This article considers this often overlooked area of social work practice and explores a range of factors emerging from a small explorative study that considers the experience of loss and bereavement for lesbian and gay elders. Discussion of issues emerging include consideration of the wider psycho-social nature of bereavement and end-of-life experiences for lesbian and gay elders, and the implications this has for social work education and practice.

The loss of a partner in later life is a key challenge to the emotional and social well-being of older people, yet it has been suggested that the experience of loss in old age is often obscured by the effects of ageism (S. Thompson, 2002). For certain groups of elders, blanket assumptions about the nature of relationships and meanings associated with loss can result in further invisibility. In particular, there is little research about the bereavement experiences and end-of-life concerns of lesbian and gay elders in the United Kingdom (Green & Grant, 2008). A focus on heterosexual relationship bereavement means that there is often a gap in the knowledge of social workers who support a diverse population of older people. As a result, practitioners may be ill equipped to deal sensitively with same-sex partner bereavement, denying individuals the support they require when they are at their most vulnerable. This article reports on a small exploratory qualitative investigation ($n = 7$) that seeks to identify bereavement and end-of-life experiences of lesbian and gay elders. Developing more understanding of these experiences can inform social work education and practice, enabling practitioners to develop sensitivity and responsiveness when meeting the needs of these vulnerable groups.

LITERATURE REVIEW

Loss and grief experiences may be universal features of human life, however, certain groups may be disadvantaged during times of bereavement if their loss is not given the social recognition it deserves. For example, assumptions that older people become accustomed to loss, due to their age and experience of multiple losses across their life course, may mean that their needs for bereavement support are overlooked (S. Thompson, 2002). For older lesbian and gay people, this lack of understanding may be compounded by inadequate social work education concerning lesbian and gay issues (Gezinski, 2009; Martinez, 2011). As a result, it is likely that social workers may not have sufficient knowledge to deal sensitively with the issues of bereavement appropriately for older lesbian, gay, bisexual and transgender (LGBT) individuals.

How one experiences bereavement and loss is affected by multiple factors, including gender, culture, ethnicity, class, age, and sexual orientation. Some of these factors will complicate the process of bereavement further, and may make individuals more vulnerable to experiences such as loneliness, isolation, and depression following bereavement. For example, Langley (2001) suggested that the closeted lives that some lesbian and gay elders lead can increase their social isolation following loss of a partner. However, the bereavement experiences of gay and nongay widowers has been described as being similar, and as individuals make sense of their life without their partner, a key aspect of this bereavement process is dealing with the "life lived without" (Hornjakevyc & Alderson, 2011, p. 820). Therefore, the process of grief for all older people involves making sense of loss through the retention and modification of emotional bonds with the deceased partner (Costello & Kendrick, 2000). However, some individuals may have limited options of support to enable them to achieve this.

It is difficult to know the precise number of older LGBT people in the UK population, although Price (2005) suggested an estimate of between 545,000 and 872,000 people over the age of 65. As the ageing population expands, it is likely that increased numbers of older LGBT people will experience the loss of their partner. There is a relative dearth of research and

literature exploring same-sex bereavement in later life or end-of-life experiences of older lesbian and gay individuals (Almack, Seymour, & Bellamy,
2010). Even less is known about the experiences of older transgender or
intersex individuals, as they get older and face the loss of their partners
(Witten & Eyler, 2012). Recent explorative research in Australia suggests that
LGBT individuals face barriers in accessing appropriate end-of-life care due
to discrimination and lack of knowledge about LGBT needs and experiences
(Cartwright, Hughes, & Lienert, 2012). Research exploring the needs of older
lesbians and gay men highlights concerns about the experience of loss of a
partner, and the lack of appropriate bereavement support available (Gay and
Grey in Dorset, 2006; Smith, McCaslin, Chang, Martinez, & McGrew, 2010).

Although human life may be punctuated by many transitions and crises,
the death of someone one loves has a significant impact on one's emotional
state and well-being (Schaefer & Moos, 2001). Grief has been described as
a multifaceted construct made up of at least three core bereavement phenomena, including nonacceptance, grief-related thoughts, and an emotional
response to loss (Futterman, Holland, Brown, Thompson, & Gallagher-
Thompson, 2010). Traditionally, the process of grief and mourning has been
depicted as a linear process with beginning, middle, and end points, com-
mencing with a stage of denial and ending with a stage of acceptance
(Worden, 1991), although Worden's later work acknowledged a process of
"readjustment" that takes in the grief and mourning process (Currer, 2007,
p. 61). More recent models recognize the dynamic nature of grief and the
oscillation back and forth between phases, as the individual comes to terms
with their life without their loved one. This ever-changing and reactive model
of grief is illustrated by the pinball model of grief (Baier & Buechsel, 2012),
which describes how individuals can quickly move between different phases
in a nonlinear process. However, for some individuals the social context of
how their loss is viewed by wider society may result in the pain and significance of their loss being overlooked. In such circumstances, their grief
experiences become disenfranchised as a result (Doka, 1989, 2002).

Doka (1989, p. 4) defined disenfranchised grief as experienced when
individuals "incur a loss that is not or cannot be openly acknowledged,
publically mourned or socially supported." Disenfranchised grief is not a
universal experience for LGBT bereavement (Shernoff, 1997), and this highlights the importance of understanding the individual context of loss, in terms
of personal, social, and cultural resilience factors available. This reinforces
the need to acknowledge the diversity of bereavement experience (Fenge
& Fannin, 2009), and the range of support available both within and outside of the LGBT community. Difficulties accessing appropriate bereavement
support emerged as one of several issues concerned with improving community support for lesbians and gay elders (Gay and Grey in Dorset, 2006).
A recent report in the United Kingdom by the National Council for Palliative
Care (2011) suggested that LGBT people may not get their end-of-life needs

recognized due to assumptions of heterosexuality. This survey found that many LGBT people are concerned that they will face discrimination from health and social care providers when they are dying, and it is likely that this will also have implications for the support their partners might receive following bereavement.

A focus on heterosexual relationship bereavement means that there is a gap in the knowledge of social workers who are supporting a diverse population of older people. Experiences across the life course, and societal attitudes toward homosexuality, contribute to individual identity development and influence how older lesbians and gay men think about themselves, and the support they might expect from health and social care providers. A key feature of the current ageing population of gay men is their shared history of HIV/AIDS as it developed in the 1980s, and the impact this had in "decimating social networks and shaping their personal and social lives" (Rosenfield, Bartlam, & Smith, 2012, p. 255). Older gay men grew up in a time when homosexuality was still illegal and criminalized, and as a consequence, many continue to live in fear of homophobia (Fredriksen-Goldsen & Muraco, 2010). A lifetime experience of homophobia, and social exclusion based on sexuality, can have a lasting impact on older LGBT people's ability to trust health and social care providers. As Fish suggested (2010, p. 309), "the historic effects of social exclusion have consequences across the lifespan and, in particular, for older LGBT people who were growing up at a time when homosexuality was criminalized." Such negative experiences may influence whether individuals feel confident about being out about their sexuality in later life, and whether they feel confident in approaching agencies who they fear might discriminate against them during times of bereavement.

The complexity of the interrelationships between biographical diversity and social context (King & Cronin, 2010) means that LGBT identity is multidimensional. Developing an understanding of this intersectionality (Yuval-Davis, 2006), allows one to consider the social divisions and identifications that may make individuals visible or invisible within their communities. This approach can enable social work to develop an understanding of the diversity of social identities within the older LGBT population. For example, LGBT people may live in dichotomous social worlds, being out in some settings but not in others (Rawlings, 2012), and living in a world where a relationship with a partner is undisclosed can mask and complicate the bereavement and grief process. For those in same-sex relationships, distress following bereavement may be increased if the nature of the relationship was hidden from family and friends (Bent & Magilvy, 2006; Rondahl, Innala, & Carlsson, 2006), or not openly acknowledged by health and social care professionals (Glacken & Higgins, 2008). Lack of acknowledgement of a same-sex relationship, or assumptions of heterosexuality, means that social work practitioners can overlook sexuality in their dealings with older service users and, as a result, may fail to provide an appropriate response. As Knocker (2012, p. 13) suggested, "Our life stories, and in particular our love stories, are not known, understood or acknowledged in the way they should be." As a result, older lesbians and gay men may experience the pain of "silent mourning" (Deevey, 2000, p. 9), and may be denied wider social acknowledgement and psychological support.

In recent years, there has been a shift in UK public policy promoting the rights of gay and lesbian people. These changes include recognition of same-sex partnerships through The Civil Partnership Act (2004), and protection against discrimination on the grounds of sexual orientation in the provision of goods and services by public bodies through The Equality Act (2006). However, despite these changes, bereavement and end-of-life care may be complicated for those older LGBT people who have experienced a lifetime of fear due to homophobia and discrimination (Rawlings, 2012). Many older lesbian and gay people may, therefore, view themselves as living a marginalized position within society (Green & Grant, 2008).

It has been suggested by Fish (2008, p. 191) that "emancipatory social work practice with LGBT people is more likely to become an achievable goal if the nature and form of sexuality oppression is commonly understood." This involves confronting the hetero-normative assumptions that have dominated both theory and practice concerning old age (Cronin, 2006). Combating discrimination and oppression related to gender or sexual orientation is enshrined within the International Federation of Social Work (IFSW, 2012) core principles. In England, the development of a Professional Capabilities Framework (Social Work Reform Board, 2010) for social work practice has highlighted the importance of understanding diversity, stating that "social workers understand that diversity characterises and shapes human experience and is critical to the formation of identity" (p. 10). It is, therefore, vital for social workers to develop an understanding of diversity not only across the ageing population, but across diverse experiences of death and bereavement.

This article hopes to contribute to the developing knowledge and understanding of older lesbian and gay bereavement needs through the consideration of findings from a small exploratory project. Due to the small sample interviewed, bisexual and transgender experience was not included in the sample group, and therefore discussion is focused on older lesbian and gay experience of bereavement.

METHODOLOGY

Sample

This small explorative study used a qualitative design, seeking to discover the bereavement experiences of older lesbians and gay men, as well as the perspectives of those supporting them during times of bereavement. It was hoped that this would help to inform the development of a larger research project. Participants were recruited using a snowball sampling strategy, as such an approach has been described as useful in identifying older lesbian and gay people for research purposes (Warner, Wright, Blanchard, & King, 2003). Details of the project were sent to local LGBT social and support groups via the Web. Respondents were either self-identified older lesbians or gay men who had experienced the loss of a same-sex partners, or workers from agencies who support older LGBT individuals during times of bereavement. The number of participants was as follows:

Bereaved: women $n = 1$ / men $n = 3$
Agencies working with older LGBT people: $n = 3$

The rationale for recruiting two distinct groups was the desire for *information-rich cases* that would provide a range of perspectives on same-sex partner bereavement. It was also anticipated that there may be a small sample size of bereaved individuals coming forward due to the sensitivity of the topic, and it would therefore be important to include the perspectives of those who support bereaved individuals, as they would also provide some information-rich cases relevant to the project. Although it was hoped to recruit an equal split between older lesbians and gay men, in the end only one older lesbian who had experienced the loss of her partner came forward.

Data Collection

The interviews were arranged to fit in with the participants' lives. Four were undertaken in the participants' homes or workplace, and three participants came into the university. All interviews were conducted by the same researcher from the university, and most interviews were an hour to an hour-and-a-half in length. Due to the emotional context of the interviews, sometimes the interviews were paused to allow the participant time to weep and then compose themselves.

Semistructured questions were used to guide the interview, but these were open ended to enable the participant to tell their own story of bereavement. For example: "Can you tell me about your experience of losing your partner?" "What were the responses of those around you to the loss of your partner?" and "What types of support did you access following the loss of your partner?" For those participants working in agencies supporting older LGBT people, questions included the following: "What is your experience of supporting those who have experienced same-sex partner bereavement?" 'What are the key issues for those who have experienced same-sex partner bereavement?" and "What types of support services are you aware of for those who have experienced same-sex bereavement?" Interviews were digitally recorded, and then transcribed. To support participants in case their participation caused undue distress, I provided wind-down time after the interview had finished (Wee, Coleman, Hillier, & Holgate, 2006). Names have been changed to protect anonymity.

Analysis

A qualitative interpretive approach was taken, using face-to-face semistructured interviews, as this was felt to be a suitable methodology to explore the sensitive topic of bereavement. It has also been suggested that qualitative inquiry holds great promise for research with older lesbians and gay men (Hash & Cramer, 2003). The aim was to obtain the participants' perceptions of their world, rather than impose my views upon them. Thematic content analysis was used to analyze the data (Miles & Huberman, 1994). I read each transcript was read at least. Codes were derived directly from the participant's responses and emerging themes were compared within cases and across cases to develop a valid understanding of the issues related to same-sex partner bereavement. This process was informed by Boyatzis (1998), who defined a theme as "a pattern in the information that at a minimum describes and organises the possible observations and at maximum interprets aspects of the phenomenon" (p. 161). As the research was exploratory in nature, it may be difficult to generalize the findings.

Ethical Approval

Ethical approval was gained through the University Research Governance Committee for a qualitative approach using semistructured interviews with older lesbian and gay respondents who had experienced the loss of a partner, and those working within specific support agencies working with them.

FINDINGS

A number of key themes arose in both the interviews with bereaved individuals and those with agencies that support them. Identity issues and concerns about prejudice and homophobia were central concerns for all participants, and these issues intersect with the five themes emerging from the study.

Undisclosed Identities

Two participants spoke of difficulties in accessing bereavement support due to the hidden or undisclosed nature of their relationship, and stories of disenfranchised grief due to undisclosed identities were also highlighted in all three agency interviews. The undisclosed nature of a relationship makes it difficult for individuals to grieve for their partners as partners and not just friends. This also means that those around them are unaware of the significance of the relationship in their lives. These stories reiterate themes identified by Almack et al. (2010) in terms of undisclosed identities and disenfranchisement. In these circumstances, grief becomes disenfranchised as the true significance of the relationship is hidden from wider view. One individual reflected upon how the 'hidden' nature of his relationship had complicated the grieving process: "I had very little support and because I wasn't out, I think that's so important to be out now in hindsight" (Edwin, loss of partner of 16 years).

As one participant clearly identified, the death of a partner can force one to *come out* when one's relationship has been hidden, and when one is already feeling very vulnerable: "The death of a partner becomes a very public thing so it's an issue and it forces you into a situation you weren't quite ready for" (Veronica, loss of partner of 28 years).

Wider issues of hidden lives may result in families not knowing or acknowledging a relationship, and denying the bereaved partner the same rights as a widow or widower would receive. For example, Penny, who has worked within the funeral business for a number of years, talked of how secret relationships mean the loss for the bereaved person remains unacknowledged: "The person who was bereaved was devastated . . . devastated by the loss, devastated that they weren't able to acknowledged what it really meant and kind of still fighting with themselves about the fact that there was this big coming out issue" (Penny, funeral practitioner with 21 years of experience).

Disenfranchised grief can also result from negative responses from faith communities concerning the validity of same-sex partnerships. Individuals may have attended church, but kept their relationship a secret. When their partner dies, they may want a faith-based funeral, but may receive a less than positive response. This situation was illustrated by Paul, who works for an LGBT older persons support agency:

> A lot of them get very anxious because they want a church funeral, a Christian funeral, and ministers will refuse because of their sexuality. . . . They might say you can't be buried in my churchyard, or they wouldn't get a Roman Catholic priest to do it because of the rules of their church, so it's very hard.

The experiences outlined by participants suggests that internalized homophobia and oppression (Thompson & Thompson, 2001) influences their feelings about being open about their sexuality (author citation), and this, in turn, contributes to the experience of disenfranchised grief. The hidden nature of relationships results in the significance of the relationship remaining unacknowledged, and their grief is subsequently disenfranchised (Doka, 1989).

Recognition of a Partnership and Disenfranchised Grief

Although having an undisclosed identity and relationship can complicate the grieving process and lead to disenfranchised grief, being *out* and in a civil partnership does not necessarily mean that individuals can access the bereavement and wider social support and recognition they require. Although it has been suggested that entering into a civil partnership can offer new kinship and extended family groups to partners (Shipman & Smart, 2007), some individuals can still find themselves socially isolated and alone following the death of their partner. Frank, who had a Civil Partnership with his partner, spoke of his desolation following the death of his partner and how he felt isolated and let down by those around him including friends and his partners family: "Oh, I've been through the mill. What else can I say? . . . And I've had no support from anybody, honest to God. I have been completely and utterly on my own" (Frank, loss of partner of 16 years).

A lack of recognition of a partnership by the wider community can negate the grief and emotions they feel, leaving them feeling isolated and bereft. However, disenfranchised grief is not a universal aspect of LGBT bereavement (Shernoff, 1997), and for some friendship groups and families of choice proved very supportive. Alex spoke positively about the support of his friends during his partner's illness and subsequent death and how this supported him to arrange his partner's funeral: "It was a non-religious ceremony and we had the coffin draped in the gay flag and I dressed outrageously in a suit covered with flowers, so we tried to make it a happy event, and it was" (Alex, loss of partner of 40 years).

Some have been able to access bereavement support in the months and years following the loss of their partner, either by reengaging with the wider gay community or by accessing private counseling. Edwin described how meeting a new gay-friendship group helped validate his feelings of loss for his partner and supported him to cope with his grief: "Oh it's wonderful; it's more than friendship; it's family; well, it's more than family."

Social networks do not remain static (Almack et al., 2010) and being able to access new groups and support can help alleviate the experience of disenfranchised grief for some. How individuals can be supported to engage with wider community support, and how LGBT communities respond to the needs of older members may warrant further exploration.

Cultural Competency Within the Health and Social Care Service Workforce

There was mixed feedback concerning the type of end-of-life and bereavement support that individuals and their partners received from health and social care providers, and the cultural competency of practitioners and agencies to deal sensitively with bereavement issues for older LGBT people. Some spoke very highly of the individualized and thoughtful support they and their partner received in terms of end-of -life care; others experienced discrimination and homophobic treatment. Veronica, who experienced the sudden and unexpected death of her partner, spoke very highly of the care both she and her partner received in the hospital setting: "I actually found that all the agencies that I had to deal with were totally professional and really helpful and supportive."

Alex spoke of positive care from the medical and health care team in his partner's end-of-life treatment and of being "very fortunate to have a doctor who was so supportive and understanding." However, his contact with social services was not so positive, and he experienced a lack of understanding of his relationship with his partner: "I think quite a few people in the council, hadn't really experience of a gay relationship like ours and found it hard to credit it as a viable relationship."

Alex's negative experience in terms of his contact with statutory social care services is somewhat surprising, given that a core social work value is to combat discrimination and oppression related to gender or sexual orientation (IFSW, 2012). However, this may confirm concerns that social work education does not adequately address LGBT issues (Gezinski, 2009; Martinez, 2011). It may equally highlight the issue of unqualified workers being increasingly employed within older people services (Lombard, 2011), who may lack the necessary knowledge and skills to work sensitively with LGBT groups. Increasingly, those working in social care agencies with older people may not have a professional social work qualification. They may, therefore, have limited training to adequately deal with issues of diversity and cultural difference in the ageing population, and this raises issues about the cultural competency across the wider health and social care workforce.

Both Frank and Edwin spoke positively of excellent end-of-life treatment within hospital settings, and of receiving recognition and validation of the importance of their relationships with their partners. However, unfortunately, Edwin's experience of his partners transfer into hospice care was not so positive, resulting in his partner being transferred back to the hospital where Edwin felt he had received more personalized and thoughtful care: "In the hospice, the person in charge was obviously very homophobic, although the care in the hospital was very positive."

This highlights the importance of end-of-life care providers remaining vigilant to heteronormative assumptions about relationships (National Council for Palliative Care, 2011), and upholding a commitment to meet the needs of the diverse community of older people.

Accessing Appropriate Bereavement Support

Two key issues arise in terms of accessing appropriate bereavement information and support. The first is the need for information and support that is readily identified as LGBT specific or friendly, and the second relates to providing accessible support for those older LGBT individuals who are not out. As Veronica suggests, this requires information to be

> Well publicized so people knew it was available, knew it was gay friendly, that it was totally discreet, because there are quite a lot of people even now, who are not out, or not fully out, so you'd want support that was both discreet and gay friendly.

Agencies need to commit to providing accurate information on what services are available both locally and nationally in terms of bereavement support, and where gaps exists; both statutory and voluntary sector agencies need to commit to service development, including consideration of how such provision can be sustainably funded.

In the months following the loss of a partner, accessing informative and appropriate professional support seemed to be difficult for the participants. Veronica spoke about trying to access support appropriate to her own needs, and encountered great difficulty in this, which compounded her feelings of loss and isolation: "I was looking for things to read just to identify with really and there was precious little. . . . There wasn't any specific support for gay people who were bereaved, and I did look."

Veronica spoke of difficulty in accessing bereavement counseling, and a concern that this would not be sensitive to her needs as a lesbian women. This highlights a potential heterosexist focus within mainstream bereavement counseling provision. As Veronica describes, "They were all very heterosexual and there was absolutely no mention of a gay relationship or partners, . . . so it didn't feel it was; it didn't feel it could be about me."

Gill, an LGBT advocacy worker, suggested that from her experience, most lesbians pay privately for bereavement counseling "because historically, the mainstream support services have actively discriminated against LGBT people." By seeking support from the private sector, the need for more appropriate LGBT bereavement services goes unrecorded and unmet by mainstream providers. Some support is forthcoming from LGBT community organizations, although access to these depends very much on geographical location, with those living in more rural communities having limited access. Frank spoke positively about eventually finding some support from an LGBT support and advocacy service: "I must say she has been brilliant, she has, although she can't be my buddy-buddy but . . . she has been there, I mean, whatever she could do she's done."

Sadly, this support was not sustainable, and when the agency lost its funding, community outreach services disappeared. Frank identified the need for more social support groups where both bereaved and lonely older gay people could meet to support each other. Fellowship groups for older gay men have developed in the United States, providing affective fellowship for socially isolated individuals (Shokeid, 2001). In the United Kingdom, local communities are increasingly looking at ways that older isolated gay and lesbian individuals can support one another through fellowship meetings. Paul describes how he helped to set up a fellowship group due to the absence of appropriate support for older gay people in the local area.

> [It] has been going 3 years now, and they are looking after each other, so if somebody is not well and somebody else will take some shopping, and they've been swapping walking sticks and all sorts of things, but it's lovely, because where do they go?

This raises the issue of support being provided from within the lesbian and gay communities to support older citizens with their bereavement support needs.

Support From Funeral Homes

All of the bereaved participants spoke very positively about the support and understanding they received from their contact with funeral homes. Alex described the funeral director as "being very supportive," and Veronica described the funeral director she had contact with as "amazing."

Funeral directors occupy a difficult space and are often caught between the colliding social worlds of the deceased person. Penny, a funeral director herself, described witnessing occasions where families took over funeral arrangements without a thought for the bereaved partner. In these instances, the funeral director can find himself or herself trying to meet the differing needs of the deceased's partner, and their biological family.

> So there were often funerals where we were negotiating with the family, who were the clients, who were the people that we, you know, legally should be negotiating with, but because um, we actually understood what the um, the wider picture was, we were also caring for the other people who had been marginalized by the clients. (Penny, funeral practitioner with 21 year experience)

Little research has been undertaken in terms of the responsiveness of the wider funeral services field and how they respond to LGBT issues, and this area appears ripe for future research. In particular, it is important for social workers to understand the wider support mechanisms that may be available from individuals across both statutory, voluntary and private sector providers.

DISCUSSION

This small-scale study has raised a number of issues concerning end-of-life and bereavement support needs of older LGBT people in the United Kingdom. There were both positive and negative experiences in the participant stories, and this raises the importance for health and social care providers to continue to focus on dignity, respect, and fairness in end-of-life care (Rawlings, 2012), and developing cultural competency to work with the needs of a diverse population of older people. The NHS National End of Life Care Programme (2012) has recently produced guidance for improving end-of-life care for LGBT people, and this identifies the importance of encouraging LGBT people to be confident in being open about their relationships and needs. However, fear of discrimination at the hands of health and social care providers is often the result of a lifetime experience of homophobia or heteronormative assumptions, and individuals will require support to begin to trust agencies with their emotional needs during end-of-life care and bereavement. Concern from individuals that they will be discriminated against (Hughes, 2009), that their needs will remain unacknowledged, alongside actual experiences of homophobic behavior, highlights the on-going importance of improving the cultural awareness and competence of health and social work practitioners.

One way that social work can respond to the unique needs of older LGBT people, during end-of-life care or bereavement, is to acknowledge the impact of "historical disadvantage" on people's fears and expectations of health and social care practice (Hughes, Ozanne, & Bigby, 2009, p. 128). Social work is in a unique position to support older LGBT individuals, as social work "brings a whole systems approach to dying," which includes community and cultural perspectives (Reith & Payne, 2009, p. 16). This approach is strengthened by a core commitment to combating discrimination and oppression linked to sexuality, which means that social work occupies a central position in being able to meet the needs of the most vulnerable and disadvantaged during times of loss and bereavement. However, as this small exploratory study suggests, to fulfill this potential social work education needs to ensure that both bereavement and LGBT issues are firmly embedded within curricula (Martinez, 2011; Walsh-Burke & Csikai, 2005). Even less is known about the experiences of other sexual minority groups including transgender and intersex individuals (Witten & Eyler, 2012), and this gap in knowledge needs to be addressed by both policy and research.

This exploratory study highlighted concerns of a small group of older lesbians and gay men concerning their bereavement experiences. A number of key issues that are pertinent to social work practice are identified, and it is important that staff members are equipped with the necessary skills and knowledge to deal sensitively with older LGBT people (Lombard, 2011). It is vital for practitioners to understand the impact of ageism, homophobia, and heterosexism on individual and group identity, and how this helps to shape bereavement experiences. To achieve this, social work education needs to broaden inclusion of LGBT issues and later life when considering diversity issues within the curriculum (Smith et al. 2010), and this theme is echoed by the IFSW (2009) who identified a need for education around ageing issues to be expanded for social workers.

A commitment to supporting older LGBT people through bereavement experiences also involves recognition of resilience factors, as well as risk factors. Older lesbians and gay men have often developed resilience by coping with a lifetime of stigma and oppression, and this may enable them to cope with some of the challenges of later life including loss (Grossman, D'Augelli, & Dragowski, 2007). This "crisis competence" (p. 117) enables negative experiences to be used as positive and affirming strengths (Kimmel, 1978). As some of the respondents in this group identified, support from within the gay community is an important element of the support available. This links to notions of fellowship groups that provide social support to often isolated individuals (Shokeid 2001). Social workers, therefore, need to develop an appreciation of the wider psycho-social nature of support that older lesbian and gay people access, including both their own resilience factors and their care networks or communities of practice (Hughes & Kentlyn, 2011), including social groups and/or families of choice (Cohen & Murray, 2006).

LIMITATIONS AND IMPLICATIONS

The small explorative nature of this study is a limitation, and research with larger LGBT samples is required to develop the knowledge base of bereavement practice. In light of the invisibility of older LGBT needs, and in particular the impact of undisclosed or disenfranchised grief, it is important to work in collaborative and empowering ways with older LGBT people (Crisp, Wayland, & Gordon, 2008), and this includes developing projects where individuals can be involved in cooperative and participative inquiry. Future research should include greater diversity with respect to geography, race/ethnicity, and gender. Issues about sampling within seldom heard communities also needs addressed. Snowball sampling can be a useful way to recruit participants, but research that is coproduced with LGBT community organizations may have better results in recruiting those seldom heard individuals, particular concerning sensitive topics such as bereavement.

REFERENCES

Almack, K., Seymour, J., & Bellamy, G. (2010). Exploring the impact of sexual orientation on experiences and concerns about end of life care and on bereavement for lesbian, gay and bisexual older people. *Sociology, 44,* 908–924.

Baier, M., & Buechsel, R. (2012). A model to help bereaved individuals understand the grief process. *Mental Health Practice, 16*, 28–32.

Bent, K. N., & Magilvy, J. K. (2006). When a partner dies: Lesbian widows. *Issues in Mental Health Nursing, 27*, 447–459.

Boyatzis, R. (1998) *Transforming qualitative information: Thematic analysis and code development*. Thousand Oaks, CA: Sage.

Cartwright, C., Hughes, M., & Lienert, T. (2012). End-of-life care for gay, lesbian, bisexual and transgender people. *Culture, Health & Sexuality, 14*, 537–548.

Civil Partnership Act. (2004). London, England: Her Majesty's Stationery Office.

Cohen, H. L., & Murray, Y. (2006). Older lesbian and gay caregivers caring for families of choice and caring for families of origin. *Journal of Human Behaviour and the Social Environment. 14*, 275–298.

Costello, J., & Kendrick, K. (2000). Grief and older people: The making or breaking of emotional bonds following partner loss in later life. *Journal of Advanced Nursing, 32*, 1374–1382.

Crisp, C., Wayland, S., & Gordon, T. (2008). Older gay, lesbian, and bisexual adults: Tools for age—Competent and gay affirmative practice. *Journal of Gay and Lesbian Social Services, 20*, 5–29.

Currer, C. (2007) *Loss and social work*. Exeter, England: Learning Matters

Deevey, S. (2000). Cultural variations in lesbian bereavement experiences in Ohio. *Journal of Gay Lesbian Medical Association, 4*, 9–17.

Doka, K. (1989). *Disenfranchised grief: Recognizing hidden sorrow*. New York, NY: Lexington Books.

Doka, K. (2002). *Disenfranchised grief: New directions, challenges and strategies for practice*. Champaign, IL: Research Press.

Equality Act. (2004). London, England: Her Majesty's Stationary Office.

Fenge, L., & Fannin, A. (2009). Sexuality and bereavement: Implications for practice with older lesbians and gay men. *Practice: Social Work in Action, 21*, 35–46.

Fish, J. (2008). Far from mundane: Theorising heterosexism for social work education. *Social Work Education, 27*, 182–193.

Fish, J. (2010). Conceptualising social exclusion and lesbian, gay, bisexual, and transgender people: the implications for promoting equity in nursing policy and practice. *Journal of Research in Nursing, 15*, 303–312.

Fredriksen, K. I., & Muraco, A. (2010). Aging and sexual orientation: A 25-year review of the literature. *Research on Aging, 32*, 372–413.

Futterman, A., Holland, J. M., Brown, P. J., Thompson, L. W., & Gallagher-Thompson, D. (2010). Factorial validity of the Texas Revised Inventory of Grief-Present Scale among bereaved older adults. *Psychological Assessment 22*, 675–687.

Gay and Grey in Dorset. (2006). *Lifting the lid on sexuality and ageing*. Bournemouth, UK: Bournemouth University & Help and Care Development Ltd.

Gezinski, L. (2009). Addressing sexual minority issues in social work education: A curriculum framework. *Advances in Social Work, 10*, 103–113.

Glacken, M. & Higgins, A. (2008). The grief experience of same sex couples within an Irish context: Tacit acknowledgement. *International Journal of Palliative Nursing, 14*, 297–302.

Green, L., & Grant, V. (2008). Gagged grief and beleaguered bereavements? An analysis of multidisciplinary theory and research relating to same sex partnership bereavement. *Sexualities, 11*, 275–300.

Grossman, A. H., D'Augelli, A. R., & Dragowski, E. A. (2007). Caregiving and care receiving among older lesbian, gay and bisexual adults. *Journal of Gay and Lesbian Social Services, 18*, 15–38.

Hash, K. M., & Cramer, E. P. (2003). Empowering gay and lesbian caregivers and uncovering their unique experiences through the use of qualitative methods. *Journal of Gay & Lesbian Social Services, 15*, 47–63.

Hornjakevyc, N. L., & Alderson, K.G. (2011). With and without: The bereavement experiences of gay men who have lost a partner to non-AIDS related causes. *Death Studies, 35*, 801–823.

Hughes, M. (2009). Lesbian and gay people's concerns about ageing and accessing services. *Australian Social Work, 62*, 186–201.

Hughes, M., & Kentlyn, S. (2011). Older LGBT people's care networks and communities of practice: A brief note. *International Social Work, 54*, 436–444.

Hughes, M., Ozanne, E., & Bigby, C. (2009). Editorial: Diversity and ageing. *Australian Social Work, 62*, 127–131.

International Federation of Social Work. (2009). *International policy on ageing and older persons.* Retrieved from http://www.ifsw.org/p38000214.html.

International Federation of Social Work. (2012). *Statement of Ethical Principles'.* Retrieved from http://ifsw.org/policies/statement-of-ethical-principles

Kimmel, D. C. (1978). Adult development and aging: A gay perspective. *Journal of Social Issues, 34*, 113–130.

King, A., & Cronin, A. (2010). Queer methods and queer practices: Re-examining the identities of older lesbian, gay, bisexual adults. In K. Browne & C. Nash (Eds.) *Queer methods and methodologies: Intersecting queer theories and social science research* (pp. 85–96). Aldershot, England: Ashgate.

Knocker, S. (2012). *Perspectives on ageing: Lesbians, gay men and bisexual.* York, England: Joseph Rowntree Foundation.

Langley, J. (2001). Developing anti-oppressive empowering social work practice with older lesbian women and gay men. *British Journal of Social Work, 31*, 917–932.

Lombard, D. (2011, July 4). College warning over misuse of personalisation. *Community Care*, 4–5.

Martinez, P. (2011). A modern conceptualisation of sexual prejudice for social work educators. *Social Work Education, 30*, 558–570.

Miles, M. B., & Huberman, A. M. (1994). *Qualitative data analysis.* Thousand Oaks, CA: Sage.

National Council for Palliative Care. (2011). *Open to all?* London, England: NCPC and the Consortium of Lesbian, Gay, Bisexual and Transgendered Voluntary and Community Organisations.

NHS National End of Life Care Programme. (2012). *The route to success in end of life care—Achieving quality for lesbian, gay bisexual and transgender people.* Retrieved from www.endoflifecareforadults.nhs.uk.

Price, E. (2005). All but invisible: Older gay men and lesbians. *Nursing Older People, 17*, 16–18.

Rawlings, D. (2012). End-of-life care considerations for gay, lesbian, bisexual, and transgender individuals. *International Journal of Palliative Nursing, 18*, 29–34.

Reith, M., & Payne, M. (2009). *Social work in end-of-life and palliative care.* Chicago, IL: Lyceum.

Rondahl, G., Innala, S., & Carlsson, M. (2006). Heterosexual assumptions in verbal and non verbal communication in nursing. *Journal of Advanced Nursing, 56*, 373–81.

Rosenfield, D., Bartlam, B., & Smith, R. D. (2012.) Out of the closet and into the trenches: Gay male baby boomers, aging and HIV/AIDS. *Gerontologist, 52*, 255–264.

Schaefer, J. A., & Moos, R. H. (2001). Bereavement experiences and personal growth. In M. S. Stroebe, R. O. Hansson, W. Stroebe, & H. Schut (Eds.), *Handbook of bereavement research: Consequences, coping, and care* (pp. 145–167). Washington, DC: American Psychological Association.

Shernoff, M. (1997). Conclusion: Mental health considerations of gay widowers. *Journal of Gay and Lesbian Services, 7*, 137–155.

Shipman, B., & Smart, C. (2007). "It's made a huge difference": Recognition, rights and the personal significance of civil partnership. *Sociological Research Online, 12*(1). Retrieved from http://www.socresonline.org.uk/12/1/shipman.html.

Shokeid, M. (2001). Our group has a life of its own: An affective fellowship of older gay men in New York City. *City and Society, 13*, 5–30.

Smith, L. A., McCaslin, R., Chang, J., Martinez, P., & McGrew, P. (2010). Assessing the needs of older gay, lesbian, bisexual, and transgender people: A service-learning and agency partnership approach. *Journal of Gerontological Social Work, 53*, 387–401.

Social Work Reform Board. (2010). *Professional capabilities framework*. London, England: Social Work Reform Board.

Thompson, N., & Thompson, S. (2001). Empowering older people, beyond the care model. *Journal of Social Work, 1*, 61–76.

Thompson, S. (2002). Older people. In N. Thompson (Ed.), *Loss and grief: A guide for human service practitioners* (pp. 162–173). Basingstoke, England: Palgrave.

Walsh-Burke, K., & Csikai, E. L. (2005). Professional social work education in end-of-life care: Contributions of the Project on Death in America's Social Work Leadership Development Program. *Journal of Social Work in End-of-Life & Palliative Care, 1*, 11–26.

Warner, J. P., Wright, L., Blanchard, M., & King, M. (2003). The psychological health and quality of life of older lesbians and gay men: A snowball sampling pilot survey. *International Journal of Geriatric Psychiatry, 18*, 754–755.

Wee, B. L., Coleman, P. G., Hillier, R., & Holgate, S. H. (2006). The sound of death rattle I: Are relatives distressed by hearing this sound. *Palliative Medicine, 20*, 171–175.

Witten, T. M., & Eyler, A. E. (Eds.). (2012). *Gay, lesbian, bisexual & transgender aging: Challenges in research, practice & policy*. Baltimore, MD: John Hopkins University Press.

Worden, W. (1991) *Grief counselleing and grief therapy—A handbook for the mental health practitioner* (2nd ed.). London, England: Routledge.

Yuval-Davis, N. (2006). Intersectionality and feminist politics. *European Journal of Women's Studies, 13*, 193–209.

Assessing Capacity for Providing Culturally Competent Services to LGBT Older Adults

JENNIFER DICKMAN PORTZ

Institute for Health Research, Kaiser Permanente Colorado, Denver, Colorado, USA,
Graduate School of Social Work, University of Denver, Denver, Colorado, USA, and
School of Social Work, Colorado State University, Fort Collins, Colorado, USA

JESSICA H. RETRUM

Department of Social Work, Metropolitan State University of Denver, Denver, Colorado, USA
and School of Public Affairs, University of Colorado Denver, Denver, Colorado, USA

LESLIE A. WRIGHT and JENNIFER M. BOGGS

Institute for Health Research, Kaiser Permanente Colorado, Denver, Colorado, USA

SHARI WILKINS

The Gay, Lesbian, Bisexual & Transgender Community Center of Colorado,
Denver, Colorado, USA

CATHY GRIMM

Jewish Family Service, Denver, Colorado, USA

KAY GILCHRIST

Services and Advocacy for Gay, Lesbian, Bisexual & Transgender Elders (SAGE)
of the Rockies Committee, Denver, Colorado, USA

WENDOLYN S. GOZANSKY

Institute for Health Research, Kaiser Permanente Colorado, Denver, Colorado, USA

This qualitative, interview-based study assessed the cultural com-
petence of health and social service providers to meet the needs of
LGBT older adults in an urban neighborhood in Denver, Colorado,
known to have a large LGBT community. Only 4 of the agencies
were categorized as "high competency"; 12 were felt to be "seeking
improvement" and 8 were considered "not aware." These results
indicate significant gaps in cultural competency for the majority

of service providers. Social workers are well-suited to lead efforts directed at improving service provision and care competencies for the older LGBT community.

INTRODUCTION

Lesbian, gay, bisexual, and transgender (LGBT) persons are at higher risk for health issues and face social and institutionalized barriers to accessing health-care and social services as they age (Fredriksen-Goldsen et al., 2011; Met Life, 2006). Related to these barriers, although older LGBT adults have disproportionately higher needs compared with their heterosexual counterparts (Cahill, South, & Spade, 2000), older LGBT community members consistently report a lack of confidence in the *gay friendliness* of service providers, which likely contributes to their lower rates of service utilization (Service and Advocacy for GLBT Elders [SAGE], 2010; Stein, Beckerman, & Sherman, 2010). This issue is not well understood and only recently has research been implemented to examine the factors associated with the lack of competence among social and health service providers when working with LGBT older adults. Although efforts are underway to counter the lack of research on the LGBT aging population and to better integrate LGBT aging issues into related public policy (Hudson, 2011), further research is needed to identify solutions regarding a lack of cultural competency among health and social service providers so that the needs of LGBT older adults can be appropriately addressed. This study contributes to addressing this gap in the literature by investigating cultural competency of health and social service organizations serving LGBT older adults in one Denver, Colorado community.

LITERATURE REVIEW

There are an estimated 2–7 million older adults in the United States who identify as LGBT; that is approximately 5–10% of the older adult population (Grant, 2010). Approximately 320,000 LGBT persons reside in Colorado, and Denver ranks 7th in the United States for percentage of LGBT households. In a 2011 survey ($N = 4,619$) conducted by Colorado's lead LGBT advocacy organization to learn more about the lives and issues faced by the state's LGBT population, One Colorado Education Fund identified that about 15% ($n = 687$) of the statewide LGBT respondents were 55 or older. When asked to identify the top five policy or social issues for LGBT people in Colorado, 52% identified increased support and services for LGBT older adults, and 42% ranked access to LGBT-welcoming healthcare. Thirty-five percent lived alone, 11% had caregiver duties for another adult or their partner, and 57% had no designated beneficiary agreement in Colorado. Thirty percent of respondents aged 65 or older ($n = 158$) were not open about their sexual orientation/gender identity with their healthcare provider (One Colorado Education Fund, 2011).

Needs and Risks

LGBT older adults are identified as a group at risk for isolation (Addis, Davies, Greene, MacBride Stewart, & Shepherd, 2009; Wallace, Cochran, Durazo, & Ford, 2011). Members of the LGBT community over the age of 50 are more likely to be single and live alone (Fredriksen-Goldsen et al., 2011). In addition, these individuals may be at higher risk of experiencing negative consequences of isolation because they are more than four times as likely as heterosexual older adults to be childless (Fredriksen-Goldsen et al., 2011). Caregiving support will likely be limited for many LGBT older adults, and LGBT persons providing care to a partner may face compounded risks related to reduced informal family supports in addition to fear of discrimination within the formal healthcare and legal systems (Fredriksen-Goldsen & Hoy-Ellis, 2007; Muraco & Fredriksen-Goldsen, 2011). This factor has several health related implications:

> Research suggests that social isolation can lead to a number of mental and physical ailments such as depression, delayed care-seeking, poor nutrition, and poverty—all factors that greatly lessen the quality of life for both LGBT older adults and elders of color. Living in isolation, and fearful of the discrimination they could encounter in mainstream aging settings, many marginalized elders are also at a higher risk for elder abuse, neglect, and various forms of exploitation. For LGBT elders of color, this social isolation might be intensified, since they might also be isolated from their racial and ethnic communities as LGBT older people and isolated from the mainstream LGBT community as people of color. (Fredriksen-Goldsen et al., 2011)

Although an initial understanding of the health needs and risks for LGBT older adults is underway, there is still much to learn. In 2011, the Institute of Medicine (IOM) and National Institutes of Health convened a group of experts to discuss ways to improve the limited evidence base on LGBT health. They put forth a research agenda focusing on demographics, social influences on health and health care inequities, interventions, and transgender-specific health needs (IOM, 2011). This agenda directly relates to examining the quality of care LGBT older adults may receive; which in several ways is directly determined by the competence of the service providers.

Additionally, The Joint Commission recently released a Field Guide for health and social service providers comprising a collation of approaches, practice examples, resources, and recommendations designed to support hospital staff in increasing quality of care by providing care that is more hospitable, safe, and inclusive of LGBT patients and families (Joint Commission, 2011). Although there is a wealth of research related to cultural competence, there is a literature gap specific to competence of health and social service provision for LGBT older adults. These recent efforts by IOM and the Joint Commission are a response to this current gap in the research and practice.

Cultural Competence

Cultural competence in social work practice is multifaceted and comprised of a combination of factors including (Cooper & Lesser, 2005, p. 71):

1. Cultural literacy or the experience from immersion in another culture,
2. Cross-cultural specific knowledge,
3. Practitioner's awareness of their own assumptions, values and beliefs, and
4. Willingness to learn and be comfortable with not being the expert in every culture.

Importantly, when cultural competence is applied at an organizational, rather than a provider level, it involves policies and procedures that are flexible and considerate of the needs, fears, and preferences of disenfranchised groups that the organization serves.

Although cultural competency is an important value of professional social work, standards are not noticeably being pursued for LGBT older adults. Studies suggest that there is a lack of culturally competent health and social services available for the older LGBT community nationwide. In many instances, social services sustain homophobic and heterosexist beliefs that provoke fear and anxiety in LGBT older adults when accessing services such as housing and healthcare (Cahill et al., 2000; Coon, 2007). LGBT seniors are five times less likely to access available public and community services due to fear of discrimination or harm (SAGE, 2010; Stein et al., 2010).

LGBT older adults and their caregivers may be apprehensive of cultural competence deficiencies among health care providers (Brotman et al., 2007; MetLife, 2006). In an extensive review of the literature examining care-seeking behavior of older LGBT individuals, Fredriksen-Goldsen and Muraco (2010) found that LGBT older adults are at increased risk of abstaining from needed care. A lack of access to care for this population has been established (Clark, Landers, Linde, & Sperber, 2001). Evidence suggests that fears experienced by LGBT seniors are warranted (Smedley, Stith, & Nelson, 2003) and the need for improved competency of services provided to the LGBT aging population is clear (Knochel, Quam, & Croghan, 2011; Meyer, 2011).

However, further examination of current cultural competencies of health-care and social service providers is needed to understand best practices for intervention.

The purpose of this study was to explore the level of cultural competence of health and social service providers to ultimately improve services for LGBT older adults in an urban neighborhood of Denver, Colorado. The study was conducted by Seniors Using Supports to Age in Neighborhoods (SUSTAIN). This community-research partnership is comprised of aging service agencies, community-based organizations, health care systems and local universities whose purpose is to understand and begin to address health, social service, and community needs of LGBT older adults in this metropolitan Denver neighborhood. The SUSTAIN partners are members of the LGBT community or straight allies with strong connections to the LGBT aging community. The vision of the partnership is to create a community where LGBT seniors are able to age in a safe and trusting environment. This article discusses findings from interviews conducted with service providers whose organizations address primary needs identified by the LGBT aging community. To better understand the level of cultural competence of local health and social service providers, the goals of this study were to: (a) describe the services of local providers, (b) better understand the consumers and staff characteristics of these organizations, and (c) explore provider perceptions of LGBT older adults' health and social needs.

METHOD

This investigation was a formative evaluation using rapid assessment techniques emphasizing a team-oriented, participatory action, and time-sensitive approach to generate information related to service provision for LGBT older adults (Beebe, 2013; Padgett, 2012; World Health Organization, 2004). Rapid assessment is commonly used to design culturally appropriate interventions for health and social problems, by focusing on local knowledge about these issues. Rapid assessment is a time efficient, team-based ethnographic approach to qualitative inquiry that can quickly develop a preliminary understanding of a problem or situation (Beebe, 2013). As a team, the SUSTAIN partnership conducted interviews with local social service, health, and faith-based organizations. All study-related procedures were approved by the Kaiser Permanente Colorado Institutional Review Board.

Recruitment

A convenience sample of local neighborhood providers was selected from a comprehensive list of providers. This list of 110 organizations was created by researching all social service, health, and faith-based providers in the geographic area, and was then organized into service categories defined by the partnership, including: legal, benefit assistance, mental health, transportation, housing, aging specific, faith-based, home services, political, senior engagement, and end-of-life care. The list was then reviewed by SUSTAIN partners to select 2–3 organizations per category to provide a broad variety of service types for interviews. With the intent to interview 30 organizations, 43 potential interview participants were initially selected based upon the following criteria: (a) unknown to the SUSTAIN partnership to be LGBT competent, and (b) provided a specific service to older adults in the Denver neighborhood under investigation. SUSTAIN participating organizations and agencies known to the partnership as particularly LGBT-friendly were excluded from participation. With the intent to interview 30 providers, the list was then distributed across six SUSTAIN partners from various organizations for the recruitment of interviewees, each responsible for the recruitment of 5 participants. Thirty potential provider participants were contacted by these SUSTAIN partners via telephone and e-mail; however, only 29 providers completed the interview.

Interviews

The interviews were completed by the six SUSTAIN partners over the phone or in-person based on the providers' preference. All of the evaluators were trained interviewers with backgrounds in either clinical or research interview techniques. To prepare for data collection, the interviewers conducted mock interviews with fellow SUSTAIN partners. Prior to the interview, participants were given an informed consent document and oral consent was obtained. The interviews were structured in format, meaning a standardized sequence of questions was utilized to increase reliability across interviewers (Patton, 1991), and were approximately 30–90 min in length. Although interviews were audio recorded to ensure accuracy in interpretation, due to the time sensitive nature of rapid assessment, field notes, rather than transcription, were utilized for data analysis. Field notes were first taken during the interviews, and were later confirmed and detailed by the interviewer when reviewing the audio recordings.

The interview guide was created collaboratively by the SUSTAIN partners. Questions were derived from SUSTAIN's previous community member needs assessment, which is currently under review for publication elsewhere. Questions inquired about consumer and staff characteristics, service provision, and LGBT cultural competency (Table 1). Specifically pertaining to competency, these questions highlighted organizations' awareness of the aging LGBT population served, friendliness of these services to older LGBT adults, and understanding of LGBT older adults' needs. Although structured in nature, the interview guide allowed the flexibility for elaboration and probing if needed.

TABLE 1 Interview Guide Summary

Consumers and staff
How would you describe your clients?
Do you have a sense of what percentage might be LGBT? What about staff?
What is the age range of LGBT clients?
What lets you know that your clients/staff are LGBT?
Does your employee benefits package equally recognize straight and LGBT partnerships?
Services
Have you thought about how welcoming your services are for LGBT older adults?
How would an older LGBT person know that you are welcoming?
Does your mission statement, intake form or marketing materials reflect that you are welcoming to the LGBT community?
Have you made any specific changes in your business to better serve the LGBT community?
How do you train your employees to be welcoming?
Serving LGBT older adults
What unique knowledge, skills or qualities do you feel you need to serve the LGBT community?
How do you keep yourself informed on LGBT community events and information?

Note. LGBT = lesbian, gay, bisexual, transgender.

Analysis

Completed interview guides and field notes were compiled for all interviews and analyzed by research assistants at Kaiser Permanente Colorado to identify key topics related to consumer and staff characteristics, services, and cultural competency. Specifically, two cycles of coding were carried out to develop final results. Structure coding, which is used to identify specific areas of inquiry, and process coding, which identifies ongoing action in response to problematic situations were first used to code based on the structured question areas and ongoing actions of agencies (Saldana, 2009). The second cycle of coding employed focused coding in which the most significant initial codes are developed into salient categories (Saldana, 2009).

Through the coding process, agencies were classified into categories based on their service type and job responsibilities to describe characteristics and services of the local providers. To better understand their consumer and staff characteristics, providers were also categorized based on the percentage of LGBT consumers and staff members that they described during the interviews. Agencies typically reported a specific percentage estimate, which were organized into categories decided by the partnership, which ranged from high (more than 70%) to medium (15–60%) to low (5% or less). None of the agencies identified having between 5–15% of LGBT consumers or staff, so this level was not included as a category. Providers that were unable to offer an estimate were labeled *unknown* or *no idea*, and providers who specifically stated the majority of their consumers were straight were assigned to the *mostly straight* category.

TABLE 2 Level of Cultural Competency Focus Code and Description

Focus Code	Description/Definition
High competence	Service provider demonstrated understanding of LGBT aging issues and implemented services appropriately. These agencies explained how older LGBT adults would know services were welcoming; used appropriate materials; made changes to better serve the LGBT community; and stayed informed on LGBT issues.
Seeking improvement	Service provider recognized the need for improving services to meet needs of LGBT older adults.
Not aware	Service provider stressed being "inclusive" but disregarded need for specific LGBT cultural competencies.

Note. LGBT = lesbian, gay, bisexual, transgender.

Focused codes were then used to explore provider perceptions about LGBT older adults' needs and providers' level of cultural competency. When discussing LGBT cultural competencies, three levels of proficiency were identified (Table 2); based on interview responses, agencies were categorized using this proficiency continuum. These categories emerged from the data, as organizations provided information and examples of their understanding, awareness, and targeted services for older LGBT adults. These qualitative categories, which ranged from high competence, or agencies demonstrating high levels of awareness for LGBT older adults, to low competence, labeled *not aware*, for organizations representing little understanding or appreciation for the needs of LGBT older adults, were used to measure the level of competency among the interviewed organizations. The level of cultural competency was then examined by agency type, service provision, percentage of LGBT consumers, and percentage of LGBT staff.

To maintain rigor throughout the analysis process, the research assistants met regularly to discuss any challenges or inconsistencies in coding. Memos were recorded throughout the analysis process to document decision making. Coding results were presented to the partnership ongoing to gain feedback and insight from experts and community partners. It is also important to note partnership presuppositions. Specifically, although SUSTAIN felt that a range of competence levels would be identified, some partners speculated that competency would be lower among faith-based organizations. No other a priori assumptions were identified by the partnership.

RESULTS

Participants

Interviewees were typically executive managers ($n = 13$), but program coordinators ($n = 7$) were also commonly interviewed. Most service providers were social service organizations, health providers, or both. However,

TABLE 3 Service Provider Characteristics

Characteristic	N	%
Profit status		
Non-profit	6	20
For-profit	4	15
Unknown	19	65
Service categories[a]		
Social service	13	45
Health	9	31
Spiritual/Religious	3	10
Legal/Business	3	10
Mental health	2	7

Note. [a]Categories are not mutually exclusive.

faith-based, business, and mental health providers were also interviewed. Although some of the organizations identified as a nonprofit ($n = 6$) or for-profit agency ($n = 4$), the majority of interviewees did not specify their nonprofit status ($n = 19$). Providers offered a variety of programming for older LGBT adults, including individual and direct services, community development, network collaboration, advocacy and public policy, outreach and education, and research services. Table 3 summarizes the provider characteristics.

Consumer and Staff Characteristics

Capturing the number of LGBT older adults receiving services was difficult, with 44% of all providers responding that they did not know the proportion of their consumers who were LGBT (Table 4). Agencies often did not inquire about sexual orientation due to antidiscrimination laws. Only three agencies asked about sexual orientation, although none of these providers tracked

TABLE 4 Service Provider Estimates of Lesbian, Gay, Bisexual, or Transgender Consumers and Staff

	N	%
Percent of clients		
High (>70%)	4	14
Medium (15–60%)	4	14
Low (5%)	6	21
Mostly straight	2	7
Unknown/No idea	13	44
Percent of staff		
High (>70%)	2	3
Medium (15–60%)	5	17
Low (5%)	6	21
Unknown	16	56

the information. Self-disclosure and self-identification were the most common ways of knowing the estimated number of LGBT individuals served by the agency. Organizations who identified higher rates of LGBT consumers of all ages often attributed their answer to the type of work in which the provider specialized (e.g., HIV case management services), the location of the agency within the specific neighborhood, or a strong referral system with LGBT specific organizations. Although most agencies did not know the number of LGBT staff, regardless of age, many organizations provided staff with same-sex partner benefits. However, some agencies did not provide benefits to same-sex partners, and two required proof of marriage for benefit provision.

Serving LGBT Older Adults

The thematic framework describing agency cultural competency processes is illustrated in Figure 1. Only a few organizations ($n = 4$) were considered proficient in their awareness, understanding, and actions to appropriately serve LGBT older adults. Labeled the *high competence* group, these providers were clearly able to explain how older LGBT adults would know their services were welcoming, used appropriate materials, made changes to better serve the LGBT community, and stayed informed regarding LGBT issues. The high competence group expressed a strong understanding of LGBT aging issues and was implementing strategies appropriately to address important needs. As such, these organizations used specific materials and outreach efforts for LGBT older adults and marketed themselves effectively to maintain a welcoming reputation. In addition to specific materials, some of these organizations included explicit statements about being open to the LGBT population in their mission statement. Because these agencies felt it was important to meet these individualized needs, they were either currently or in the process of adopting strategies, such as training and documentation protocols, to improve the competence and inclusivity of their agency.

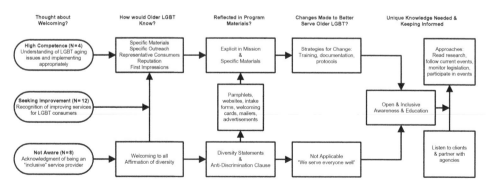

FIGURE 1 Thematic framework.

These were the same agencies that specifically followed current research, monitored legislation, and participated in events related to LGBT issues.

Most organizations ($n = 12$) were *seeking improvement*. These providers used only a few welcoming practices and, during the interview, most recognized several areas in need of improvement. The organizations classified as *not aware* ($n = 8$) stressed being inclusive but disregarded that LGBT older adults have distinct needs. The providers reported that they were welcoming to all diverse groups and stressed the use of diversity statements and antidiscrimination clauses within organization materials. The *not aware* group did not see a reason to make changes to their current practices and expressed that all persons were treated fairly and the same, regardless of specific characteristics.

Competency by agency type, service provision, and percentage of LGBT consumers and staff members varied (Figure 2). Half of the nonprofit organizations were classified as *seeking improvement* and the other half were *not aware*, whereas the majority of for-profit organizations were classified as *seeking improvement*. The largest grouping of *not aware* was among unknown nonprofit status organizations. Seven social service agencies and only one health agency were identified as *not aware*, but all mental health and legal/business providers were *seeking improvement*. The three spiritual/religious organizations interviewed were represented across all three levels of competency. The majority of providers who were unable to provide an estimate of LGBT consumers ($n = 9$ agencies) and staff

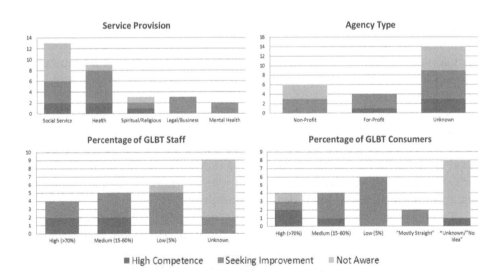

FIGURE 2 Lesbian, gay, bisexual, and transgender cultural compentency by service provider characteristics. Due to the small sample size the frequency (n) was provided for each category. The categories of service provision are not mutually exclusive.

($n = 7$ agencies) were considered *not aware*, however one agency specifying a high number of LGBT consumers was also classified as *not aware*.

DISCUSSION

This interview-based study of service providers for older adults in a metropolitan area of Denver known to have a large LGBT community revealed a broad spectrum of services and practices. Few participating agencies were categorized as having high competence to address the needs of LGBT older adults. Similar findings have been presented for aging network services in Michigan, revealing a lack of services specific to LGBT older adults and little outreach to this population (Hughes, Harold, & Boyer, 2011). However, regardless of competency classification, all providers interviewed expressed interest in partnering with SUSTAIN in ongoing work to address health and social service barriers. Thus, our results indicate a role for social work practitioners in increasing awareness of and education about culturally competent and sensitive service provision for the aging LGBT community.

The findings from these data and conversations with community stakeholders and policy makers have confirmed that the majority of organizations lack appropriate focus on the specific needs of the LGBT aging population. Social workers, whether they are community or clinical practitioners, are uniquely suited to work with communities and providers to ensure that culturally competent services are available. A few topic areas that social workers can hone their focus of practice are worth mentioning here. First, navigating and coaching older adults to identify LGBT-friendly providers is a role that social workers should seek out. As those most often providing case management services aimed at keeping older adults in their homes and maintaining independence, social workers can advocate that services be modified in a way to attend to the unique needs of LGBT older adults. Social workers can collaborate with provider agencies to identify ways to increase socialization and decrease isolation for this vulnerable population. Social workers can also work with communities to identify unique health and social service priorities based on neighborhood assessments and recommend subsequent interventions. For example, recommending competency training for providers who lack cultural proficiency for LGBT older adults.

Training provided to area agencies on aging (aging network organizations) around LGBT aging issues is limited. However, agencies with such training are significantly more likely to have services and outreach to the older LGBT community (Knochel, Croghan, Moone, & Quam, 2012). Therefore, LGBT aging curricula must first be available to social work students. This topic might best be suited for diversity or aging practice courses. Recent research suggests that LGBT aging training should provide useful and valuable information, a safe enviornment for deeper understanding and self-relflection, and incorpeate older LGBT instructors (Rogers, Rebbe, Gardella, Worlein, & Chamberlin, 2013).

Project Visibility is one example of a group that has received local as well as national accolades for providing LGBT aging specific cultural education to nursing homes, assisted livings, home care agencies, and other senior service agencies in Colorado. Project Visibility highlights the fears of "going back in the closet" and "being invisible" when LGBT older adults have to go to a nursing home or assisted living situation (Project Visibility, n.d.). Even with this wonderful resource available locally, we found many local agencies stuck in the treat-everybody-the-same mindset are unlikely to be open to these education opportunities. Social workers can increase organizations' awareness of LGBT older adult consumers, identify inadequate services, advocate for openly LGBT employees, and utilize welcoming marketing materials.

Many of the providers interviewed could not specify the sexual orientation of their client population. When agencies are unaware of the populations they serve, they are also likely to be unfamiliar with the specialized needs of diverse and vulnerable populations. Antidiscrimination policies restricted providers from inquiring about sexual minority status, and LGBT older adults are unlikely to disclose this information (One Colorado Education Fund, 2011; SAGE, 2010; Stein et al., 2010); however, agency-level policies can be put in place to enhance the provision of individualized competent services. Specifically, policies and procedures that are flexible and considerate of the needs, fears, and preferences of disenfranchised groups that the organization serves (Cooper & Lesser, 2008). However, Hughes et al. 2011 identified an agency-level resistance to provide LGBT specific services to aging adults. Addressing the reluctance of health and social service agencies to increase awareness of the expanding LGBT aging population and discomfort with LGBT issues must be addressed.

As an initial step toward providing culturally competent services for LGBT older adults, social workers must address issues of LGBT older adults' awareness of their services by improving the welcoming nature of the organization and ensuring the acceptability and accessibility of their services to LGBT older adults. Overall, there are several recommendations for macro social work practitioners that can serve as a guide for the provision of culturally competent services for LGBT older adults (Coon, 2003; Joint Commission, 2011; Lee & Quam, 2013; SAGE, 2010), including: (a) provide LGBT older adult competency training, (b) develop and adopt LGBT aging specific nondiscrimination policies, (c) collaborate with aging and LGBT supportive organizations to develop improved service standards, (d) increase onsite LGBT older adult specific services, and (e) improve opportunities for LGBT older adults to engage in services, such as volunteering and equal employment, and participate in decision making processes relevant to LGBT older adults' needs.

In addition to improvements in macro practice, clinical social workers can develop cultural competencies for older LGBT adults through the use of reflective practice to learn about their lives and concerns (Lee & Quam, 2013). Social workers should first adopt an LGBT-affirming attitude, avoiding assumptions about sexual orientation and gender identity, and working within the spectrum of *openness* (Concannon, 2007; Joint Commission, 2011). Use of open-ended and gender-neutral language in assessment questions, forms, and when speaking with consumers is essential, as is listening to individual descriptions of sexual orientation, relationships, and partnership (Concannon, 2007; Coon, 2003; Joint Commission, 2011). By providing informed, open-minded and supportive care, social workers are likely to offer enhanced culturally competent services for LGBT older adults.

Several study limitations should be acknowledged. First, the list of local aging service providers developed by the SUSTAIN partnership was meant to be highly representative, but not comprehensive, and the final choice of providers interviewed was determined by convenience, rather than random selection. This study was also limited to a specific region of a metropolitan area that has unique demographic characteristics that may influence the types of providers serving the area and thus may impact generalizability. However, it should be noted that this community was targeted due to a higher percentage of LGBT persons suggesting that our findings could represent a best case scenario for a high likelihood of cultural competency. Finally, the number of LGBT older adults actually receiving services through these local agencies remains poorly captured.

Overall, although some providers demonstrated high levels of competency and welcoming strategies, most providers need assistance in improving service provision for LGBT older adults. Further research exploring the specialized needs of this population is required to inform best practices with LGBT older adults. Social workers should collaborate with health and social service agencies and at-risk communities to enhance welcoming and sensitive services through awareness and education efforts.

ACKNOWLEDGMENTS

We acknowledge the support of additional SUSTAIN community partners: Debra Angell, Carlos Martinez, Rene Hickman, and William Lundgren.

FUNDING

This work was supported by NIH/NCATS Colorado CTSI Grant Number UL1 TR000154. Contents are the authors' sole responsibility and do not necessarily represent official NIH views.

REFERENCES

Addis, S., Davies, M., Greene, G., MacBride Stewart, S., & Shepherd, M. (2009). The health, social care and housing needs of lesbian, gay, bisexual and transgender older people: A review of the literature. *Health & Social Care in the Community*, *17*, 647–658.

Beebe, J. (2013). *Rapid assessment process*. Retrieved from http://www.rapid assessment.net/

Brotman, S., Ryan, B., Collins, S., Chamberland, L., Cormier, R., Julien, D., & Richard, B. (2007). Coming out to care: Caregivers of gay and lesbian seniors in Canada. *Gerontologist*, *47*, 490–503.

Cahill S., South K., & Spade J. (2000). *Outing age: Public policy issues affecting gay, lesbian, bisexual and transgender elders*. The Policy Institute of the National Gay and Lesbian Task Force Foundation. Retrieved from http://www. thetaskforce.org/downloads/reports/reports/OutingAge.pdf

Clark, M. E., Landers, S., Linde, R., & Sperber, J. (2001). The GLBT Health Access Project: A state-funded effort to improve access to care. *American Journal of Public Health*, *91*, 895–896.

Concannon, L. (2007). Developing inclusive health and social care policies for older LGBT citizens. *British Journal of Social Work*, *39*, 403–417.

Coon, D. W. (2003). *Lesbian, gay, bisexual and transgender (LGBT) issues and family caregiving*. San Francisco, CA: Family Caregiver Alliance, National Center on Caregiving.

Coon, D. W. (2007). Exploring interventions for LGBT caregivers. *Journal of Gay & Lesbian Social Services*, *18*(3), 109–128.

Cooper, M. G., & Lesser, J. G. (2005). *Clinical social work practice: an integrated approach*. Boston, MA: Pearson Education.

Fredriksen-Goldsen, K. I., & Hoy-Ellis, C. P. (2007). Caregiving with pride. *Journal of Gay & Lesbian Social Services*, *18*(3–4), 1–13.

Fredriksen-Goldsen, K. I., Kim, H. J., Emlet, C. A., Muraco, A., Erosheva, E. A., Hoy-Ellis, & Petry, H. (2011). *The aging and health report: Disparities and resilience among lesbian, gay, bisexual, and transgender older adults*. Institute for Multigenerational Health. Retrieved from http://caringandaging.org/wordpress/wp-content/uploads/2011/05/Full-Report-FINAL-11-16-11.pdf

Fredriksen-Goldsen, K. I., & Muraco, A. (2010). Aging and sexual orientation: A 25-year review of the literature. *Research on Aging*, *32*, 372–413.

Grant, J. M. (2010). *Outing age: Public policy issues affecting gay, lesbian, bisexual and transgender elders*. The Policy Institute of the National Gay and Lesbian Task Force Foundation. Retrieved from http://www.thetaskforce.org/downloads/reports/reports/outingage_final.pdf

Hudson, R. B. (Ed.). (2011). Integrating lesbian, gay, bisexual, and transgender older adults into aging policy and practice [Special issue]. *Public Policy Aging Report*, *21*(3).

Hughes, A. K., Harold, R. D., & Boyer, J. M. (2011). Awareness of LGBT aging issues among aging servies network providers. *Gerotological Social Work*, *54*, 659–677.

Institute of Medicine. (2011). *The health of lesbian, gay, bisexual, and transgender people: Building a foundation for better understanding*. Retrieved from http://www.iom.edu/Reports/2011/The-Health-of-Lesbian-Gay-Bisexual-and-Transgender-People.aspx

The Joint Commission. (2011). *Advancing effective communication, cultural competence, and patient- and family-centered care for the lesbian, gay, bisexual, and transgender (LGBT) community: A field guide*. Retrieved from: http://www.jointcommission.org/assets/1/18/LGBTFieldGuide.pdf

Knochel, K. A., Croghan, C. F., Moone, R. P., & Quam, J. K. (2012). Training, geography, and provision of aging services to lesbian, gay, bisexual, and transgender older adults. *Journal of Gerontological Social Work, 55*, 426–443.

Knochel, K. A., Quam, J. K., & Croghan, C. F. (2011). Are old lesbian and gay people well served? Understanding the perceptions, preparation, and experiences of aging services providers. *Journal of Applied Gerontology, 30*, 370–389.

Lee, M. G., & Quam, J. K. (2013). Comparing supports for LGBT aging in rural versus urban areas. *Journal of Gerontological Social Work, 56*, 112–126.

MetLife Mature Market Institute. (2006). *Out and aging: The MetLife study of lesbian and gay baby boomers*. Retrieved from https://www.metlife.com/assets/cao/mmi/publications/studies/mmi-out-aging-lesbian-gay-retirement.pdf

Meyer, H. (2011). Safe spaces? The need for LGBT cultural competency in aging services. *Public Policy & Aging Report, 21*(3), 24–27.

Muraco, A., & Fredriksen-Goldsen, K. (2011). "That's what friends do": Informal caregiving for chronically ill midlife and older lesbian, gay, and bisexual adults. *Journal of Social and Personal Relationships, 28*, 1073–1092.

One Colorado Education Fund. (2011). *Invisible: The state of LGBT health in Colorado*. Retrieved from http://www.one-colorado.org/wp-content/uploads/2012/01/OneColorado_HealthSurveyResults.pdf

Padgett, D. K. (2012). *Qualitative and mixed methods in public health*. Thousand Oaks, CA: Sage.

Patton, M. Q. (1991). *Qualitative research and evaluation methods*. Thousand Oaks, CA: Sage.

Project Visibility. (n.d.) *Training schedule and information*. Retrieved from http://www.bouldercounty.org/family/seniors/pages/projvis.aspx

Rogers, A., Rebbe, R., Gardella, C., Worlein, M., & Chamberlin, M. (2013). Older LGBT adult training panels: An opportunity to educate about issues faced by the older LGBT community. *Journal of Gerontological Social Work, 56*, 580–595.

Saldana, J. (2009). *The coding manual for qualitative researchers*. Thousand Oaks, CA: Sage.

Service and Advocacy for GLBT Elders. (2010). *Movement advancement project and services and advocacy for gay, lesbian, bisexual and transgender elders*. Retrieved from http://www.lgbtmap.org/policy-and-issue-analysis/improving-the-lives-of-lgbt-older-adults

Smedley B. D., Stith A. Y., & Nelson A. R. (Eds.). (2003). *Unequal treatment: Confronting racial and ethnic disparities in health care*. Washington, DC: National Academies Press.

Stein, G. L., Beckerman, N. L., & Sherman, P. A. (2010). Lesbian and gay elders and long-term care: Identifying the unique psychosocial perspectives and challenges. *Journal of Gerontological Social Work, 53,* 421–435.

Wallace, S. P., Cochran, S. D., Durazo, E. M., & Ford, C. L. (2011). *The health of aging lesbian, gay and bisexual adults in California.* Los Angeles, CA: UCLA Center for Health Policy Research.

World Health Organization. (2004). *A guide to rapid assessment of human resources for health.* Retrieved from http://www.who.int/hrh/tools/en/Rapid_Assessment_guide.pdf

Working With LGBT Older Adults: An Assessment of Employee Training Practices, Needs, and Preferences of Senior Service Organizations in Minnesota

RAJEAN P. MOONE

Moone Consulting, Minneapolis, Minnesota, USA

JOHN G. CAGLE

School of Social Work, University of Maryland–Baltimore, Baltimore, Maryland, USA

CATHERINE F. CROGHAN

Croghan Consulting, Roseville, Minnesota, USA

JENNIFER SMITH

Gerontology Department, Bethel University, St. Paul, Minnesota, USA

As the population ages and LGBT older adults become more visible among senior service providers, the need for cultural competency training will grow. Although this training is a relatively new phenomenon, curricula exist. These are generally in person for 2- to 8-hr durations. Training to Serve embarked on a study to investigate preferences in cultural competency format and duration. One-hundred and eighty-four Minnesota service providers participated in the online survey. The majority (90%) were interested in participating in LGBT cultural competency training. Results suggest a preference for shorter duration and online formats. Implications for curricula development and future research are included.

As the nation prepares for the rapid increase in older adults, it is also preparing to serve a more racially, ethnically, and culturally diverse population

(Vincent & Velkoff, 2011) including lesbian, gay, bisexual, and transgender (LGBT) people. This recognition of diversity has prompted interest in providing staff training to create culturally appropriate/competent care that goes beyond the binary discussion of race and ethnicity to include sexual orientation and gender identity (Parker, 2010). However, it can be hard for a service provider to allocate scarce funds to address the needs of a population that is rarely included in federal research and is not part of the US Census.

The lack of Census data has left demographers with the difficult and sometimes controversial task of estimating the number of LGBT persons (Gates, 2012). Demographers at the Williams Institute estimate 3.8% of the US population identify as LGBT (Gates, 2011), which suggests that there are currently about 1.5 million LGBT adults age 65 and older. Other estimates place this subpopulation as high as 4 million (Movement Advancement Project & Service and Advocacy for GLBT Elders, 2010). In 2010, the Administration on Aging funded the establishment of a National Resource Center on LGBT Aging (NRC; http://www.lgbtagingcenter.org) which signaled Federal acknowledgement that LGBT older adults are a key part of the current population. Furthermore, a growing body of research points to health disparities that suggest a greater need for support services (Fredriksen-Goldsen et al., 2011; Institute of Medicine, 2011).

Although the Older Americans Act (OAA, 2006) entitles LGBT older adults to services that allow them to age with dignity, such as housing, long-term care, home care, and community-based services, it is unclear whether providers are ready (i.e., culturally competent) to work with these clients. A 2010 national survey of the OAA-funded network of area agencies on aging and state units on aging found them generally unprepared to meet the needs of LGBT older adults (Knochel, Croghan, Moone, & Quam, 2012) and educational opportunities at national Aging Network conferences have been lacking (Moone & Cagle, 2011). Further, multiple regional and local studies suggest few providers are prepared to work with LGBT clients (Knochel, Quam, & Croghan, 2011; Logie, Bridge, & Bridge, 2008; Willging, Salvador, & Kano, 2006).

As the LGBT aging population grows, so will the need for culturally competent aging service providers who truly understand the unique needs of this population. This investigation adds to the relatively limited number of studies on LGBT aging cultural competency training.

Robert Berger, in *Gay and Gray* (1982), noted that LGBT advocates and researchers began making the tie between successful aging and LGBT-aging cultural competency training (CCT) in the 1970s and early 1980s. By 1993, the American Society on Aging's Lesbian and Gay Aging Issues Network (Freedman & Martinez, 1994) had made recommendations to the White House Conference on Aging that included "funding professional education to increase understanding and sensitivity broadening the scope of targeted populations to include gay men and lesbians" (p. 1). This call for culturally competent services is underscored by the many reports of LGBT community fears of being discriminated against when accessing services (Brotman, Ryan, & Cormier, 2003; Croghan, Mertens, Yoakam, & Edwards, 2003; Croghan, Moone, & Olson, 2012; de Vries, 2006; Grant, Mottet, & Tanis, 2011; Hughes, 2009; MetLife, 2010) and observations by service providers themselves that LGBT clients may not receive culturally appropriate and welcoming services (Jackson, Johnson, & Roberts, 2007; Knochel et al., 2012; Knochel et al., 2011).

Early training efforts were mostly local. However, *Rainbow Train*, which began in 1999 at the instigation of the Seattle Commission for Sexual Minorities and with a coalition of local professional individuals and agencies, began development of a standardized curriculum for elder sexual minority sensitivity training for care providers that could be replicated and marketed across the country (Rainbow Train, 2003). Replication of the Rainbow Train curriculum required the training of at least two local trainers and 24 hr of train-the-trainer contact before replication would be licensed. It also required both initial and annual relicensing fees.

Five years later, three additional curricula were introduced: *Project Visibility*, developed by the Boulder County Colorado Aging Services Division (2004); *No Need to Fear, No Need to Hide*, developed by Seniors Active in a Gay Environment (renamed Services and Advocacy for GLBT Elders) and the Hunter College Brookdale Center on Aging (2004), New York City; and *Understanding and Caring for Lesbian and Gay Older Adults*, developed by the Council for Jewish Elderly, Center for Applied Gerontology (2004), Chicago.

Both the Council for Jewish Elderly curriculum and the Boulder County Aging Services curriculum have been updated and are publically available for purchase. Two more recently-marketed curricula are also available: From *Isolation to Inclusion: Reaching and Serving the Lesbian, Gay, Bisexual and Transgender Seniors*, developed by Openhouse (2009) and *A Caring Response for LGBT Clients: CCT Using Gen Silent a Documentary Film*, published jointly by Virginia Commonwealth University, The LGBT Aging Project, and MAD STU Media, LLC (2011).

The NRC, funded by a 3-year grant from the US Department of Health and Human Services, developed four curricula that are not available for sale or general distribution, and are limited to presentation by NRC-certified trainers. They include two 4-hr trainings for aging services providers and two 4-hr trainings for LGBT organizations (Paraprofessional Healthcare Institute & Services and Advocacy for GLBT Elders, 2011).

There are a number of training initiatives that use curricula that they have developed or purchased or some combination thereof. Among these are Friendly House (n.d.), Portland, OR; *Heale Curriculum* for nursing professionals developed at the Howard Brown Center (n.d.), Chicago; Los Angeles Gay and Lesbian Center Seniors Services (n.d.); Training to Serve (n.d.), Minneapolis–St. Paul; and Transgender Aging Network (2013), Milwaukee.

Although there has been much activity in development and marketing LGBT cultural competency training curricula across the United States., only one state, California, currently mandates such training through the California Health Facilities Training Bill (2008). Therefore, almost all workplace LGBT-aging CCT occurs on a voluntary basis. Employers must recognize the need for staff training and choose to dedicate valuable resources to support training.

Although recent studies report that service providers were interested in learning more about LGBT aging issues (Knochel et al., 2012; Knochel et al., 2011), we could find no published record of curriculum developers seeking the employers' perspective regarding the length of time and mode of training that would best fit their workplace.

To address this question, we partnered with Training to Serve in an online survey of aging service providers to understand their current LGBT CCT practices and perceptions of training formats best suited to the workplace.

Training to Serve was founded in 2009 and dedicated to providing resources and training for senior service providers to ensure LGBT people receive welcoming, respectful, and competent care. It grew from the results of the Twin Cities (Minneapolis–St. Paul) 2002 LGBT Aging Needs Assessment Survey (Croghan et al., 2003) and a 2007 provider readiness survey conducted by the University of Minnesota and Metropolitan Area Agency on Aging (Knochel et al., 2011). These studies found strong interest on the part of the LGBT community in seeking services from providers that were trained in LGBT aging issues, and that area senior service providers were not very ready to work with the LGBT community but were interested in being trained. Training to Serve is a largely Board-driven organization with minimal contracted staff for administrative functions, and offers a menu of fee-for-service trainings presented across the region with primary focus in the Twin Cities Metro Area. It began charging fees for their initial training products and offered discounts to organizations that ordered more than one training session for their staff. Training to Serve quickly found there was considerable demand for a shorter product and began offering a 1-hr session. Although the pricing structure created an incentive for longer training, with each additional hour of training having a lower cost to the employer, Training to Serve recognized that the primary cost to the employer was not the training fee, but the lost productivity and/or replacement cost of placing an employee in the training chair.

As a result of these observations, the Training to Serve Board of Directors commissioned research to characterize the structural requirements of LGBT-aging CCT, and better understand the demands and needs of their target market, the senior service provider. The study explores providers' opinions of the length and modalities of LGBT CCT that best match their workplace. This information will be used to inform future CCT curricula development.

METHODS

In response to Training to Serve directives, our project team conducted a statewide marketing survey to assess the current CCT activities and needs of agencies serving older adults. This study and its procedures were submitted for IRB review through Bethel University and determined to be *not human subjects research* and, therefore, were considered exempt from review according to 21 CFR 56.104. The primary intent of the project was to conduct a routine market analysis for the purposes of informing quality assurance for Training to Serve's training products. Data were collected from senior service providers in Minnesota using a Web-based self-report survey. To solicit service provider participation, Care Providers of Minnesota, Central Minnesota Council on Aging, Land of the Dancing Sky Area Agency on Aging, Metropolitan Area Agency on Aging, Minnesota River Area Agency on Aging, and Minnesota Association of Senior Services sent a link to their contact lists. These e-mail lists are considered proprietary and, as a result, the sampling frames could not be reviewed by the research team for duplicative contacts. Thus, the exact number of unique e-mail contacts was unknown; however, the total population of unique e-mail contacts was estimated to be between 500 and 1,000 based on membership status or funding status. To ensure that multiple respondents were not providing information about a single organization, the final dataset was examined to eliminate redundant cases based on agency name.

The survey was developed by the Training to Serve project team and distributed to the combined e-mail list. The survey took approximately 15 min to complete and was made available to potential respondents during February 2012. Potential participants were offered a chance to win a $50 gift card to encourage participation. Partner organizations reviewed and approved study protocols prior to the initiation of the study.

Participants

Participants were 184 agency representatives. The unit of analysis for this study, however, was at the agency-level, rather than the individual-level. Thus, demographic characteristics about individual respondents were not collected. Agencies were included if they: (a) provided services to persons aged 60 or older in 2011 and (b) were located within the state of Minnesota.

When multiple respondents provided information about a single agency, we only included the first completed survey from that agency in the final analytic sample.

Measures

The survey presented respondents with a variety of questions about their organization, including agency type, number of employees, services area, and number of older adults served in 2011. Respondents were also asked whether they currently serve lesbian, gay, and bisexual (LGB) older adults, as well as whether they have received any training related to serving this population. A similar series of questions were asked relating to transgender older adults. These questions were asked separately from LGB for two primary reasons. First, previous research suggests that sexual orientation (LGB) is both conceptually and empirically different from gender identity (T; see Croghan et al., 2012; Fredriksen-Goldsen, et al., 2011). Second, Training to Serve wanted to identify any similarities and differences between these related but distinct populations who identify based on sexual orientation (LGB) and gender identity (T). Survey questions also asked respondents about training-related preferences, including: preferred training duration (ranging from less than 1 hr to 4 or more hr); format (conference call, in person, online or Webinar, video/DVD, or interactive video conference); and content (cultural change consultation, customized consultations, legal and HR advice, marketing advice, resources).

Analysis

We explored variable frequencies (N and %) to describe agency characteristics. To analyze associations with categorical data, we used a series of chi-square tests. These bivariate tests for differences were used to answer the following research questions:

1. Did preferences for training differ based on agency size?
2. Did preferences for training differ based on agency service area (metro, rural, or statewide)?
3. Did agencies that currently serve LGBT older adults have differing training practices?

Alpha levels were set at the conventional $p = .05$. Prior to the analysis, 23 cases were removed from the dataset. Twenty of the excluded cases were duplicate responses from the same organization; two reported that they did not serve any older adults in 2011; and one case was eliminated because the respondent only answered the first question.

RESULTS

Data were provided on 184 separate senior service agencies. Table 1 summarizes agency characteristics, current service population, present CCT content, and preferences. The majority of agencies were small (< 20 employees), home- and community-based service providers, and served a metropolitan area. Few agencies (only 17.4%) reported that they currently provide LGBT-related content in their employee training. Many providers (46–56%) reported that they were unsure whether their organization served LGBT older adults.

Although a minority of respondents (22%) indicated that they were interested in a formal consultation/technical support regarding LGBT older adults, 90% indicated a preference for LGBT cultural competency training of some type. The preferred training format, which was indicated by 70% of respondents, was an online training or Webinar. In-person training was the second leading format preference, which was indicated by 59% of the sample. A majority of respondents (64%) indicated that their staff would be able to attend a 1- to 2-hr cultural competency training.

Did Preferences for Training Differ Based on Agency Size?

The association between agency size and whether current employee training includes LGBT content was not statistically significant. However, large agencies (those with > 100 employees) were more likely to request in-person trainings than small or mid-size agencies ($\chi^2 = 7.282$, $df = 2$, $p = .026$). More specifically, 42% ($n = 45$) of agencies with > 100 employees indicated a preference for in-person trainings, compared to 26% ($n = 28$) of mid-size agencies and 32% ($n = 35$) of small agencies. Other associations between agency size and preferred training format (e.g., conference call, online/Webinar, video-based for television, interactive video conference) were not statistically significant. Because this variable contained multiple response options, separate analyses were conducted on each possible response, but none were statistically significant. The association between agency size and staff training time was also not statistically significant.

Did Preferences for Training Differ Based on Agency Services Area (Metro, Rural, or Statewide)?

Respondents from nonmetropolitan areas were less likely to indicate a preference for in-person training than respondents from metropolitan or mixed service areas ($\chi^2 = 16.850$, $df = 2$, $p < .001$). Fifty-seven percent ($n = 62$) of agencies serving metropolitan areas indicated a preference for in-person training; only 28% ($n = 30$) of agencies covering nonmetro areas and 15%

TABLE 1 Description of Older Adult Service Agencies in the Study Sample ($N = 184$)

Characteristic	N	Percent
Agency type		
Adult day program	9	4.9%
Care management	12	6.5%
Government or AAA	8	4.3%
Healthcare		
Hospice/palliative care	5	2.7%
Skilled nursing facility	16	8.7%
Other healthcare	11	6.0%
Health plan	4	2.1%
Home and community based service	61	33.1%
Housing	37	20.1%
Senior center	12	6.5%
Elder law/legal	5	2.7%
Other	4	2.1%
Number of employees		
1–20	72	39.1%
21–100	63	34.2%
101+	49	26.6%
60+ individuals served in 2011		
1–50	35	19%
51–100	17	9.2%
101–500	50	27.2%
501–1000	17	9.2%
1000+	42	22.8%
Don't know	23	12.5%
Service area		
Metro	87	47.3%
Non-metro	74	40.2%
Entire state	23	12.5%
Currently serves lesbian, gay, and bisexual consumers		
Yes	80	43.5%
No	19	10.3%
Don't know	84	45.7%
Missing	1	0.5%
Currently serves transgender consumers		
Yes	38	20.7%
No	42	22.8%
Don't know	103	56%
Missing	1	0.5%
Staff training currently includes lesbian, gay, bisexual, and transgender (LGBT) content		
Yes	32	17.4%
No	117	63.6%
Don't know	25	13.6%
Missing	10	5.4%
Interested in consultation/technical support regarding LGBT older adults		
Yes	42	22.8%
No	30	16.3%
Don't know	99	53.8%
Missing	13	7.1%

($n = 16$) of statewide agencies reported a preference for in-person trainings. Geographic service area was not related to any other training format—nor to whether the agency currently had training with LGBT content. The association between service area and staff training time was also not statistically significant.

Did Agencies That Currently Serve LGBT Older Adults Have Differing Training Practices?

Although few agencies currently offered training content on working with LGBT older adults, the agency clientele was associated with current training practices. For example, agencies that reported currently serving LGB clients were associated with offering LGBT training content ($\chi^2 = 6.739$, $df = 1$, $p < .009$). Respondents whose agency knowingly provides services to LGB older adults were more likely to currently have staff education programs with LGBT content. Conversely, those who indicated that they do not currently serve LGB older adults were more likely to be from agencies that do not currently provide LGBT training. Note that these results should be interpreted with caution, because low cell counts violated the assumptions of the chi-squared test. The results were similarly associated for agencies serving transgendered persons ($\chi^2 = 5.823$, $df = 1$, $p = .016$).

DISCUSSION

As noted in previous research, Knochel et al. (2012) found that most aging-service providers are untrained and potentially unprepared to understand the unique needs and challenges of a burgeoning LGBT older population; however, nearly 80% of providers were interested in receiving LGBT aging cultural competency training. These results strongly support the idea that community organizations across the country should offer and/or develop LGBT-aging CCT. Juxtaposed with Knochel and colleagues' (2012) work, our literature review and examination of LGBT curricula and provider preference depict products that do not meet preferences.

The results of this study depict a service provider landscape that prefers LGBT-aging CCT lasting 2 hrs or less and delivered online. Clearly, this sharply contrasts with the body of available training products that use an in-person trainer or self-directed model of teaching and are designed for delivery in 2-hr, half-day, or full-day time frames.

Nonmetropolitan-based respondents were less likely to prefer an in-person format. This likely is due to the additional expense of travel to a training session that most often occurs in metropolitan areas and suggests a particular need for online training opportunities. There are a wide range of agency types and sizes that could potentially influence the ability to partici-pate in training. As a result, a number of analyses were run based on factors related to agency size, location, and experience serving LGBT clients.

Upon reflection, the development of many curricula may have taken place without consulting the target market, the service provider employer, to ensure development of training products that will be accepted into the work environment (Croghan, 2011). The real cost to providers is not the training, itself, which is often offered at no cost, but the investment in staff time and loss of productivity by participation in training. Understanding the needs of the employer and workplace can inform future curricula development initiatives. Fortunately, LGBT CCT training organizations are beginning to recognize the need to not only update curricula content, but to also rethink format and duration of training products. Project Visibility reports that they plan to develop an online training module for sale to the public (N. Grimes, personal communication, March 15, 2013), and Training to Serve developed three computer-based training modules for a client in 2012 and plans to create a product for general use.

This study also reaffirmed the critical relationship between serving LGBT older adults and training on LGBT aging. Those organizations that know-ingly serve LGBT older adults are more apt to conduct LGBT CCT. On the other hand, most organizations do not ask whether their clients are LGBT during assessments or intake (Knochel et al., 2012). This is not surprising, because LGBT older adults are not easily identifiable and many individu-als may choose to not disclose. Although we are not suggesting that all providers should ask about sexual orientation and gender identity, it is important to note that disclosure can lead to positive mental and physi-cal health outcomes (Fredriksen-Goldsen et al., 2011). Whether providers of senior services should inquire about a client's sexual orientation or gen-der identity will depend on the client's unique needs and service context. However, LGBT CCT is designed to help providers understand that LGBT older adults have unique needs and challenges, and ignoring their sexual orientation and gender identity can, in fact, isolate and do more harm than good. As noted by the *Fenway Guide to LGBT Health*, published by the American College of Physicians (2007), LGBT individuals experience health disparities as a direct result of the discrimination and ignorance of sexual orientation and gender identity by providers.

Future Research

These results show that organizations prefer online training with a duration of 2 hrs or less. However, beyond the development of these types of prod-ucts, one might ask, "Who, then, are the several thousand service providers that have received LGBT aging cultural competency training in current for-mats, and what motivated them to seek training?" Current CCT initiatives may be reaching only the proverbial *low-hanging fruit* or professionals already inclined to understand care issues relating to LGBT older adults. Research exploring how to reach the less motivated provider is needed.

Further, the efficacy of shorter duration and virtual formats needs to be explored within the context of CCT. Although an online training format allows for cost-effective dissemination of curriculum content across a large and diverse geographic area, the comparative effectiveness of Web-based education (e.g., vs. in-person, booklet-based, or hybrid) has been the subject of debate (e.g., see Lai, Wong, Lie, Lui, Chan, & Yap, 2012). Thus, future research is needed to determine the ideal means of training content delivery particularly as it relates to CCT.

Conclusion

More than 30 years after aging advocates and researchers began drawing the connection between targeted CCT and successful LGBT aging, there are a variety of curricula on the market, as well as one national and numerous local/regional training programs being offered to service providers. The challenge is to ensure the availability of effective products that fit the unique demands of the workplace. Our study sheds light on the CCT practices, needs, and preferences among a sample of senior service organizations. Findings may help to inform and improve future training initiatives in these environments where almost all LGBT-aging CCT is voluntary.

REFERENCES

American College of Physicians. (2007). *The Fenway guide to LGBT health*. Washington, DC: Author.

Berger, R. (1982). *Gay and gray*. Urbana, IL: University of Illinois Press.

Brotman, S., Ryan, B., & Cormier, R. (2003). The health and social service needs of gay and lesbian elders and their families in Canada. *Gerontologist, 43*, 192–201.

Boulder County Aging Services. (2004). *Project Visibility: Awareness and sensitivity training manual for service providers of lesbian, gay, bisexual and transgender elders*. Boulder, CO: Author.

Council for Jewish Elderly Center for Applied Gerontology. (2004). *Understanding and caring for lesbian and gay adults: Frontline worker sensitivity training system*. Chicago, IL: Author.

Croghan, C. (2011). *Assessing interest in LGBT cultural competency training*. Retrieved from http://www.asaging.org/blog/assessing-interest-lgbt-cultural-competency-training

Croghan, C., Mertens, A., Yoakam, J., & Edwards, N. (2003, April). *GLBT Senior Needs Assessment*. Poster presented at the Aging in America Conference, Chicago, IL.

Croghan, C., Moone, R., & Olson, A. (2012) *Twin Cities LGBT aging needs assessment survey*. Minneapolis, MN: Greater Twin Cities United Way and PFund Foundation.

de Vries, B. (2006). Home at the end of the rainbow. *Generations, 29*(4), 64–69.

Fredriksen-Goldsen, K. I., Kim, H.-J., Emlet, C. A., Muraco, A., Erosheva, E. A., Hoy-Ellis, C. . . . Petry, H. (2011). *Aging and health report: Disparities and resilience among lesbian, gay, bisexual, and transgender older adults*. Seattle, WA: Institute for Multigenerational Health.

Freedman, M., & Martinez, C. (1994). LGAIN breaks new ground: Policy recommendations submitted to the White House Conference on Aging. *OutWord Newsletter, Lesbian and Gay Aging Issues Network, American Society on Aging, 1*(2), 1.

Friendly House. (n.d.). *SAGE metro Portland*. Retrieved from http://www.friendlyhouseinc.org/programs/gay-and-grey/

Gates, G. J. (2011). *How many people are lesbian, gay, bisexual and transgender?* Retrieved March 26, 2013 from http://williamsinstitute.law.ucla.edu/wp-content/uploads/Gates-How-Many-People-LGBT-Apr-2011.pdf

Gates, G. J. (2012). LGBT Identity: A demographer's perspective. *Loyola of Los Angeles Law Review, 45*, 693–714.

Grant, J. M., Mottet, L. A., & Tanis, J. (2011). *Injustice at every turn: A report of the national transgender discrimination survey*. Retrieved from http://www.thetaskforce.org/downloads/reports/reports/ntds_full.pdf

Health Facilities Training Bill, CA-SB 1729 (2008).

Howard Brown Center. (n.d.). *Nurses HEALE curriculum*. Retrieved from http://howardbrown.org/hb_services.asp?id=1936

Hughes, M. (2009). Lesbian and gay people's concerns about ageing and accessing services. *Australian Social Work, 62*, 186–201.

Institute of Medicine. (2011). *The health of lesbian, gay, bisexual and transgender people: Building a foundation for better understanding*. Washington, DC: National Academies Press.

Jackson, N. C., Johnson, M. J., & Roberts, R. (2008). The potential impact of discrimination fears of older gays, lesbians, bisexuals and transgender individuals living in small to moderate sized cities on long-term health care. *Journal of Homosexuality, 54*, 325–339.

Knochel, K. A., Croghan, C. F., Moone, R., & Quam, J. (2012). Training, geography and provision of aging services to lesbian, gay, bisexual, and transgender older adults. *Journal of Gerontological Social Work, 55*, 426–443.

Knochel, K. A., Quam, J. K., & Croghan, C. F. (2011). Are old lesbian and gay people well served? Understanding the perceptions, preparation, and experiences of aging service providers. *Journal of Applied Gerontology, 30*, 370–389.

Lai, C. K. Y., Wong, L. F., Lie, K. H., Lui, W., Chan, M. F., & Yap, L. S. Y. (2012) Online and onsite training for family caregivers of people with dementia: Results from a pilot study. *International Journal of Geriatric Psychiatry, 28*, 107–108.

Logie, C., Bridge, T. J., & Bridge, P. D. (2008). Evaluating the phobias, attitudes, and cultural competence of Master of Social Work students toward the LGBT populations. *Journal of Homosexuality, 53*, 201–221.

Los Angeles Gay and Lesbian Center Seniors Services. (n.d.). *Senior services*. Retrieved from http://laglc.convio.net/site/PageServer?pagename=YW_Seniors_Program

MetLife. (2010). *Still out, still aging: The MetLife study of lesbian, gay, bisexual and transgender baby boomers*. Westport, CT: MetLife Mature Market Institute.

Moone, R., & Cagle, J. G. (2011). A content analysis of Aging Network conference proceedings. *Educational Gerontology, 37*, 955–1008.

Movement Advancement Project & Services and Advocacy for GLBT Elders. (2010). *Improving the lives of LGBT older adults*. Retrieved March 26, 2013 from http://www.sageusa.org/uploads/Advancing%20Equality%20for% 20LGBT%20Elders%20%5BFINAL%20COMPRESSED%5D.pdf.

Older Americans Act, 42 U.S.C. § 35. (2006).

Open House. (2009). *From isolation to inclusion: Reaching and serving lesbian, gay, bisexual and transgender seniors*. San Francisco, CA: Rainbow Adult Community Housing.

Paraprofessional Healthcare Institute & Services and Advocacy for GLBT Elders. (2011). *Improving the quality of services and supports offered to LGBT adults*. New York, NY: Author.

Parker, V. (2010). The importance of cultural competence in caring for and working in a diverse America. *Generations, 34*(4), 97–102.

Rainbow Train. (2003). *Rainbow train: Sexual/gender minority sensitivity trainings for providers of health and social services for elders* [Brochure]. Seattle, WA: Author.

Senior Action in a Gay Environment & Brookdale Center on Aging of Hunter College. (2004). *No need to fear, no need to hide*. New York, NY: Author.

Training to Serve. (n.d.). *Training to Serve curriculum*. Retrieved from http://www. trainingtoserve.org

Transgender Aging Network. (2013). *Training and events*. Retrieved from http:// www.forge-forward.org/aging/

Vincent, G. K., & Velkoff, V. A. (2010). *The next four decades: The older population in the United States: 2010 to 2050* [Current Population Reports, P25–1138]. Washington, DC: US Census Bureau.

Virginia Commonwealth University, The LGBT Aging Project, & MAD STU Media, LLC. (2011). *A caring response for LGBT clients: Cultural competency training using Gen Silent*. Richmond, VA: Author.

Willging, C. E., Salvador, M., & Kano, M. (2006). Unequal treatment: Mental health care for sexual and gender minority groups in a rural state. *Psychiatric Services, 57*, 867–870.

Assessing the Efficacy of LGBT Cultural Competency Training for Aging Services Providers in California's Central Valley

VALERIE L. LEYVA, ELIZABETH M. BRESHEARS,
and ROBIN RINGSTAD

Social Work Department, California State University, Stanislaus, Turlock, California, USA

This study reviews the outcomes of a cultural competency training for aging services providers regarding lesbian, gay, bisexual, and transgender (LGBT) older adults. Results indicate that participants significantly increased their knowledge, skills, and positive attitudes about working with LGBT older adults, with men and non-LGBT individuals reporting the most gain. Recommendations for future research include determining which factors influence the enduring effects of this type of training and developing a standardized instrument for measuring such success. Legislative and policy changes targeted at requiring this type of cultural competency training for all direct service providers are considered.

With the demographic rise in the number of older adults in the United States, there will likely be a concurrent rise in the number of older adults who identify as lesbian, gay, bisexual, or transgender (LGBT). A recent Gallup poll estimates the LGBT adult population in the United States (18 years old and older) to be around 9 million individuals and to be evenly distributed across the country (Gates & Newport, 2013). This affirms previous findings that LGBT adults reside in 99% of the counties in the United States, and represent about 3.5% of the adult population (Gates, 2011; Gates & Ost, 2004). Included in this statistic is the LGBT older adult population.

Most adults in the United States have some sense of their trajectory of aging and how they will be cared for in old age. However, the life-course of LGBT older adults is understudied. Multiple trajectories may exist based on the variability of factors related to exploring one's sexual orientation or gender identity at different life stages (Herdt, Beeler, & Rawls, 1997; Muraco, LeBlanc, & Russell, 2008). Older adults with an LGBT identity may experience trajectories that add multiple dynamics not experienced by non-LGBT elders. For example, in 2013, a 75-year-old gay man would have been 31 years old when the Stonewall protest occurred in 1969 (National Association of Social Workers [NASW], 2012). The Stonewall riots became a symbol for the gay liberation movement when police attempted a raid at the Stonewall Inn bar to arrest the gay and lesbian patrons and the gay community fought back. The protestors were joined by hundreds and battled the police for 3 days (Haber, 2009; NASW, 2012). Such memories or life experiences are likely to impact LGBT elders differently than non-LGBT elders of a similar age.

Numerous systemic oppressions historically and currently target LGBT individuals (NASW, 2012). A few of the many legislative actions that reveal how policies have impacted the lives or livelihoods of older adults who are LGBT are illustrated in the following by continuing the example of our 75-year-old gay man. In 1975 (at 37 years old), he would have witnessed Congress removing the ban on employing homosexuals in federal jobs. In 1996, at age 56, he would have seen Congress pass the federal Defense of Marriage Act (DOMA) allowing states to restrict marriage to one man and one woman.

At 63 years old, our representative gay man would have observed Vermont becoming the first state to pass legislation recognizing a civil union between two same-sex people. In 2003, at age 65, he would have witnessed the Supreme Court ruling that sodomy laws were unconstitutional. At age 71 (in 2009), he would have observed Congress pass hate crime legislation that made it a federal crime to assault or attack an individual because of his or her LGBT status (NASW, 2012). At age 75, he would have observed the US Supreme Court strike down key provisions of DOMA (*United States v. Windsor*, 2013) and the affirmation of legal same-sex marriage in 16 states and domestic partnership in an additional five (Freedom to Marry, 2013).

How social injustice and oppression, such as that illustrated in the preceding example, factor into life trajectories of today's LGBT older adults is unique to each individual's lived experiences. However, all LGBT elders in the United States live in a social environment that, numerous times, has demonstrated moral condemnation as evidenced by discriminatory laws. Additionally, should they need services, they must seek them from a health and medical system that often pathologizes or ignores individuals' LGBT status (Blumenfeld, 2010). The decisions of these older adults regarding public and private disclosure of sexual orientation or gender identity are built on a lifetime of cultural stigma and on laws by which they could be punished for their openness and honesty (Blumenfeld, 2010; Stein, Beckman, & Sherman, 2010). Younger age-related cohorts of LGBT adults are likely to have vastly different experiences of aging with an LGBT identity. It is apparent that the social environment can dramatically impact the experience of aging as an LGBT individual. Issues related to family and personal relationships can also significantly influence the lives of LGBT older adults as they age. Connections to family and meaningful relationships in the lives of LGBT elders may differ significantly from the experiences of their non-LGBT age-related cohort members, particularly in relationship to patterns of caring and being cared for in old age. For example, rather than being cared for in community settings by family members, as is true for nearly 80% of the general population, current studies of LGBT older adults suggest that they will use residential care facilities in greater numbers than their non-LGBT cohort members (Grossman, D'Augelli, & Dragowski, 2007). Preparing social service and healthcare providers to meet the routine and unique needs of this population is an immediate and growing challenge (Brotman, et al., 2007; Haber, 2009; Hughes, Harold, & Boyer, 2011; Knochel, Croghan, Moone, & Quam, 2012; Lee & Quam, 2013).

The geographically dispersed population of LGBT older adults in the United States face aging in the context of a patchwork of laws, rights, and service accessibility that typically varies according to state-level legislative and budget imperatives (Jacobsmeier, DiSarro, Lewis, & Taylor, 2012). This may range from jurisdictions that provide culturally competent, comprehensive care for this population, to jurisdictions wherein providers are unaware that they are even serving LGBT older adults in their agencies (de Vries, 2007; Quam, Croghan, & Knochel, 2011). The lack of knowledge, skills, and awareness regarding this population leads to many LGBT older adults avoiding medical, social service, and long-term care providers, rather than exposing themselves to discrimination and inadequate care (Brotman et al., 2007; Grant, Mottet, & Tanis, 2010; Knochel et al., 2012).

The Older Californian Equality and Protection Act (AB2920) was passed by the California General Assembly in 2006 to address the gap in knowledge, skills, attitudes, and awareness of service providers about LGBT older adults in California (Equality California [EQCA], 2006). AB2920 mandates that sexual orientation and gender identity be included in the factors considered by Area Agencies on Aging (AAA) when conducting needs assessments and area plans (EQCA, 2006). The inclusion of this mandate has been addressed in a number of ways by the various AAAs in California. One county undertook a multimethod needs assessment to determine how LGBT older adults perceived that their needs were being met across eight domains of service provision (Smith, McCaslin, Change, Martinez, & McGrew, 2010). Results revealed that most participants providing an opinion on the

LGBT-friendliness of these domains indicated that the services were generally perceived as unfriendly or unwelcoming.

Given these findings and those of similar studies across the United States (Brotman et al., 2007; Cahill, South, & Spade, 2000) another AAA in the Central Valley of California was guided by a *power-with* ethic. This county AAA created a community advisory board consisting of LGBT individuals, community stakeholders, LGBT and senior advocacy groups, and agencies that fall within the AB2920 purview. *Power-with* (as opposed to *power-over*) represents a construct that aligns with social work's values and ethical principles. Power-over (Berger, 2005; Dahl, 1957) is the traditional, hierarchical approach to decision making based on control and dominance. As Foucault (1982) pointed out, exercising power of this type "is not a function of consent" (p. 788). In contrast, power-with, implemented by this Central California AAA, is an "empowerment model where dialogue, inclusion, negotiation and shared power guide decision making" (Berger, 2005, p. 5). The power-with approach pursues social change through a non-oppressive and social justice underpinning. The director of this AAA sought to enhance well-being among the older LGBT population by seeking engagement of those most impacted.

The advisory group adopted the name *LGBT Roundtable* and evolved into a coalition that included representatives from the county AAA, Commission on Aging, American Association of Retired Persons/AARP, California Rural Legal Assistance, the Central Valley Stonewall Democratic Club, an affiliate congregation of the Metropolitan Community Church, local business representatives and a local university social work department, among others. The LGBT Roundtable members chose to focus on developing a cultural competency training program to address the mandates included in AB292 and pooled their knowledge, community connections, and resources to accomplish this task. The Roundtable chose a title that aptly reflected their commitment and the intent of the training: *The Special Needs of LGBT Seniors: Developing Understanding, Empathy, and Respect*.

CULTURAL COMPETENCY TRAINING EVENT

The overall purpose of the cultural competency training curriculum developed by the LGBT Roundtable was to improve service providers' knowledge, skills, and attitudes (KSAs) regarding the cultural norms of LGBT older adults in the region, the forms of discrimination and maltreatment experienced by this group, and the current legal rights and key legal concerns they may have. The day-long event focused on four general areas: (a) basic information and terminology pertinent to LGBT older adults; (b) legal issues faced by this population; (c) how to assist LGBT older adults in accessing culturally competent, long term residential care; and (d) how to make service environments more LGBT friendly. The objectives included enabling participants to acquire the knowledge, skills, and attitudes to create and promote services and policies that were LGBT-older-adult-friendly, to competently serve them in skilled nursing and other residential facilities, to assist them in obtaining access to avenues of recourse when faced with discrimination, and to identify and use a broad range of resources to improve their quality of life.

The cultural competency training was developed as a 1-day event and targeted toward a broad range of service providers who were likely to encounter LGBT older adults during the course of their employment. These providers included social workers, counselors, nurses, first responders, senior services ombudsmen, skilled nursing and other residential care facility managers and staff members, and religious leaders. LGBT Roundtable members felt a critical part of the training was to include LGBT older adults willing to share their lived experiences of discrimination and challenges of heteronormativity, homophobia, and the intersection of ageism and heterosexism in each of the workshop areas addressed. These LGBT elders indicated that they chose to reveal their concerns and vulnerability so that providers would know them as real people and to increase providers' awareness of the active presence of discrimination in this region and its lingering effects on this population.

The training consisted of four workshops, each conducted by a panel of experts. The sessions were interspersed with personal accounts by LGBT elders relating to each of the workshops, in areas such as living with and losing a partner, adverse experiences with housing, health care, employment, social stigma, and other ordeals.

The first workshop of the day, *LGBT 101*, served as a general overview of LGBT history, culture, and terminology. It prepared participants for the subsequent workshops by clarifying terms and introducing the major themes to be addressed during the training. The second workshop, *Making Services/Agencies More LGBT Friendly*, was facilitated by members of the local Transgender Law Center. It included information on practical ways in which agencies could make changes in paperwork and their physical environments to welcome LGBT clients. In addition, this workshop included substantial information on the life-long discrimination experienced by transgender older adults and ways in which to sensitively and competently serve this population.

Third, special concerns of *Long-Term Care* were addressed as related to LGBT older adults who receive services through skilled nursing facilities. The fourth panel presentation, by several local attorneys, was designed to assist participants in learning about current *Legal Issues and What We Need to Know to Advocate*, including state laws regarding estate planning and pension survivorship rights. During lunch, a vignette exercise was used to facilitate dialog among participants to increase empathy and awareness of their biases in working with this population. A question and answer session by a panel of LGBT older adults rounded out the day.

All participants were given a binder of materials that included articles on LGBT and aging, links to web sites, examples of LGBT-friendly forms, pictures of LGBT welcoming environments, and an extensive list of resources to access for information and services related to LGBT and aging in both community and residential settings. Additionally, all participants were asked to complete a pretest and posttest regarding their KSAs and awareness of LGBT older adult issues, and were asked if the LGBT Roundtable could contact them in the future for additional interviews and feedback.

METHODS

The LGBT Roundtable adopted a participatory approach in designing, delivering, and assessing the cultural competency training curriculum and event. The Roundtable met as a whole to plan each workshop, identify desired outcomes, and establish the specific objectives to be measured. The group decided to utilize a pretest and posttest model to see if changes could be accomplished in the identified areas of KSAs and awareness within the context of the 1-day training event.

At the time the event was developed (spring, 2011) few studies specific to older adult LGBT cultural competency training existed. To develop a valid and reliable assessment tool, studies of cultural competency training regarding LGBT issues in general were utilized to create the instrument for this event (Brotman et al, 2007; Greytak & Kosciw, 2010; Landers, Mimiaga, & Krinsky 2010; Pearson, 2003; US Department of Health and Human Services, 2001). Questions were crafted to target KSAs and awareness regarding service provision to LGBT older adults in the region. The pretest included demographic questions and 25 KSA and awareness questions rated on a 5-point Likert scale ranging from 1 (*strongly agree*) to 5 (*strongly disagree*). The posttest included 23 KSA items using the 5-point Likert scale, plus two qualitative open-ended questions exploring how participants would implement what they learned at the workshop. Awareness items were included on the pretest to determine current policies and practices in participants' service agencies and participants' conscious biases in working with an LGBT older adult population. The awareness items were not repeated at posttest, and were not included in the analysis of pretest and posttest changes.

Given the challenges of measuring various characteristics among this population, all demographic questions were open-ended, requiring participants to write-in a response, rather than affirm a predetermined definition (Gates, 2011). This enabled all participants to describe themselves in personally accurate ways and still enabled the grouping of this information into meaningful categories for data analysis. LGBT Roundtable members reviewed all questions for face and content validity, and edited some items to tailor them to regional concerns. Initial analysis of this instrument yielded an overall Cronbach's alpha of 0.75, which is an acceptable level of internal consistency given the complex nature of the constructs being measured (Tavakol & Dennick, 2011). Finally, the training event was audited in-vivo by a member of the LGBT Roundtable to insure that the information for each item was explicitly covered during the course of the training segments. Items not covered were introduced into the question and answer session at the end of the day.

RESULTS

The goal of the LGBT Roundtable was to reach out to those who provided direct services to LGBT older adults. Those who attended the event were a mix, however, of these service providers and a significant contingent of LGBT older adults who identified themselves as service users ($n = 29$, 25.2%). The presence of this group of service users may be due to this being only the second event of this type in this region. In addition, some of the LGBT older adults who were invited to serve on the various panel presentations throughout the day also completed surveys and contributed to the total number of service users who responded.

Of the 123 participants, 115 completed the pretest and 112 completed the posttest. The demographic questions only appeared on the pretest, but the questionnaires were numbered to allow matching of pretest and posttest results of individual participants. The ages of the participants ranged from 22 to 80 years old with a mean age of 50.57 years. Of those reporting an ethnic or racial affiliation, a little over half of the participants identified as White or Anglo ($n = 65$, 56%), with the rest of the participants representing a diversity of ethnic and racial groups common to this region (Hispanic or Latino, $n = 17$, 14.8 %; African America or Black, $n = 12$, 10.4%; Mexican or Mexican American, $n = 7$, 6.1%; Asian, $n = 6$, 5.1%; mixed race or ethnicity, $n = 3$, 2.6%; and American Indian, $n = 1$, 0.9%). Not surprising in a training program targeted to service providers, 67.8 % ($n = 78$) of the participants had a Bachelor's or a Master's degree, and the participants' median income was $65,000 per year. Only 12 participants indicated that they did not subscribe to or practice any religion (10.5%). The remaining participants ascribed to one of over 16 different religious faiths or denominations, with Catholic ($n = 29$, 25.2%) and Christian ($n = 22$, 19.1%) being the most common.

The sexual orientation category contained a variety of self-identified statuses. During data analysis, these were broadly recoded as non-LGBT ($n = 70$, 60.9%), lesbian ($n = 17$, 14.8%), gay man ($n = 9$, 7.8%), and bisexual ($n = 3$, 2.6%). A significant percentage of the participants declined to answer this question ($n = 15$, 13.0%). Of those participants answering the question regarding gender identification, 84 identified as women (73%) and 29 as men (25.2%). Interestingly, despite numerous participants identifying themselves as transgender in various presentations, panels, and discussion periods throughout the day, only one individual did so at the time of the pretest (0.9%). This could indicate that participants did not feel comfortable reporting a transgender identity in writing, even on an anonymous survey, but became more comfortable throughout the day as they experienced the activities. Demographic questions were not repeated at the time of posttest, so there is no way to know how they might have self-reported gender identity at the end of the event.

Univariate analysis was used to determine participants' level of KSA on all individual items, both at the time of pretest and posttest. Individual items were scored on a scale of 1 to 5, and some items were reverse coded for analysis so that lower scores indicated more knowledge, more skills, and a more positive attitude about LGBT issues, and higher scores indicated less knowledge, less skill, and a less positive attitude about LGBT issues. Items were then combined to create total scale scores for each of the areas being examined. The area of knowledge included 8 items, resulting in a total possible score of 8 to 40. The skills category, with 6 items, had a total possible score of 6 to 30. The attitude category included 5 items, and had a total possible of 5 to 25.

After total scores were determined, paired samples t-tests were used to determine whether scores in each area differed at times of pretest and posttest. The mean knowledge score at pretest was 20.14 ($SD = 4.01$) and at posttest was 18.19 ($SD = 3.17$). With a $t = 6.21$ ($df = 63$) and a p-value of .000, results indicated that these scores significantly differed and that participants gained knowledge as a result of participation in the training. The mean skills score at pretest was 15.28 ($SD = 3.24$) and at posttest was 12.17 ($SD = 3.00$). With a $t = 8.10$ ($df = 77$) and a p-value of .000, results indicated that the skill scores also significantly differed and that participants had increased skills as a result of participation in the training. Finally, the mean attitude scores at pretest was 9.13 ($SD = 2.88$) and at posttest was 8.30 ($SD = 2.43$). With a $t = 2.91$ ($df = 78$) and a p-value of .005, results indicated that these means statistically differed and that participants had more positive attitudes at the conclusion of the training.

In addition to examining differences in total scores,independent samples t-tests were conducted to determine whether participants' scores differed based either on gender or on sexual orientation. Men and women were compared in terms of their scores on all pretest and posttest scales. Statistically significant differences ($t = 2.12$, $p = .037$, $df = 100$) were found in terms of men's and women's attitudes about LGBT issues at pretest, with women reporting more positive attitudes ($M = 8.82$, $SD = 2.80$) than men ($M = 10.21$, $SD = 2.84$). At posttest, both women ($M = 7.97$, $SD = 2.29$) and men ($M = 8.87$, $SD = 2.71$) indicated more positive attitudes regarding LGBT older adults than they had at pretest. Although women still reported slightly more positive attitudes at posttest than men, and men reported an increase in positive attitudes regarding LGBT older adults, the statistically significant pretest differences between men and women were no longer evident at posttest.

Participants' scores on all pretest and posttest scales were also compared based on self-identified sexual orientation. Because of the small number of responses in two categories (bisexual and those who declined to answer), sexual orientation was recoded into a dichotomous variable of lesbian/gay or heterosexual. Independent samples t-tests were used to compare participants' scores at pretest and posttest. Results revealed that participants' scores significantly differed on all three of the pretest scales—knowledge, skills, and attitudes—based on whether participants identified as lesbian/gay or heterosexual. Table 1 reports the t-test results and statistical significance of differences in mean scores of lesbian/gay and heterosexual participants in each of the scale areas. Lesbian/gay participants' scores were consistently lower than heterosexual participants on each scale. This indicates, not surprisingly, that lesbian/gay individuals had more knowledge, more skills, and more positive attitudes about LGBT older adults than did heterosexual participants. However, both knowledge and attitudes changed considerably for heterosexual participants during the course of the training, with heterosexual participants reporting more knowledge ($M = 17.90$, $SD = 3.48$) and a more positive attitude ($M = 8.18$, $SD = 2.47$) at the conclusion of the training. As a result, scores of heterosexual participants more closely mirrored those of lesbian/gay participants, and no significant differences between these two groups were found at posttest. In the area of skills in working with LGBT issues, both lesbian/gay and heterosexual training participants improved their scores from pretest to post test. The two groups continued to differ in level of skill, however, with lesbian/gay participants reporting significantly more skills at the conclusion of the training ($M = 10.23$, $SD = 3.01$) than heterosexual participants ($M = 12.50$, $SD = 2.81$).

TABLE 1 Results of Lesbian/Gay and Heterosexual Training Participants' Pretest and Posttest Knowledge, Skill, Attitude (KSA) Scores

	Lesbian/Gay		Heterosexual			
	M	SD	M	SD	t	p
Pretest knowledge	17.95	3.63	20.40	4.35	2.32	.023*
Pretest attitudes	10.33	5.21	13.92	4.63	3.56	.001*
Pretest skills	13.21	3.23	15.94	3.06	3.69	.000*
Posttest knowledge	17.06	3.10	17.90	3.48	.89	.379
Posttest attitudes	7.64	1.97	8.18	2.47	.91	.365
Posttest skills	10.23	3.01	12.50	2.81	3.07	.003*

*$p < .05$

DISCUSSION

These results clearly indicate that the individuals who attended a 1-day cultural competency training improved their KSAs regarding working with LGBT older adults. Despite nearly half (47%) of the participants indicating attendance at prior cultural competency training regarding LGBT issues, most participants indicated that they gained additional skills from the current training, enabling them to create more LGBT friendly environments in their service agencies.

These results replicate the single published results of cultural competency training regarding LGBT older adults in the United States (NRC, 2012). The NRC cultural competency training resulted in increased knowledge regarding the experiences of LGBT older adults, increased knowledge of the medical and mental health needs of this population, and increase awareness of the ways in which service providers could make their service agencies more LGBT friendly. The NRC training also resulted in more positive attitudes and acceptance of LGBT older adults, and increased skill in the ability to confront bias against this population when it was encountered in service settings.

A hallmark of the LGBT Roundtable cultural competency training reported on in this study was the use of panels of LGBT older adults who described their experiences of ageism and homophobia when attempting to access services, vignettes of actual events that took place in this region, and the inclusion of poetry and other narratives from LGBT older adults. Previous research on the acceptance of the LGBT population indicates it is familiarity and identification with LGBT individuals that results in attitude change (Herek & Glunt, 1993). It is possible that using first-person accounts of discrimination and service barriers sensitized participants to the real experiences of this population.

In spite of the positive changes in KSAs among participants in this study, a further review of the posttest scores revealed a few areas that indicate the need for additional focus or clarification at future training events. Among the knowledge items measured in this study, there remained challenges among participants in understanding differences between California law that is LGBT-affirmative and the active presence of discrimination in spite of these laws. For instance, there are multiple laws in place to protect LGBT California residents against discrimination in the workplace and in healthcare settings. Although this topic was discussed and clarified during the training event, only 19.3% of participants affirmed the presence of these laws on the posttest. Additionally, two of the skill items appeared to demonstrate a shift in personal awareness of the presence of homophobia and heteronormativity in the workplace. Although 21.0% of the participants indicated at pretest that they assumed that some of their clients and coworkers were LGBT, this number increased to 45.6% at posttest. Similarly, at pretest 46.4%

of the participants indicated that discussions about LGBT issues were normalized or destigmatized at their workplaces, yet only 25.9% indicated the same at posttest. Perhaps, during the course of the event, participants became more aware of their own unconscious hetero-normative practices and the challenges of sustaining a truly bias free workplace.

Finally, this event was accomplished with a small group of like-minded individuals (12–15) on a limited budget ($2,000 plus in-kind donations). The recent development of cultural competency training curricula regarding LGBT older adults and the online accessibility of these programs make this type of training reasonably replicable across the United States (NRC, 2012).

LIMITATIONS

A limitation of this study, and all such studies of LGBT older adult cultural competency training at this time, is the lack of a standardized and widely available instrument to measure participant changes in KSAs when working with this population. As the primary goal of the LGBT Roundtable was to design a cultural competency curriculum that was locally relevant, rather than developing a sophisticated assessment tool, questions were adopted from existing scales and edited to create the tool used to measure the results of our training event. These items originated in studies of cultural competency training regarding LGBT youth (Greytak & Kosciw, 2010), LGBT older adults (Brotman et al., 2007; Landers et al., 2010), and LGBT populations in general (Pearson, 2003; US Department of Health and Human Services, 2001). Developing a standardized assessment tool is clearly a needed advancement in the study of this population.

IMPLICATIONS

Although it is encouraging to find that individuals attending cultural competency training demonstrate increased knowledge, skill, and awareness of working with LGBT older adults, this does not insure that their agencies will engage in a correlational shift in service provision. Prior studies have found that positive attitudes of individual service providers toward LGBT older adults and the skills to serve this population do not necessarily translate into agency or institutional support (Hughes et al., 2011). Furthermore, there is a reported difference in the experiences of urban and rural LGBT older adults that may well be replicated in the mixed urban and rural region of the LGBT Roundtable (Lee & Quam, 2013). Individual service providers in similar regions will need to be advocates within their service agencies to develop a culture of competence in serving this population.

Although it was an initial goal of the LGBT Roundtable to target entry-level personal care aides, such as certified nurse assistants and patient technicians, with this training, few such providers attended. At the time of this study, there was no state-level requirement for this group to obtain any training specific to cultural competency with LGBT older adults. As a result of this gap, several members of the LGBT Roundtable partnered with an already existing effort in California to generate legislation to require this type of training. Although this legislation was enacted, the final bill (AB663) only requires cultural competency training for skilled nursing home and assisted living center directors, and not direct care staff (EQCA, 2013). Despite this limitation, it is hoped that this legislation becomes a pathway to increasing cultural competency with LGBT older adults across these residential facilities.

Additionally, although we were able to detect shifts in KSAs in a pretest and posttest administered on a single day, the longer-term effects of this type of training have yet to be explored. Research to determine the factors that will produce enduring changes in KSAs is another area for exploration. Finally, refinement of the instrument used to assess this type of training should continue. A growing body of tools and evidenced-based practices will help insure a better quality of service and service accessibility for this historically marginalized population.

REFERENCES

Berger, B. K. (2005). Power over, power with, and power to relations: Critical reflections on public relations, the dominant coalition, and activism. *Journal of Public Relations Research, 17*, 5–28. doi:10.1207/s1532754xjprr1701_3

Blumenfeld, W. J. (2010). Heterosexism: Introduction. In M. Adams, W. J. Blumenfeld, C. Castañeda, H. W. Hackman, M. L. Peters, & X. Zúñiga (Eds.), *Readings for diversity and social justice* (2nd ed., pp. 371–376). New York, NY: Routledge.

Brotman, S., Ryan, B., Collins, S., Chamberland, L., Cormier, R., Julien, D., . . . Richard, D. (2007). Coming out to care: Caregivers of gay and lesbian seniors in Canada. *Gerontologist, 47*, 490–503. doi:10.1093/geront/47.4.490

Cahill, S., South, K., & Spade, J. (2000). *Outing age: Public policy affecting gay, lesbian, bisexual and transgender elders*. New York, NY: Policy Institute of the National Gay and Lesbian Task Force Foundation. Retrieved from http://www.thetaskforce.org/reports_and_research/outing_age_2010

Dahl, R. A. (1957). The concept of power. *Behavioral Science, 2*, 201–215. doi:10.1002/bs.3830020303

de Vries, B. (2007). LGBT couples in later life: A study in diversity. *Generations, 31*(3), 18–23.

Equality California. (2006). *AB2920 fact sheet*. Retrieved from http://www.eqca.org/site/apps/nlnet/content2.aspx?c=kuLRJ9MRKrH&b=4025853&ct=5198079

Equality California. (2013). *AB663 fact sheet*. Retrieved from http://www.eqca.org/site/pp.asp?c=kuLRJ9MRKrH&b=8629791

Foucault, M. (1982). The subject and power. *Critical Inquiry, 8*, 777–795. doi: 10.1086/448181

Freedom to Marry. (2013). *Where state laws stand.* Retrieved from http://www. freedomtomarry.org/states/

Gates. G. (2011). *How many people are lesbian, gay, bisexual, and transgender?* Retrieved from http://williamsinstitute.law.ucla.edu/category/research/page/5/

Gates, G., & Newport, F. (2013, February). *Gallup special report: New estimates of the LGBT population in the United States.* Retrieved from http://www.gallup.com/ poll/160517/lgbt-percentage-highest-lowest-north-dakota.aspx?version=print

Gates, G., & Ost, J. (2004). *The Gay and Lesbian Atlas.* Washington, DC: Urban Institute Press.

Grant, J., Mottet, L., & Tanis, J. (2010). *Injustice at every turn: A report of the National Transgender Discrimination Survey.* Retrieved from http://www.transequality. org/PDFs/NTDSReportonHealth_final.pdf

Greytak, E., & Kosciw, J. (2010). *Year one evaluation of the New York City Department of Education "Respect for All" training program.* New York, NY: Gay, Lesbian and Straight Education Network. Retrieved from http://www.glsen. org/research

Grossman, A., D'Augelli, A., & Dragowski, E. (2007). Caregiving and care receiving among older lesbian, gay, and bisexual adults. *Journal of Gay and Lesbian Social Services, 18*, 15–38. doi:10.1300/J041v18n03_02

Haber, D. (2009). Gay aging. *Gerontology & Geriatrics Education, 30*, 267–280. doi:10.1080/02701960903133554

Herdt, G., Beeler, J., & Rawls, T. (1997). Life course diversity among older lesbians and gay men: A study in Chicago. *Journal of Gay, Lesbian, and Bisexual Identity, 2*, 231–246.

Herek, G., & Glunt, E. (1993). Interpersonal contact and heterosexuals' attitudes toward gay men: Results from a national survey. *Journal of Sex Research, 30*, 239–244. doi:10.1080/00224499309551707

Hughes, A., Harold, R., & Boyer, J. (2011). Awareness of LGBT aging issues among aging services network providers. *Journal of Gerontological Social Work, 54*, 659–677. doi:10.1080/01634372.2011.585392

Jacobsmeier, M., DiSarro, B., Lewis, D., & Taylor, J. (2012). Content and complexity in policy reinvention and diffusion: Gay and transgender-inclusive laws against discrimination. *State Politics & Policy Quarterly, 12*, 75–98.

Knochel, K., Croghan, C., Moone, R., & Quam, J. (2012). Training, geography, and provision of aging services to lesbian, gay, bisexual, and transgender older adults. *Journal of Gerontological Social Work, 55*, 426–443. doi:10.1080/01634372.2012.665158

Landers, S., Mimiaga, M., & Krinsky, L. (2010). The open door project task force: A qualitative study on LGBT aging. *Journal of Gay and Lesbian Social Services, 22*, 316–336. doi:10.1080/10538720903426438

Lee, M. G., & Quam, J. (2013). Comparing supports for LGBT aging in rural versus urban areas. *Journal of Gerontological Social Work, 56*, 112–126. doi:10.1080/01634372.2012.747580

Muraco, A., LeBlanc, A., & Russell, S. (2008). Conceptualizations of family by older gay men. *Journal of Gay and Lesbian Social Services, 20*, 69–90. doi:10.1080/ 10538720802178957

National Association of Social Workers. (2012). *Social work speaks: NASW policy statements, 2012–2014*. Alexandria, VA: NASW Press.

National Resource Center on LGBT Aging. (2012). *Cultural competency training results: February 2011–February 2012*. Retrieved from www.lgbtagingcenter. org/resources/download.cfm?r=532

Pearson, Q. (2003). Breaking the silence in the counselor education classroom: A training seminar on counseling sexual minority clients. *Journal of Counseling and Development, 81*, 292–300. doi:10.1002/j.1556-6678.2003.tb00256.x

Quam, J., Croghan, C., & Knochel, K. (2011). Are old lesbian and gay people well served?: Understanding the perceptions, preparation, and experiences of aging services providers. *Journal of Applied Gerontology, 30*, 370–389.

Smith, L., McCaslin, R., Chang, J., Martinez, P., & McGrew, P. (2010). Assessing the needs of older gay, lesbian, bisexual, and transgender people: A service-learning and agency partnership approach. *Journal of Gerontological Social Work, 53*, 387–401. doi:10.1080/01634372.2010.486433

Stein, G., Beckerman, N., & Sherman, P. (2010). Lesbian and gay elders and long-term care: Identifying the unique psychosocial perspectives and challenges. *Journal of Gerontological Social Work, 53*, 421–435. doi:10.1080/01634372.2010.496478

Tavakol, M., & Dennick, R. (2011). Making sense of Cronbach's alpha. *International Journal of Medical Education, 2*, 53–55. doi:10.5116/ijme.4dfb.8dfd

United States v. Windsor, 133 S. Ct. 2675 (2013)

US Department of Health and Human Services, Substance Abuse and Mental Health Services Administration. (2001). *A provider's introduction to substance abuse treatment for lesbian, gay, bisexual, and transgender individuals*. Retrieved from http://store.samhsa.gov/product/A-Provider-s-Introduction-to-Substance-Abuse-Treatment-for-Lesbian-Gay-Bisexual-and-Transgender-Individuals/SMA12-4104

"I Want to Know More About Who We Are": New Directions for Research With Older Lesbians

PAIGE AVERETT, ASHLEY ROBINSON, CAROL JENKINS,
and INTAE YOON

School of Social Work, East Carolina University, Greenville, North Carolina, USA

Previous literature has consistently discussed reoccurring issues with conducting research in the gay and lesbian community and, for the purposes of this article, particularly the older lesbian community. Issues with sampling, including gaining access, ethical considerations, and conceptual definitions are ongoing struggles repeated within the literature. This article provides the experience of a research team in conducting such research and presents the viable solutions and ongoing barriers, as well as newer considerations that future research must take into account. In addition, this article provides the viewpoint of 189 older lesbians on the future research needs within their community.

The lesbian, gay, bisexual, and transgender (LGBT) and gerontological research communities acknowledge older lesbians as an invisible and often ignored population, at triple the threat of marginalization and oppression (Averett & Jenkins, 2012; Bayliss, 2000; Fullmer, Shenk, & Eastland, 1999; Gabbay & Wahler, 2002; Healey, 1994; Healy, 2002; Jacobson & Samdahl, 1998; Shenk & Fullmer, 1996; Wojciechowski, 1998). This invisibility is experienced not only in general society, but also within the research community. Two literature reviews, which in combination have examined the research conducted on lesbian gerontology over the past 30 years (1979–2010), have found an ongoing lack of research focused on this population and more gaps than knowledge (Averett & Jenkins, 2012; Gabbay & Wahler, 2002). Gabbay and Wahler, in their review of the literature from 1979 to 1997, found only 11 empirical articles focused exclusively on older lesbians. In our follow-up review of articles from 1997 to 2010, we found 13 empirical articles (Averett & Jenkins, 2012). Thus, as of 2010, there were approximately 24 empirical articles published within the past 30 years that focused solely on the older lesbian population. As well, it is important to note that even within these 24 empirical studies, there were many limitations and continual discussion of the need for more research.

There are numerous reasons for this dearth of research, including societal issues that seemingly filter into the research community, such as heterosexism, sexism, and ageism, which lead to a lack of interest in the topic, a lack of concern for this specific population, and a lack of funding that supports the research needs. In addition, there are many difficulties by researchers in accessing and conducting research with this specific population. Several articles have discussed these ongoing issues and called for specific research to be conducted within the LGBT aging and older lesbian populations (Averett & Jenkins, 2012; Donahue & McDonald, 2005; Gabbay & Wahler, 2002; Grossman, 2008; Jacobson, 1995; Martin & Knox, 2000; Meyer & Wilson, 2009). In response to this call, we conducted a nationwide online survey and completed the largest study to date specifically on older lesbians (Averett, Yoon, & Jenkins, 2011). We, too, experienced difficulties and had many limitations within our study. However, our experience also provided new reflections on the existing problems within the literature, potential solutions, new directions for future research, and the feedback of our participants on what researchers should do next. Thus, this article's purpose is to contend with the issues of sampling, gaining access, ethical considerations, and conceptual definitions of researchers studying the older lesbian population. We provide the experience of our research team in conducting such research, the viable solutions and ongoing barriers, and newer considerations that future research may well take into account, both from the perspective of the research team and 189 older lesbian participants.

SAMPLING ISSUES

The most consistently cited problem with the existing literature on older lesbians (and LGBT aging research in general) is related to issues with sampling (Averett & Jenkins, 2012; Donahue & McDonald, 2005; Gabbay & Wahler, 2002; Grossman, 2008; Jacobson, 1995; Meyer & Wilson, 2009; Parks, Hughes, & Werkmeister-Rozas, 2009). However, very few suggestions for practical ways to address these sampling issues exist. Similar to problems with the sampling found in much of the LGBT research literature (Meyer & Wilson, 2009), the participants of older lesbian studies tend to be Caucasian; of high socioeconomic status (SES); high education level; located in urban clusters; and, similar to those in gerontology samples, middle-aged or young-old, rather than the old-old (Jacobson, 1995; Grossman, 2008).

We intentionally utilized an online methodology in an attempt to reach more rural and racial minority older lesbians (Averett et al., 2011). Most of the critiques of the literature point to the use of convenience samples that have both an urban bias and a bias toward participants who are involved with support organizations (Jacobson, 1995; Meyer & Wilson, 2009). Our methodology did provide more suburban, rural, and isolated participants who were not connected to a physical LGBT community (over half of our sample). Although many of our participants were connected online to LGBT community resources, a slight majority of them were not connected to actual community centers, groups, or even informal circles of older lesbians (over half of our sample). Thus, we were able to hear about the lives of women who are not typically represented in the research. This points to the use of online methods in particular to access suburban, rural, and isolated participants.

Racial Identity

Racial sexual minorities are greatly underrepresented in the older lesbian samples (Averett & Jenkins, 2012; Donahue & McDonald, 2005; Gabbay & Wahler, 2002; Grossman, 2008; Jacobson, 1995; Meyer & Wilson, 2009). Although we did reach more racial minorities than previous studies, the overall percentage (13% of our sample or $n = 43$) was still very small and not significant enough for analysis purposes (Averett et al., 2011). This was despite our very intentional attempt to access and connect with online racial minority lesbian communities. Although we communicated with several online racial minority lesbian groups, we found resistance to promoting the study.

Particularly, an older Black lesbian gatekeeper from one of the online communities shared (informally and after data collection was completed) several very specific issues that future researchers should take into consideration (personal communication, April 4, 2011). First, and not surprising, was that a relationship of trust and ongoing communication must exist before contacting a racial minority lesbian group for research purposes. Although we were successful in building relationships and connections with several online lesbian communities at the beginning of data collection, it became apparent that, due to a large mistrust of researchers, as well as confidentiality and privacy concerns, attempts to connect with racial minorities once a study is initiated is much too late. As has been documented in literature on outreach and engagement, there is a needed level of commitment of time and energy to develop relationships, prior to a focus on scholarship, to access these groups (Fogel & Cook, 2006). Researchers attempting to study racial minority lesbians must engage with minority groups and build relationships of support and connection prior to attempting to conduct research.

Second, and also not surprisingly, there is a need for similar racial minorities to be members of the research team when conducting research with racial minorities. Specifically, we were told that because we were Caucasian and did not have an African American on our research team, we were less likely to gain access to African American lesbian groups (personal communication, April 4, 2011). As members of quadruple minority status, at high risk of oppression, misrepresentation, and misuse, we were informed that these groups of women want to be assured that their beliefs, experiences, and voices are well represented, respected, and understood. Their belief is that, in part, they can be more assured of this if there is someone of their similar identity representing them on the research team.

Third, the African American older lesbian gatekeeper brought to our attention that the women she knows would prefer to be paid or to receive compensation of some sort to be research participants (personal communication, April 4, 2011). Specifically, it was stated that, unlike the concerns of some that financial incentives can create undue influence (Grady, 2005), compensation is viewed by older African American lesbians as a form of respect and equity for their time and energy as participants. This anecdotally supports Grant and Sugarman's (2004) statement that research incentives can be useful in overcoming barriers in recruitment, specifically in accessing racial minorities. Future researchers should consider the use of incentives and the resulting ethical considerations in order to complete research with racially diverse older lesbians.

SES AND AGE

Also, our hope was that an online methodology might provide more variety in SES and age. We were aware that online methods typically produce middle- and upper-middle-class participants (Matsuo, McIntyre, Tomazic & Katz, 2004) and younger participants (Duffy, Smith, Terhanian, & Bremer, 2005), but there has been reconsideration of these critiques as home computers become more widespread, as well as increasing free access to the Internet at a variety of sources (public libraries, community centers, etc.) and as the baby boomers become more technologically savvy while continuing to age. However, we found that our online method was still limited in accessing these underrepresented groups. One potential solution for accessing the old-old would be sampling that is intentional to assisted living and nursing home facilities. Of particular use could be research with existing lesbian-only retirement and LGBT-friendly aging facilities. To our knowledge, there has been no research conducted specifically in these settings. Although this sampling falls prey to the aforementioned issues of sampling within established communities, it could provide different demographics in terms of age. Although a smaller possibility, sampling within nursing homes in certain states that are known to be more LGBT friendly (see http://www.sageusa.org/ for a database), could possibly result in finding lower SES participants. There are aging facilities across the country that accept lower-income individuals, and in light of the recent mandate by the Secretary of Health and Human Services, Kathleen Sebelius, facilities must provide equal rights to same-sex couples and LGBT residents (http://www.hhs.gov/lgbt/health-objectives-2012.html). Reaching older participants and those from a lower SES could provide potentially much different information than that which currently exists. Currently, researchers know very little about old-old and low SES older lesbians (Averett & Jenkins, 2012; Donahue & McDonald, 2005; Gabbay & Wahler, 2002; Jacobson, 1995). However, a specific benefit of utilizing an online survey that is important to note is that we were able to sample across the country and had representation from 41 states and the District of Columbia (Averett et al., 2011). This was low in cost and provided the most diverse location sampling of a study on older lesbians to date (Averett & Jenkins, 2012). Additionally, online methodology has the potential for reaching an international sample without extra cost. Without attempting to, we had respondents from several other countries that we then had to exclude from our final analysis. In the current age of decreased funding, increased competition, and ongoing lack of interest in funding LGBT aging research, online methods, despite their limitations, should be considered.

Gender/Sex and Sexual Identity

The previously discussed need for similar racial identity representation on the research team is also found in connecting with lesbian groups in general. One of our main relationships in conducting our research was with the Old Lesbians Organizing for Change (OLOC). OLOC requires that a member of the research team identify as lesbian before they will promote studies on their Web site (http://www.oloc.org/researchrules.php). Additionally, they encourage and prefer the use of older lesbians as research team members or consultants. Although past literature has called for researchers to include older lesbians in participatory studies (Jacobson, 1995), none of the literature we are aware of has acknowledged the reality that some of the difficulty in accessing these groups is a result of the different racial and sexual identities of the researchers themselves. Gates and Kelly (2013) acknowledged the ongoing focus by the research community on the representation of the LGBT community as "disenfranchised, marginalized, and oppressed," which, they stated, supports a stigmatizing attitude in broader society (p. 69). The inclusion of both LGBT and racial minority community members within the research team is key to rethinking and critically examining potentially oppressive and stagnant research paradigms.

As pointed out in our literature review (Averett & Jenkins, 2012), there is a need for studies that separate male and female participants and/or that pay particular attention to gender differences, as there have been studies that have shown great differences between the aging experiences of the two (Donahue & McDonald, 2005; Pugh, 2005). Yet, most studies will discuss LGBT aging and issues and then have predominantly gay male samples and little to no lesbian, bisexual, or transgender participants and no analysis by gender/sex or sexual identity (Averett & Jenkins, 2012; Gabby & Wahler, 2002; Donahue & McDonald, 2005). Similarly, research has also pointed out the differences in the aging experience via various race and ethnicities and the need to consider each racial/ethnic identity separately (Calasanti & Slevin, 2001).

Rethinking Sampling

The aforementioned sampling issues, those of setting, location, race, sexual identity, gender, and age, will likely be ongoing challenges for researchers. However, we have attempted to provide suggestions for various ways to improve and address these issues. We believe it important to note that all of these issues will not be fixed or possible to address in a single study. We also do not believe that they always need to be, for several reasons.

In terms of sexuality research on LGBT populations, there is great difficulty in conceptualization and term use (Parks et. al., 2009). Martin and Knox (2000) stated that random sampling is impossible, because "studies cannot obtain a true random sample of lesbians or gay men because there is no conceivable sampling frame for them" (p. 54). Some have suggested that one way to address this is via explicit definitions when conducting and reporting LGBT research (Parks et.al., 2009). Yet we find this problematic. Our experience, and the experience of some researchers, is that there is great difficulty in exact definitions by sexual minority participants, let alone by sexuality researchers. These difficulties are found in attempts to define sexual orientation (Averett, Yoon, & Jenkins, 2012; Kehoe, 1989; Nichols, 2004), sexual behavior (Averett, Moore, & Price, 2013; Averett, Yoon & Jenkins, 2012; Claasen, 2005; Diamond, 2000; Kehoe, 1989), and identity (Brown, 1995; Diamond, 2000; Kehoe, 1989; Nichols, 2004) and all are subject to change several times within a lifetime (Diamond, 2000; Martin & D'Augelli, 2009), as the continuum approach to sexual orientation suggests. Interestingly, the current trend is away from traditional sexual orientation and gender labels and toward the all-encompassing term *queer*. However, there is also movement toward an ever-increasing spectrum of labels such as pansexual, asexual, genderfluid, genderfuck, genderqueer, omnigendered, etc. This movement will create increasing difficulty for researchers in terms of specificity, detail, and conceptualization, which then will continue to thwart attempts at random sampling and achieving generalizability.

There is also difficulty in the gerontology literature in defining and capturing "aging" and "older" (Averett & Jenkins, 2012; Denton & Spencer, 2002). Researchers use a variety of markers and different human development theories or sampling decisions in choosing age ranges in their studies. The literature on these concepts varies a great deal in definitions and use, and there is little consistency or clarity. Even with the simple word use of being older, it is difficult to find consistency among researchers. A cursory examination of gerontology literature and our own specific examination in the older lesbian research (Averett & Jenkins, 2012) found a variety of terms and language use (i.e. aging, older, old, aged, elder, elderly, etc). In our study (Averett et al., 2011), we followed Neugarten's (1974) widely used theory of the *young-old*. Neugarten argued that the young-old include those aged 55 due to the lowering age of retirement. Based on this, we specified an age minimum of 55 in our call for participants, but our participants did not heed this and those younger than 55 responded to the survey and in such numbers that we could not discard the data. This speaks to the refusal of particularly the older lesbian women who participated in our study as unwilling to fit into categories, as was revealed in our data analysis that is discussed further in the following section.

Feminist, lesbian, social work, and aging researchers often call for respect of the large differences between identities and the need to discard the search for grand narratives of Truth and generalizable knowledge, which is attempted through perfect sampling techniques. Instead, these scholars seek specific and tailored truths that respect and honor the large variety of human experiences (DeVault, 1999). There is a need for a shift in the critiques to move away from a focus on representative and random samples to critiques that are based on social justice, participant power in the process, representation, and trustworthiness (Brown & Strega, 2005). Social work researchers, in particular, should be at the forefront of considering these aspects of research with the aging LGBT population. For these reasons, we sought to hear specifically from our participants about their experiences as participants. The following provides qualitative data collected on their experience of the survey.

METHODS

In addition to our experiences, reflections, and the anecdotal feedback on the research issues within the older lesbian and LGBT communities, we also collected data from our study participants on the topic. As described in full detail in our original article, our study included an online survey of 115 questions and had 456 older lesbian participants (Averett et al., 2011).

For this study, we examined the last question of the survey, which asked the participants in an open-ended, unlimited text box to provide any comments they had about the questionnaire. One hundred and eighty-nine women (48% of participants) responded to this particular question. Two members of the research team independently analyzed this data, looking for themes and similarities in responses. The researchers then met and found they had very similar resulting themes and that the women were very clear in their responses. The following provides the major themes found in the participants' responses.

FINDINGS AND REFLECTIONS

Conceptual Issues/Dislike of Labels

A consistent message from the participants was that they felt that they generally did not fit the options provided and/or did not like their lives and experiences being reduced to "boxes." As one participant stated, "These do not reflect my reality." Others shared, "The questions are too confining and somewhat off the mark," and "One size does not fit all." This was an interesting finding to us, as we provided as many options as possible for each question, and to provide any possible missing options, we also always included an *other* unlimited space, text box for each question. One participant even noted this and seemed to understand our intention. She shared "Good questions and I'm delighted you have given room for personal comments. Not all questions apply to all people."

However, we were not entirely surprised to receive the feedback that, "Some choices don't allow for a full range of answers." Consideration of the existing literature, discussed herein, which has cited ongoing conceptual problems and difficulty with operational definitions of sexual minorities and aging, explains this experience. Older lesbians (and many LGBT community members) do not easily fit into neat categories (Averett, Moore, & Price, 2013; Frye, 1992). Thus, social work researchers should consider the limitations of surveys of any sort when conducting research within the LGBT community. For a community who defies definition and does not fit into boxes, it is not necessarily, then, a good fit to try to understand them via those methods.

Interview Us!

Thus, it was not surprising that for many of the participants, the issue was with the data collection being via a survey and quantitative method. As was stated by a participant, "I think the questions are pretty general, which is probably typical of a survey. But I am not sure how the results will really describe the experiences of growing old as a lesbian." One very pointedly stated, "I don't think that surveys are very useful for anything other than statistics." Another wrote, "As with any survey, there isn't much room for shades of gray." This leads to the idea that the women prefer to be interviewed, and many stated just that. Participants shared, "Good, but you need much more details. I supposed that will be handled via personal interviews, eh?" Another asked, "Are you doing face-to-face interviews also?" and another stated, "I could see a need for more in-depth research in the future." Another simply stated, "You need to talk to me!" This idea of their desire for talking directly to researchers, rather than completing surveys, was supported via our request for e-mail addresses to contact them for follow-up studies and the fact that 276 women (60% of the participants) provided their e-mail addresses. Thus, older lesbians could potentially be more responsive and likely to be research participants if they are talked to directly, and this direct conversation supports the continued use of qualitative methods in future research. In addition, it seems likely that mixed-method studies, ones that combine surveys with follow-up interviews, would be useful and provide the data that both researchers and participants value.

Future Research Directions

The older lesbian women provided many topics that they felt needed to be explored in future research studies. These include, but are not limited to, the following: friendships, military experiences, pets, coming out stories, online relationships, domestic violence, romantic/emotional relationships, and occupation/careers. It is interesting to note that the participants provided several directions that are not covered in the current older lesbian literature (Averett & Jenkins, 2012). Thus, future social work researchers may find that by exploring these topics, they will find willing participants.

Share the Results

The largest, most robust and consistent message from the participants in regards to feedback on the questionnaires was an overwhelming "I would like to hear the results." As one participant shared, "I want to know more about who we are." Another stated, "I would be interested in the results when this is done," and another asked, "Will we be able to see the results?"

This theme points to an important ethical issue for social work researchers studying in the LGBT community: the need to give back the information to the participants. As mentioned earlier, we gained access to the OLOC online community via their very specific and challenging research rules (http://www.oloc.org/researchrules.php). This access provided us with the majority of our participants. We are aware of this due to our survey including a question that asked how the women found the survey and the overwhelming response being "OLOC" or mention of their Web site. As a result of our ongoing communication and connection to several of the leaders of OLOC, but most specifically Sharon Raphael, PhD, we committed that our results and manuscripts would be provided to the OLOC leadership for their use and dissemination. In addition, a team member travelled to a regional gathering to present and discuss some of the data with the membership. Dr. Raphael shared that of all the research that OLOC has approved, ours was the only that has followed through and maintained communication after data collection was complete (personal communication, July 7, 2011). We suggest that part of the difficulty in accessing sexual minorities as participants in research studies is due to the lack of effort and ethical drive of research teams in maintaining communication and relationships with gatekeepers and community groups. Social work researchers, more than any other social science, are called to change this practice and must commit not only to the publication of research, but also to practical dissemination back to the populations being discussed. Most LGBT community centers do not have access to research journals or have use for the data in its academic form. Researchers have a responsibility to participants to share what they learn with them and to respect their interest in knowing more about who they are.

Our Own Limitations

Earlier we discussed some of the limitations of our study, such as the inability to reach racial minorities in any significant numbers, the high SES, and low age of our participants. The pros and cons of online use have been discussed earlier and in our other manuscripts (Averett et al., 2011). Additionally, as we have in other manuscripts (Averett et al., 2011, 2012), we acknowledge that having OLOC as the main source of participants meant that we also had responses from women who tended to be more politically and socially engaged. This, as well as their SES and educational level, potentially provides a context for understanding their reaction to being categorized and their desire for seeing the results. Women with different demographics may provide very different experiences with researchers. Researchers will not know until they begin to locate and access these groups.

CONCLUSION

We have attempted to provide new directions and perspectives on the often-discussed difficulties in older lesbian and LGBT research. In addition to examining the problems in the literature, we have also provided potential solutions, new directions for future research, and the feedback of our participants on what social work researchers should consider. Specifically, there is a need to redirect from a focus on representative sampling towards a more tailored and anti-oppressive focus on individuality and clear differences in experience. As well, future social work research with LGBT populations must respect the communities and individuals who make up our participant pools.

What is needed next are studies that consider the interests of the participants, include members on the research team, and provide the results back to the participants. Then the participants will know that they, too, have ownership in the research and thus be willing to be involved in further studies.

ACKNOWLEDGMENT

We thank Dr. Sharon Raphael, OLOC Research Gatekeeper, for her knowledge, expertise, and commitment to research on old lesbians.

REFERENCES

Averett, P., & Jenkins, C. (2012). A review of the literature on older lesbians: Implications for education, practice, and research. *Journal of Applied Gerontology, 31,* 537–561.

Averett, P., Moore. A., & Price. L. (2013). *Virginity definitions and meaning among LGBT students.* Manuscript submitted for publication.

Averett, P., Yoon, I., & Jenkins, C. (2011). Older lesbians: Experiences of aging, discrimination and resilience. *Journal of Women & Aging, 23,* 216–232.

Averett, P., Yoon, I., & Jenkins, C. (2012). Older lesbian sexuality: Identity, sexual behavior, and the impact of aging. *Journal of Sex Research, 49,* 495–507.

Bayliss, K. (2000). Social work values, anti-discriminatory practice and working with older lesbian service users. *Social Work Education, 19,* 45–53.

Brown, L. (1995). Lesbian identities: Concepts and issues. In A. D'Augelli & C. Patterson (Eds.), *Lesbian, gay and bisexual identities over the lifespan: Psychological perspectives.* (pp. 3–24). New York, NY: Oxford University.

Brown, L., & Strega, S. (Eds.). (2005). *Research as resistance: Critical, indigenous, & anti-oppressive approaches.* Toronto, Canada: Canadian Scholars Press.

Calasanti, T., & Slevin, K. (2001). *Gender, social inequalities, and aging.* New York, NY: Almira.

Denton, F., & Spencer, B. (2002). Some demographic consequence of revising the definition of "old age" to reflect future changes in lift table probabilities. *Canadian Journal on Aging, 21,* 349–356.

DeVault, M. (1999). *Liberating method: Feminism and social research.* Philadelphia, PA: Temple University Press.

Diamond, L. M. (2000). Sexual identity, attractions, and behavior among young sexual-minority women over a 2 year period. *Developmental Psychology, 36,* 241–250.

Donahue, P., & McDonald, L. (2005). Gay and lesbian aging: Current perspectives and future directions for social work practice and research. *Families in Society, 86,* 359–366.

Duffy, B., Smith, K, Terhanian, G., & Bremer, J. (2005). Comparing data from online and face-to-face surveys. *International Journal of Market Research, 47,* 615–640.

Fogel, S., & Cook, J. (2006). Considerations on the scholarship of engagement as an area of specialization for faculty. *Journal of Social Work Education, 42*, 595–606.

Frye, M. (1992). *Willful virgin: Essays in feminism 1976–1992*. Freedom, CA: Crossing Press.

Fullmer, E., Shenk, D., & Eastland, L. (1999). Negating identity: A feminist analysis of the social invisibility of older lesbians. *Journal of Women & Aging, 11*(2/3), 131–148.

Gabbay, S., & Wahler, J. (2002). Lesbian aging: Review of a growing literature. *Journal of Gay & Lesbian Social Services, 14*(3), 1–21.

Gates, T., & Kelly, B. (2013). LGB cultural phenomena and the social work research enterprise: Toward a strengths-based, culturally anchored methodology. *Journal of Homosexuality, 60*, 69–82.

Grady, C. (2005). Payment of clinical research subjects. *Journal of Clinical Investigation, 115*, 1681–1687.

Grant, R., & Sugarman, J. (2004). Ethics in human subjects research: Do incentives matter? *Journal of Medicine and Philosophy, 29*, 717–738.

Grossman, A. (2008). Conducting research among older lesbian, gay, and bisexual adults. *Journal of Gay & Lesbian Social Services, 20*(1/2), 51–67.

Healey, S. (1994). Diversity with a difference: On being old and lesbian. *Journal of Gay & Lesbian Social Services, 1*(1), 109–117.

Healy, T. (2002). Culturally competent practice with elderly lesbians. *Geriatric Care Management Journal, 12*(3), 9–13.

Jacobson, S. (1995). Methodological issues in research on older lesbians. *Journal of Gay and Lesbian Social Services, 3*, 43–56.

Jacobson, S., & Samdahl, D. (1998). Leisure in the lives of old lesbians: Experiences with and responses to discrimination. *Journal of Leisure Research, 30*, 233–255.

Kehoe, M. (1989). *Lesbians over 60 speak for themselves*. New York, NY: Harrington Park Press.

Martin, J., & D'Augelli, A. (2009). Timed lives: Cohort and period effects in research on sexual orientation and gender identity. In W. Meezan & J. Martin (Eds.), *Handbook of research with lesbian, gay, bisexual, and transgender populations*. (pp. 190–207). New York, NY: Routledge.

Martin, J., & Knox, J. (2000). Methodological and ethical issues in research on lesbians and gay men. *Social Work Research, 24*, 51–59.

Matsuo, H., McIntyre, K., Tomazic, T., & Katz, B. (2004). The online survey: Its contributions and potential problems. *Proceedings of the Survey Research Methods section of the American Statistical Association*. Retrieved from http://www.amstat.org/sections/srms/proceedings/y2004f.html

Meyer, I., & Wilson, P. (2009). Sampling lesbian, gay, and bisexual populations. *Journal of Counseling Psychology, 56*, 23–31.

Nichols, M. (2004). Lesbian sexuality/female sexuality: Rethinking "lesbian bed death." *Sexual and Relationship Therapy, 19*, 363–371.

Neugarten, B. (1974). Age groups in American society and the rise of the young old. *Annals of American Academy of Sciences, 415*, 187–198.

Parks, C., Hughes, T., & Werkmeister-Rozas, L. (2009). Defining sexual identity and sexual orientation in research with lesbians, gay men, and bisexuals. In

W. Meezan & J. Martin, (Eds.). *Handbook of research with lesbian, gay, bisexual, and transgender populations* (pp. 71–99). New York, NY: Routledge.

Pugh, S. (2005). Assessing the cultural needs of older lesbians and gay men: Implications for practice. *Practice, 17,* 207–218.

Shenk, D., & Fullmer, E. (1996). Significant relationships among older women: Cultural and personal construction of lesbianism. *Journal of Women & Aging, 8*(3/4), 75–89.

Wojciechowski, C. (1998). Issues in caring for older lesbians. *Journal of Gerontological Nursing, 24*(7), 28–33.

Breaking Barriers and Building Bridges: Understanding the Pervasive Needs of Older LGBT Adults and the Value of Social Work in Health Care

SHILOH D. ERDLEY

Department of Sociology, Social Work and Criminal Justice, Bloomsburg University of Pennsylvania, Bloomsburg, Pennsylvania, USA and Nephrology Department, Geisinger Medical Center, Danville, Pennsylvania, USA

DONALD D. ANKLAM

Harrisburg, Pennsylvania, USA

CHRISTINA C. REARDON

Nonprofit Evaluation, Services and Training Program (NEST), Temple University, Harrisburg, Pennsylvania, USA

Given the rise in the aging population and the increased use of health care services, there is a demand for awareness and training that targets underserved populations such as older lesbian, gay, bisexual, and transgender (LGBT) adults. Older LGBT adults are 5 times less likely to access health care and social services (King, 2009). Ethically responsible health service delivery is needed to capitalize on the strengths and capabilities of older LGBT adults and is vital for combating existing health disparities. Social workers aim to prevent ongoing gaps in care for older LGBT adults that can lead to negative individual and social consequences.

BACKGROUND AND SIGNIFICANCE

Older adults are among the fastest-growing age group in the United States, and it is anticipated that more than 37 million older Americans will be expected to manage more than one chronic condition by 2030 (American Hospital Association, 2007). Older adults often require specialized services and professional expertise that addresses their comorbid medical problems, and these adults also confront challenges with social resources and support systems. Many older adults who do not receive adequate health care are at risk for hospitalizations, nursing home admission, low quality of care, and death (Kramarow, Lubitz, Lentzner, & Gorina, 2006; Wolinsky, Callahan, Fitzgerald, & Johnson, 1992). Aging minorities, including lesbian, gay, bisexual, and transgender (LGBT) adults, often face additional hardships including isolation, financial stress and social inequities that make managing their medical and mental health problems challenging (Cahill & South, 2002; Heck, Sell, & Gorin, 2006; Mayer et al., 2008; Morrison & Dinkel, 2012). Furthermore, the risk of suicide is estimated to be two to four times higher than that of heterosexual individuals in this population (Climent, Ervin, Rollings, Plutchik, & Batinelli, 1977; Morrow, 2008; Saghir & Robins, 1973; Saunders & Valente, 1987).

Despite the specialized needs of older LGBT adults, there has been little empirical consideration given to defining potential health disparities that exist for this aging subpopulation. Previous research regarding race-based health disparities indicates a strong relationship between higher mortality, chronic illness, and declining health in minorities and suggests that multiple areas of diversity such as age and sexual orientation may lead to increased risk for negative individual outcomes (Barker, 2008; National Research Council, 2006). As a result, efforts aimed at uncovering disparities in LGBT elders should involve a deeper understanding of individual, social and health service-delivery determinants of care.

Increased awareness of the characteristics and needs of older LGBT adults is needed to ensure best practices in health care institutions. The lack of studies of the LGBT community has led to wide variations in estimates of the size of this population. In his 1948 book, *Sexual Behavior in the Human Male,* Alfred Kinsey proposed that 10% of the public is LGBT (Robison, 2002). More recent estimates suggest that between one and 3.5 million older adults self-identify as lesbian or gay men in the United States, and that this number is expected to double by 2030 given the aging of the baby boomers (N. Jackson, Johnson, & Roberts, 2008).

Despite a recent trend among researchers to learn more about the needs of older LGBT individuals, many methodological problems and individual barriers present significant obstacles to understanding the needs of this population (Blando, 2001; Kochman, 1997; McFarland & Sanders, 2003; Orel, 2004). According to Gay and Lesbian Medical Association (2001), the main cause of this inability to quantify the population is a fear that many people have of disclosing their sexuality. Also, sexuality is a subjective idea, and many people may have feelings for someone of the same sex but do not consider themselves to be gay or lesbian. Most surveys ask a person about their sexual behavior, not their sexual orientation; therefore, the information obtained may not be an accurate snapshot of this community. The lack of studies looking into the actual numbers, combined with the reluctance of many LGBT individuals to disclose their sexuality, makes it hard to get exact numbers. Additionally, most available studies have been conducted in urban settings and often involve a homogeneous limited sample (Butler & Hope, 1999; Kehoe, 1986; Wahler & Gabbay, 1997).

Limited information exists about older LGBT adults' experiences accessing the health care system. LGBT elders are medically underserved and at higher risk for health problems than their heterosexual counterparts (Morrison & Dinkel, 2012). These risk factors, alone, suggest the need for direct interventions and policies that will result in better outcomes for LGBT clients such as improved access to care and increased awareness of the medical needs of this population. Recent efforts have been made regarding changes in the health care law for federal and state government research projects to involve more inclusive data covering the issues faced by the aging community, including the needs of older LGBT adults (National Gay and Lesbian Task Force, 2010; Sebelius, 2011). Although this signifies an expanded awareness of the growing and diverse needs of the aging population, more concentrated efforts that focus on the specific needs of older LGBT adults will be needed to ensure that the culture of health care institutions reflects the diverse needs of every older adult.

Responsiveness to the growing needs of this population is vital to ensure that health service delivery reflects the core values of cultural competency. Medical social workers and various other health care professionals are situated at the center of service delivery for this population; however, it is unclear how well prepared and aware health and social service practitioners are regarding the needs of LGBT elders. Furthermore, homophobia and heterosexism are well documented among these practitioners (Berkamn & Zinberg, 1997; Cochran, Peavy, & Cauce, 2007; Harris, Nightengale, & Owen, 1995; Swank & Raiz, 2008) and are believed to be a result of limited educational material and field work experiences concentrating on LGBT content and oppression, particularly in the field of social work (Bergh & Crisp, 2004; Fredriksen-Goldsen, Woodford, Luke, & Gutierrez, 2011; Longres & Fredriksen, 2000; Morrow & Messinger, 2006). Although the Council on Social Work Education (CSWE; 2013) and the National Association of Social Workers (2013) promote the development of culturally competent curriculum and practice to ensure social justice and to foster diversity, awareness of the needs of older LGBT population and visibility of older LGBT individuals in health care systems remains low (Butler, 2004; McFarland &

Sanders, 2003). A heightened focus on this area of practice at the curricula and field-work level of education, combined with faculty preparedness and development, may further strengthen the training of new graduates and prepare them for being advocates for older LGBT adults in health care settings. Additionally, collaborative advocacy among health care providers will be the vehicle through which equality and justice will be achieved for LGBT elders. Furthermore, social workers who support this process will have opportunities to foster nondiscriminatory practices in health care settings. Actions that will reframe interventions, programs, and procedures to include the needs of older LGBT adults should be based upon a clear understanding of health determinants. Such advocacy in this area of practice is a necessary step toward uncovering unknown health disparities in this population.

The focus of this article is to examine the individual, social, and service delivery determinants of health in older LGBT adults and the current state of awareness and preparedness of health care social workers regarding LGBT elder issues. Additionally, this article discusses implications for practice, including future suggestions on how health and social service practitioners can collaboratively provide gay-affirmative practices in hopes to improve quality of health and life in this population. This article will serve as the initial groundwork for future studies aimed at understanding perceptions, attitudes, and practices of social workers in health care organizations and will build upon existing work focused on uncovering health disparities in aging LGBT adults.

INDIVIDUAL AND SOCIAL DETERMINANTS

Historical Synopsis of Homosexuality

The first law regarding any prohibition of homosexuality can be traced back to a 1697 Massachusetts law that addressed sodomy. It referred to "the detestable and abominable sin of buggery [anal sex] with mankind or beast, which is contrary to the very light of nature" (Koerner, 2002). The word *homosexual* was first used in 1869 by an Austro-Hungarian advocate for sexual rights, K. M. Kertbeny, who used it to describe those with a "healthy love for their own sex" (Eisenbach, 2006, p. 222). Shortly after, a professor of psychiatry in Berlin, Germany, Carl Westphal, used the word *homosexual* in a case history of a woman whom he diagnosed as having "contrary sexual feelings" (Eisenbach, 2006, p. 222). For the next 100 years, the term *homosexual* was used as a label for a disease or sickness. It was not until April 1974 that the American Psychological Association removed homosexuality as a disease from its *Diagnostic and Statistical Manual of Mental Disorders* (Eisenbach, 2006), despite the existing empirical evidence that negated any association between psychological aberrations and homosexuality (Christie & Young, 1986; Hart et al., 1978; Newman, Dannenfelser, &, Benishek 2002;

Saghir, Robins, Walbran, & Gentry, 1970; Siegelman, 1972). Notwithstanding progress in the mental health arena, controversy continues to surround recent changes to the DSM-5 that classify *gender dysphoria*, previously named *gender identity disorder*, as a mental disorder (American Psychiatric Association, 2013).

The historical social construction of the term *homosexuality*, along with the associated connection to illness by professionals, provided the building blocks for continued stigma against homosexual communities at the onset of the AIDS epidemic. The AIDS epidemic was first reported in 1981 and, from that point forward, the disease would be linked to the gay male community, as the origins of the disease in the United States were traced to a French-Canadian gay flight attendant named Gaetan Duga. Ignorance surrounding the disease and the discriminatory views toward homosexuals during this period led to a misleading focus on sexual orientation, rather than the disease itself, and ultimately resulted in the disease being named gay-related immunodeficiency disease or GRID. This epidemic occurred during the Reagan administration, which did little to address the growing concern. Consequently, cuts in funding by the Reagan administration and a lack of media coverage regarding this epidemic forced many in the LGBT community to begin forming support networks. Organizations such as the Gay Men's Health Crisis were formed to address many of the needs that health care professionals and lawmakers were not addressing (Eisenbach, 2006). According to the documentary *Before Stonewall* (Center for Study of Filmed History, 1985), many doctors refused to treat AIDS patients initially, because they perceived that AIDS was a gay disease primarily concentrated among males. AIDS and the gay male community would go on to share this linked history that continues to influence service delivery and perceptions of the gay male community today.

Older LGBT persons faced significant societal and political stigma prior to the modern gay rights movements (Grossman, 2008; Orel, 2006). The silencing of this generation regarding sexuality grew out of the fears that the wider society imposed. Many older LGBT persons hid their sexuality for fear of discrimination that could have potentially negative individual and familial consequences such as job loss, harassment, shaming, and death. The use of electroshock therapy to treat homosexuality and overt discrimination by medical professions further compounded and reinforced disapproval and isolation in this population (Flaxman, 2001). Many older LGBT adults lived during a time in history when they were afraid for their safety and often remained silent and isolated to survive.

These views continue to be salient for many older adults today. A 2010 study performed by Services and Advocacy for Gay, Lesbian, Bisexual, and Transgender Elders (SAGE) showed that this history of discrimination has led many LGBT elders to distrust persons in authority. Because health care providers often are perceived as authority figures, many LGBT elders are skeptical that they will receive adequate care from health care professionals (SAGE, 2010). These belief systems continue to permeate the gay community and are evidenced in reports that LGBT elders use health care services at a lower rate than their heterosexual counterparts (King, 2009; Stein, Beckerman, & Sherman, 2010). Despite past and present attempts to reduce discriminatory practices against LGBT adults, homophobia and heterosexism remain a salient part of American mainstream culture (Morrow, 2008).

Information regarding the history of homosexuality in health care is scant. What is known is that the traditional medical model of care is designed to meet the needs of heterosexual patients and that existing medical assessment and care models have resulted in reduced access to care, poor communication, and decreased quality of care for older LGBT adults (DeHart, 2008; Morrison & Dinkel, 2012; Saulnier, 2002). It is not clear if negative outcomes for older LGBT adults result from obvious discriminatory practices or because most interventions involve a heterosexist approach. Results from Saulnier's (2002) focus group with 33 lesbian and bisexual women suggest that provider heterosexist attitudes alone influenced health care decisions. In focus groups with older LGBT adults in the Midwest, Orel (2004) also uncovered the fact that health care experiences among this population varied depending upon whether or not the older adult was out or remained closeted. Orel found that older adults who felt comfortable enough to be open with their physician and health care providers about their sexual orientation had more positive experiences than the older adults who remained silent. Research suggests that beyond obvious discriminatory practices, there are various systemic and individual factors that affect health care outcomes for older LGBT adults (Clover, 2006; Mayer et al., 2008; Morrison & Dinkel, 2012).

The intersection of systemic and individual factors continues to contribute to the experiences of practitioners and older LGBT adults in health care settings. The health care climate—including culture, economy, and traditional practices—has resulted in a complex world where, although diversity is more openly discussed, culturally sensitive practices are by no means consistently integrated. Although every practitioner and health care organization may have their goals set on best practices, change at the most effective level must take into consideration interventions that result in sustainable practices that provide equality to all. Furthermore, for change to take place, individual accountability and openness on the part of the older LGBT adult is essential. A generational shift combined with a changing political climate may aid in helping older LGBT adults overcome many of the challenges faced by previous generations and may potentially lead to more positive health care outcomes.

Despite the changing social context and increased efforts to study and report current practices, older LGBT adults continue to be faced with many challenges in health care settings. A shift in a more open LGBT community provides hope for advocacy for older LGBT adults; however, overcoming social injustices and personal fears will require increased awareness and collaboration among individuals, communities, and health care leaders. Although older LGBT adults face unique challenges specific to their environment, many are faced with similar barriers to care including, but not limited to ageism, homophobia, heterosexism, isolation, and financial stress (Cahill & South, 2002; Clover, 2006; McFarland & Sanders, 2003). An understanding of these barriers will help to reduce discriminatory practices in health care and further promote improved access to care for this marginalized population.

Ageism

It is not uncommon for elders, whether they are heterosexual or homosexual, to experience some form of ageism. Often when one is considered old, he or she is considered "less attractive, less important, and less useful; therefore, less worthy of attention and resources" (Cahill, South, & Spade, 2000). For the LGBT community, specifically gay men, this idea of what is old seems to develop earlier than in heterosexual or lesbian society. Often, "old" for homosexual men is considered to be 35, while "later life" is considered to begin at age 44 (Meisner & Hynie, 2009).

In the larger LGBT community, ageism is a real problem. Community support groups often are age-segregated. Despite the existence of LGBT support/advocacy centers for young people, few centers exist for the elder community. Some factors that may influence coping with ageism among older LGBT adults include prior exposure to extreme adversity and generational differences. Adaptive styles of coping in older LGBT adults can be attributed to what Kimmel (1978) referred to as "crisis competency" (p. 117) and involves a higher level of preparedness for discrimination that develops out of past traumas. As a result of past stigmas associated with homosexuality, older LGBT adults may be better prepared than their heterosexual counterparts to deal with the current effects of ageism (Berger & Kelly, 1996; Cohler & Hostetler, 2006). Although the current LGBT aging population has been named the *silent generation*, the history of discrimination, injustice, and adversity among this group provides a stronger mental framework for managing present forms of injustice such as ageism (Berger & Kelly, 1996; Butler, 2004; Cohler & Hostetler, 2006). However, the baby boomer LGBT population also may face adversities such as ageism with an open and assertive style, given the generational characteristics and societal and political times that have led to increased support systems for this group (Crisp, Wayland, & Gordon, 2008; MetLife Mature Market Institute, 2006). An understanding of the generational gaps between aging LGBT elders and how the coping styles of these groups intersect with social injustices such as ageism will aid in the development of more efficient and effective health care interventions and programs.

Homophobia/Heterosexism

Existing literature indicates that past discriminatory practices against LGBT patients leads to perceived and actual homophobia that perpetuates problems with accessing adequate health care (Berkman & Zinberg; 1997; Brotman, Ryan, & Cormier, 2003; Morrison & Dinkel, 2012). Most gay adults have experienced homophobia and heterosexism. Heterosexism is defined as "a belief system that values heterosexuality as superior to and/or more 'natural' than homosexuality" (Morin & Garfinkle, 1978, p. 30). As per Herek (1992), homophobia is the fear or hatred of lesbian and gay people. Despite the growing need for, and access to, social and community programs, LGBT elders are not likely to use such resources for fear of discrimination. Research suggests that the culture of heterosexist institutions and LGBT adults' perceptions of these institutions results in decreased use of services (Behney, 1994; Cahill & South, 2002; Knochel, Croghan, Moone, & Quam, 2012). An understanding of the effects of homophobia and heterosexism in the health care setting is essential for overcoming discriminatory practices.

In a report released in 2001, health disparities among LGBT people included negative attitudes toward LGBT adults and a lack of training among health care professionals (Gay and Lesbian Medical Association, 2001). An example of this is the intake forms used by most practitioners. These forms often do not take into consideration any person who does not fall into the norm. For instance, when the form asks for marital status, it does not take into consideration those persons who may be in committed relationships with someone of the same sex. The following excerpt is an example of how a heterosexual framework in practice affects same-sex couples.

> Paul and Carter are a gay couple in their mid-fifties. Carter is an office manager of their podiatry clinic, and his partner Paul is the podiatrist. Describing medical forms he has completed in the past, Carter stated, "None of those boxes applied to me and my monogamous relationship of 28 years" (Carter, personal communication, February 20, 2011).

> Paul commented that even people who are widowed have no box to check on most intake forms (Paul, personal communication, February 20, 2011).

Although there are often blank spaces for individuals to fill in regarding their marital status, these medical forms lack the ability to capture an adequate history of the LGBT patient.

This overall disregard for identifying differences among older adults in health care can affect how LGBT adults perceive their medical problems. Often, health care professionals use health education materials such as pamphlets, books, or audiovisual aids that do not include language or illustrations inclusive of LGBT persons. Also, health professionals may use language relating to patients' support systems that does not take into account their relationships or partnerships. In addition, "even if a provider is culturally sensitive to the LGBT population, that provider should not assume all providers are" (Burch, 2008, p. 192). This approach to practice can create feelings of mistrust among older LGBT adults resulting in decreased compliance with health care treatment (Addis, Davies, Greene, MacBride-Steward, & Shepherd, 2009; Mayer et al., 2008).

Changing the lens of practice for health care professionals will aid in the development of culturally sensitive services. Posting rainbow stickers in offices and offering LGBT nonprofit pamphlets in medical clinics are small steps that providers can take to address diversity among their patients and to improve the comfort level of older LGBT clients (Gay and Lesbian Medical Association, 2006). A better understanding of the effects of homophobia and heterosexism on LGBT elders in health care is needed to improve practice. Training and education for professionals should address the inherent biases that exist among professionals and further include guidelines for practice that promote nondiscriminatory approaches to care.

Isolation

In addition to the heteronormative view in health care practice, barriers to adequate health care for LGBT elders include isolation and invisibility of this population (Jeyasingham, 2008; Pugh, 2005;). Unlike their heterosexual peers, older LGBT adults are more likely to live alone and rely on friends or informal caregivers for support later in life (Adelman, Gurevitch, de Vries, & Blando, 2006; Stein et al., 2010).

Research demonstrates a need for an increased focus on social supports for gay and lesbian older adults as they age. However, obtaining social supports is particularly challenging for rural older LGBT adults because smaller communities are characterized as having limited education, less visibility, and fewer networking options (Butler & Hope, 1999: McFarland & Sanders, 2003). Additionally, access to and availability of LGBT organizations is minimal in rural communities. Overcoming isolation is easier in urban settings where the visibility of the gay community is heightened and where programs and support services that specifically meet the needs of LGBT elders are more likely to exist (Butler, 2004, SAGE; 2010). Several factors, including the impact of stress related to stigma, discrimination, and finances, can lead to isolation (Kuyper & Fokkema, 2010; LGBT Movement Advancement Project & SAGE, 2010; Stein et al., 2010). In the following interview, many of these factors leading to isolation are evident.

In a recent interview, Dale,[1] a 60-year-old retired government employee living in rural Pennsylvania, discussed a number of issues preventing him

---

[1]   Name changed to protect privacy.

from receiving adequate health care, but he primarily spoke about the effects of isolation. Dale lives in a small town and does not have access to a larger LGBT community. The distance he must travel to be connected to older LGBT individuals is not feasible, given his age and his income. Not unlike many older LGBT adults, Dale is single and has limited financial and family resources. He retired early from the US government and is not yet able to collect Social Security. His options for support are limited, and his feelings of isolation are compounded by the heterosexual culture that surrounds him. "I used to be on the go all the time just because I have no one to come home to; but now, I'm finding it harder to do that due to some health concerns" (Dale, personal communication, February 22, 2011). He leaves the radio on all day so that there is some noise when he walks in the door and to make it seem as if he is not really alone.

The consequences of isolation in LGBT elders are not well known. Research suggests that isolation in older LGBT adults can lead to negative social and individual outcomes, including poor medical and mental health (Diaz, Ayala, Bein, Henne, & Marin, 2001; Kuyper & Fokkema, 2010). For older LGBT adults, isolation involves a complex process characterized by stigma, discrimination, and social inequities that influence financial and community resources (Butler, 2004; Cahill, 2002; Cahill et al., 2000; Phillips & Marks, 2006). To reduce isolation among aging LGBT adults and increase access to services, health care institutions will benefit from adopting culturally competent approaches that focus on provider attitudes and training (Anetzberger, Ishler, Mostade, & Blair, 2004; Brotman et al., 2003; Crisp et al., 2008). More information is needed to understand and combat the effects of isolation in LGBT elders.

Poverty

"Systemic discrimination coupled with a lack of uniform relationship recognition increases the risk of poverty for same-sex couples, their children, and the growing number of LGBT older adults" (Maril & Estes, 2013, p. 7). Traditional means for financial support, including Social Security and pension plans, present problems for LGBT adults. Although significant progress has been made for same-sex couples at both the state and federal level, financial benefits and federal protections that come with marriage do not exist for same-sex couples nationwide. Same-sex couples that will benefit from these advocacy efforts include those who reside in the 14 states plus the District of Columbia where same-sex marriage is legal. These couples will also benefit from the recent overturning of the Defense of Marriage Act (DOMA); an act that prevented same-sex couples from receiving the federal protections that come with marriage for heterosexual couples. Although this landmark decision by the Supreme Court marks continued success for overcoming existing social injustices faced by same-sex couples, this decision does not change the present discriminatory practices in states where same-sex marriage is illegal. Furthermore, the decision did not overturn section 2 of DOMA, which still gives power to states to discriminate against same-sex couples that are married legally in other states (LGBT Organizations Fact Sheet Series, 2013).

As a result of the remaining discriminatory laws, many couples remain financially at risk, with no access to the benefits available to heterosexual couples. These benefits include medical benefits from a spouse's employer, Social Security benefits from a spouse, inheritance of estates without having to pay any taxes, Medicaid and long-term care, Family Medical Leave (FMLA) to care for a spouse, sponsorship of a foreign-born spouse for citizenship, and veteran's spousal benefits (LGBT Organizations Fact Sheet Series, 2013; SAGE, 2010).

The lack of recognition of LGBT families can lead to profound financial consequences for LGBT elders, and this practice has been described as the "most blatant and costly example of institutional heterosexism in federal policy" (Butler, 2004, p. 36; Cahill et al., 2000). Beyond the strain that results from being targeted as a marginalized individual in society, the consequences of financial stress can be physically and emotionally destructive. Older LGBT adults residing in states where same-sex marriage is not recognized as legal may be at risk for negative physical and mental health problems as a result of limited access to financial resources. The areas where these couples may be affected most significantly involve support from FMLA benefits, Social Security, Medicaid spousal protection laws, and property inheritance taxes. Many of these older LGBT adults in caretaking roles who remain employed due to the economic downturn or as a result of lack of access to state and federal benefits can be faced with the hardship of being unable to leave work because they are not eligible for FMLA benefits. In many cases, the older adult may have no other option but to leave their job to care for their partner, which could result in loss of employment, decreased health and potentially the loss of home, property, and savings (SAGE, 2010).

Older LGBT adults often rely on Social Security as their most important financial safety net, not unlike their heterosexual counterparts. However, LGBT elders who pay into Social Security identically to their heterosexual peers are not equal when it comes to its benefits if they are not residing in a state that respects their marriage. Due to this discrimination, older LGBT adults have lower incomes and decreased opportunities to save for disability and retirement (Maril & Estes, 2013). Under these circumstances, when a gay or lesbian partner dies, the surviving partner is not entitled to survivor benefits, as a heterosexual spouse would be. It is estimated that the lack of spousal Social Security income costs an LGBT elder $14,076 a year (SAGE, 2010).

Same-sex couples residing in states that do not recognize their union may also experience financial strain and stress related to planning for long-term care because they are not entitled to the same spousal protection laws as heterosexual married couples. The couples residing in these states may, at some point, have to sell their home to pay for their partner's care in the nursing facility if they were relying on Medicaid as the provider. Although the overturning of DOMA has provided spousal protection in these circumstances for same-sex couples residing in states where their marriage is legal, many older married LGBT couples do not have this protection, placing them at risk for poverty or potentially providing an incentive to not seek necessary services that a long-term care facility provides. Many same-sex couples will continue to reside in states where their unions are not recognized and their need for long-term care planning and skilled care will be unavoidable, making attention to this matter vital.

As stated in SAGE (2010), allowing LGBT people to legally marry would be the single most helpful solution to protect this vulnerable population. Spouses then could receive the death benefits afforded to heterosexual spouses, such as access to Social Security and pensions. They would not suffer tax penalties from inheriting estates and property. The protections afforded spouses under Medicaid and long-term living would be available to all. Ultimately, the hope for same-sex marriage is to achieve the ends that are provided to heterosexual couples, which is an important first step toward overcoming the economic inequities LGBT elders face. State-conferred marriage rights and a full repeal of all sections of DOMA under the Respect for Marriage Act are needed to ensure that every legally married same-sex couple receives protections, resources, and programs that are equal to that of all married couples in the United States.

Despite the resiliency of many LGBT elders, the various social and economic injustices faced by this population can have detrimental effects on mental and physical health. Health care providers and institutions serve as gatekeepers for the aging population, especially for minority groups such as older LGBT adults. However, for service delivery to promote health in minority aging populations, practice must be rooted in a culturally competent interdisciplinary approach with a specific focus on the individual and social determinants of health.

HEALTH-SERVICE DELIVERY DETERMINANTS

Health care agencies have extensive opportunities to engage with older adults and to provide support, education, and meaningful resources that promote adequate quality of life. Unfortunately, bias in health care is widespread. Research demonstrates that increased risks for adverse physical and mental health outcomes have been linked to discriminatory practice and perceptions of unfair treatment (Boardman, 2004; Brown et al., 2000; J. S. Jackson et al., 1996; Krieger, 1990, Krieger & Sidney, 1996). Additionally, few health care providers have training on the aging population and are even less likely to engage in culturally competent practice with aging LGBT adults (Barker, 2008; Institute of Medicine, 2008; Kochman, 1997; LGBT Movement Advancement Project & SAGE, 2010; Weinick, Zuvekas, & Drilea, 1997).

Optimal delivery of health care involves practice and interventions designed around the specific needs of the population served (C. V. Johnson, Mimiaga, & Bradford, 2008; Mayer et al., 2008; Stein et al., 2010). Effective service-delivery models in health care involve good communication and culturally sensitive practices and further aim to balance individual capacity with environmental opportunity (Compton & Galaway, 1989; Ryan, Meredith, MacLean, & Orange, 1995; World Health Organization, 1984).

Health care service delivery outcomes for older LGBT adults are not well known. However, literature suggests that both overt and subtle forms of oppression may contribute to health disparities within this group (Dinkel, Patzel, McGuire, Rolfs, & Purcell, 2007; Morrison & Dinkel, 2012). Heterosexist and homophobic health care practice often lead to underused and ineffective interventions (Barker, 2008; Cahill & South, 2006; Dehart, 2008; Morrison & Dinkel, 2012). Research further suggests that older LGBT adults perceive fear of discrimination and lack of understanding from health care providers as significant barriers to accessing care (McFarland & Sanders, 2003). In a 2006 survey on the LGBT community by MetLife Mature Market Institute, 19% of respondents reported "little or no confidence that medical personnel would treat them with dignity and respect as LGBT individuals in old age" (MetLife Mature Market Institute, 2006, p. 14). Another cutting-edge report, published in 2009 and led by the National Senior Citizens Law Center in collaboration with the National Center for Lesbian Rights, Lambda Legal, the National Center for Transgender Equality, the National Gay and Lesbian Task Force, and SAGE) (2011) surveyed 769 individuals to examine issues faced by older LGBT adults in longer-term care facilities. Results from this report highlighted several areas of mistreatment and discrimination experienced by this group, including harassment by residents and staff members, negation of care and refusal of staff members to recognize assignment of medical power of attorney of same-sex partners.

The MetLife report, the National Senior Citizens Law report on long-term care, and other self-report surveys identify serious gaps in care that could have potentially devastating outcomes for older adults. These reports further indicate that aging LGBT adults often do not disclose their sexual orientation for fear that they will be confronted with prejudice and biased treatment by their providers (M. J. Johnson, Jackson, Arnette, & Koffman, 2005; Stein & Bonuck, 2001). Failure to disclose sexual orientation or avoidance of health care institutions for fear of discrimination also has implications for family members, caretakers, partners, and providers (Brotman, 2007; Stein & Bonuck, 2001). Ultimately, the unmet physical and mental health needs of older LGBT adults will result in increased demands on the individual and society. Health and social service practitioners need to be more informed and participate in education and training aimed to reduce practice barriers that diminish patient quality of life for older LGBT adults (McFarland & Sanders, 2003; Stein et al., 2010).

RELEVANCE TO SOCIAL WORK

Social workers can play a pivotal role in ensuring that older LGBT adults receive the necessary resources to overcome individual, social, and health-service delivery barriers to health. As a profession, social workers strive to advocate for older LGBT adults and have the ability to work collaboratively with other members of the health care team. Furthermore, social workers' positions in the health care industry in home care, hospitals, long-term care facilities, rehabilitations centers, and community agencies provide expansive opportunities for collaborative interventions with institutions, various health care professionals and clients.

Best practice in health care should involve interventions that balance the interpersonal needs of clients with practitioner awareness and preparedness that is rooted in culturally sensitive practice. Effective competency training should address the importance of service delivery that provides for a safe and comfortable environment promoting trust and meaningful communication between provider and patient. This approach will allow LGBT elders to live out the rest of their lives without fear and anxiety over their sexual orientation regardless of their living environment and will promote increased comfort and access to health care (Stein et al., 2010). Such approaches to practice will require significant attention to areas of self-awareness, education, and the promotion of organizational and policy changes based on quality initiatives and empirical data.

Self-awareness is an important step to ensuring that health care practices promote health in older LGBT adults and includes self-affirmation and respect for aging LGBT adults. The existence of bias against LGBT older adults presents a significant barrier to health and well-being. These biases exist among all health care professionals—including social workers—and often are subtle and indirect. Reports from LGBT elders suggest that health and social service practitioners need to be more knowledgeable about the lifestyles and needs of older LGBT adults (McFarland & Sanders, 2003; Orel, 2004; Stein & Bonuck, 2001).

A second, and equally important, focus on change should center on education, training, and social policy. The goal of social work education is to prepare professionals to understand the various systemic issues associated with sexual orientation and gender expression and to be leaders in promoting social and economic justice for subjugated populations such as older LGBT adults (CSWE, 2013). Ideally, social workers' training provides for linkage of underserved populations to systems that will promote health and well-being. The core values of the social work profession promote cultural competency in practice and provide workers with the skills to empower clients to advocate for individual, societal and policy change.

Although social work education and professional organizations promote culturally competent curricula and policies, little is known regarding implementation and sustainability of this approach to practice as it relates to older LGBT adults (Frederiksen-Goldsen et al., 2011; Jeyasingham, 2008; Martinez, 2011). Some studies regarding social workers' attitudes toward gay and lesbian individuals exist, but fewer studies involve practice behaviors of social workers with this population (Crisp, 2006). Further, lack of evidence exists as it relates to training specifically regarding older rather than younger LGBT individuals. Martin et al. (2009) uncovered that most social work programs lack the ability to formally assess competency levels of students in providing LGBT services but focused their study primarily on LGBT youth. In their study, Logie, Bridge, and Bridge (2007) found that almost half of the social work graduate students surveyed perceive that they are ill prepared to provide culturally competent practice to LGBT individuals and their families, thus suggesting that the value of education is more concentrated in practice behaviors rather than practice knowledge. It is suggested that this potential gap in preparedness for social work students regarding LGBT adults may be attributed to faculty development and attitudes, limited fieldwork opportunities with LGBT adults, and the unfortunate reality that LGBT elders represent a multifaceted area of practice involving sexual orientation and age that has been historically invisible in the American culture (Frediken-Goldsen et al., 2011).

Additional limitations to understanding the practice behaviors of social workers with older LGBT adults include poor research response rates by social workers and sparse availability of validated instruments to measure attitudes and behaviors (Crisp, 2006). One available tool to help overcome these limitations is known as the Gay Affirmative Practice (GAP) scale. This scale is a rapid assessment instrument that has beneficial uses for all health care professionals and evaluates the degree to which professionals engage in affirmative practice with gay and lesbian individuals (Crisp, 2006; Crisp et al., 2008). Davies (1996) defined GAP as practice that "affirms a lesbian, gay, or bisexual identity as an equally positive human experience and expression to heterosexual identity" (p. 25).

GAP models of intervention are a good fit for social workers because they align with the core values of social work and include attention to the person in the environment, empowerment, and cultural competency (Crisp, 2006). The use of self-evaluation tools and conceptual frameworks such as GAP by all health care professionals will aid in the assessment and improvement of practice with older LGBT adults. Although advocacy efforts at the education and practice level provide a solid foundation for culturally competent practice with older LGBT adults, much work is needed to ensure that social work practitioners in all settings consistently practice and prepare for the changing needs of aging LGBT adults. Furthermore, mandated review and assessment of attitudes and behaviors regarding older LGBT adults at the undergraduate level utilizing validated instruments such as the GAP would help to ensure consistency across social work programs nationwide.

Finally, social workers are needed to promote research and training to address the rapidly growing needs of the LGBT aging community. Without appropriate competency training and research, many health care professionals lack the tools to address the health concerns of the LGBT community. These include mental health disorders—in particular depression, eating and body image disorders, anxiety, and suicide—as well as substance abuse (Burgard, Cochran & Mays, 2005; Drabble, Midanik, & Trocki, 2005; Mayer et al., 2008; Meyer, 2003; Stein et al., 2010). Transgender individuals can encounter issues related to hormone replacement therapy and sexual reassignment surgery (Mayer et al., 2008). Despite the specialized needs of older LGBT adults, guidelines for care are not broadly known or communicated. Future research will be pivotal in guiding and developing evidence-based practices in this area of care.

Social workers' frontline access to LGBT elders makes incorporating cultural competencies with behaviors a priority. Social work education and training should prepare social workers to be instruments of change and leaders in various social and health care institutions, but will only reach this goal when all social work programs recognize the value of infusing LGBT aging issues throughout undergraduate- and graduate-level coursework. Social workers are a valuable resource for older LGBT adults and other health care professionals. The profession's commitment toward self-awareness and advocacy for underserved populations like aging LGBT is essential for reducing health disparities among this population.

IMPLICATIONS FOR PRACTICE

Future research on the aging population should expand beyond lesbian and gay older adults to include individuals of diverse ethnic backgrounds, socioeconomic status, and sexual orientations. More information is needed regarding health disparities associated with ethnicity and varied sexual orientations, including bisexual and transgendered adults. The health and well-being of the LGBT aging community is affected by access to health care and social service care programs. The future of the aging LGBT population will depend greatly upon continued provisions of health and social service programs that aim to overcome the marginalization of this population.

Best practices and models of care for LGBT elders in health care settings should involve efforts to overcome barriers to treatment, strive to build bridges between providers, and aim to define existing disparities among LGBT elders. Models of care should acknowledge the existing individual, social, and health-service delivery determinants of health that often involve significant barriers for older adults in the health care environment. A deeper understanding of how isolation, poverty, discrimination, invisibility, and distrust can lead to negative individual outcomes will provide a foundation for building valuable connections between providers, consumers, and the community. However, to sustain long-term positive changes that embody LGBT affirmative services in health care, all providers should strive to engage in the following practices: (a) self-awareness and utilization of LGBT affirmative practice tools such as the GAP; (b) annual education forums that address the needs of older LGBT adults, including sexuality in old age; (c) collaboration with other health care providers, community elder care organizations, and LGBT communities to identify the specific needs of clients; and (4) trust-building initiatives that aim to reduce the oppressive nature of the organizational setting.

Beyond education, quality improvement programs and collaboration among health care professionals, empirical evidence regarding outcomes of models of care for LGBT elder will aid in understanding and provide future data to replicate and enhance programs that serve as the gold standard of care for this population. Additionally, as advocacy efforts continue to increase in the areas of social service and in local, state, and federal programs and policies, the hope will be that aging LGBT adults will feel more comfortable discussing their sexual identity and their personal experiences, thus overcoming many of the methodological shortcomings that have existed for decades in this area of research.

The rise in the aging population coupled with poor health care could have potentially crippling consequences for older LGBT adults, their families, and the health care system. Equal access to health care should never be compromised regardless of race, ethnicity, gender, income, or sexual orientation, and services should always promote cultural humility and dignity. Although efforts aimed at reducing discriminatory practices in health care exist, collaborative efforts and organizational culture must continue to engage in practice that aims to overcome the various systemic and societal factors that contribute to poor quality of care for LGBT elders.

FUTURE GOALS

Future goals include research aimed at uncovering the following: (a) perceptions and attitudes of social workers and administrators in health and residential settings, (b) health disparities among older LGBT adults, and (c) practice interventions in rural versus urban health care settings. As a part of this research, we hope to address potential correlations between these environments and individual health outcomes. It will be important for research to examine the current needs of older LGBT adults in health and residential care settings. Efforts will need to be extended beyond education and awareness to include needs assessments of older LGBT adults in both rural and urban settings. A clear picture of the needs of this population as they relate to context will provide valuable insight into effective interventions to ensure positive outcomes for aging adults. A specific next step from this project will include collaboration with social work students and community aging programs to survey and examine the needs of older LGBT adults and health care professionals in a seven-county region in central Pennsylvania. These assessments will be used to better understand the needs of the stakeholders in a rural setting so as to best identify more meaningful and effective interventions that embody culturally sensitive practices. Additionally, an intergenerational approach to research that focuses on collaboration between students, providers, the community, and clients will help to strengthen and sustain present and future efforts aimed at eliminating discriminatory practices against older LGBT adults.

REFERENCES

Adelman, M., Gurevitch, J., de Vries, B., & Blando, J. (2006). Openhouse: Community building and research in the LGBT aging population. In D. Kimmel, T. Rose, & S. David (Eds.), *Lesbian, gay, bisexual, and transgender aging: Research and clinical perspectives* (pp. 247–264). New York, NY: Columbia University Press.

Addis, S., Davies, M., Greene, G., MacBride-Steward, S., & Shepherd, M. (2009). The health, social care and housing needs of lesbian, gay, bisexual and transgender older people: a review of the literature. *Health and Social Care, 17,* 647–658.

American Hospital Association. (2007). *When I'm 64: How Boomers will change health care.* Chicago, IL: American Hospital Association, First Consulting Group.

American Psychiatric Association. (2013). *Diagnostic and statistical manual of mental health disorders* (5th ed.). Arlington, VA: American Psychiatric Publishing.

Anetzberger, G., Ishler, K., Mostade, J., & Blair, M. (2004). Gray and gay: A community dialogue on the issues and concerns of older gays and lesbians. *Journal of Gay & Lesbian Social Services, 17*(1), 23–41.

Barker, R. M. (2008). Gay and lesbian health disparities: Evidence and recommendations for elimination. *Journal of Health Disparities Research and Practice, 2,* 91–120.

Behney, R. (1994). The aging network's response to gay and lesbian issues. *Outword: Newsletter of the Gay and Lesbian Aging Issues Network of the American Society on Aging, 1*(2), 2.

Berger, R. M., & Kelly, J. J. (1996). Gay men and lesbians grown older. In R. P. Cabaj & T. S. Stein (Eds.), *Textbook of homosexuality and mental health* (pp. 305–316). Washington, DC: American Psychiatric Association.

Bergh, N. V. D., & Crisp, C. (2004). Defining culturally competent practice with sexual minorities: Implications for social work education and practice. *Journal of Social Work Education, 40*, 221–238.

Berkman, C., & Zinberg, G., (1997). Homophobia and heterosexism in social workers. *Social Work, 42*, 319–335.

Blando, J. (2001). Twice hidden: Older gay and lesbian couples, friends, and intimacy. *Generations, 25*, 87–89.

Boardman, J. D. (2004). Health pessimism among Black and White adults: The role of interpersonal and institutional maltreatment. *Social Science and Medicine, 59*, 2523–2533.

Brotman, S., Ryan, B., Collins, S., Chamberland, L., Cormier, R., Julien, D., & Richard, B. (2007). Coming out to care: Caregivers of gay and lesbian seniors in Canada. *Gerontologist, 47*, 490–503.

Brotman, S., Ryan, B., & Cormier, R. (2003). The health and social service needs of gay and lesbian elders and their families in Canada. *Gerontologist, 43*, 192–202.

Brown, T. N., Williams, D. R., Jackson, J. S., Neighbors, H. W., Torres, M., Sellers, S. L., & Brown, K. T. (2000). Being Black and feeling blue: The mental health of consequences of racial discrimination. *Race & Society, 2*, 117–131.

Burch, A. (2008). Health care providers' knowledge, attitudes, and self-efficacy for working with patients with spinal cord injury who have diverse sexual orientations. *Physical Therapy, 88*, 191–197.

Burgard, S. A., Cochran, S. D, & Mays, V. M. (2005). Alcohol and tobacco use patterns among heterosexually and homosexually experienced California women. *Drug and Alcohol Dependence, 77*(1), 61–70.

Butler, S. S. (2004). Gay, lesbian, bisexual, and transgender (GLBT) elders: The challenges and resilience of this marginalized group. *Journal of Human Behavior in the Social Environment, 9*, 25–44.

Butler, S., & Hope, B. (1999). Health and well being for late middle-aged and older lesbians in a rural area. *Journal of Gay & Lesbian Social Services, 9*(4), 27–46.

Cahill, S. (2002). Long term care issues affecting gay, lesbian, bisexual and transgender elders. *Journal of Geriatric Care Management, 12*(3), 4–8.

Cahill, S. R., & South, K. (2002). Policy issues affecting lesbian, gay, bisexual, and transgender people in retirement. *Generations, 26*, 49–54.

Cahill, S., South, K., & Spade, J. (2000). *Outing age: Public policy issues affecting gay, lesbian, bisexual and transgender elders*. Retrieved from http://www.thetaskforce.org/downloads/reports/reports/OutingAge.pdf

Center for Study of Filmed History (Producer). (1985). *Before Stonewall: The making of a gay and lesbian community* [Videotape]. New York, NY: First Run Features.

Christie, D., & Young, M. (1986). Self-concept of lesbian and heterosexual women. *Psychological Reports, 59*, 1279–1282.

Climent, C. E., Ervin, F. R., Rollings, A., Plutchik, R., & Batinelli, C. J. (1997). Epidemiological studies of female prisoners. *Journal of Nervous and Mental Diseases, 164*, 25–29.

Clover, D. (2006). Overcoming barriers for older gay men in the use of health services: A qualitative study of growing older, sexuality and health. *Health Education Journal, 65*, 41–52.

Cochran, B. N., Peavy, K. M., & Cauce, A. M. (2007). Substance abuse treatment providers' explicit and implicit attitudes regarding sexual minorities. *Journal of Homosexuality*, *53*, 181–207.

Cohler, B. J., & Hostetler, A. J. (2006). Gay lives in the Third Age: Possibilities and paradoxes. *Annual Review of Gerontological and Geriatrics*, *26*, 263–281.

Compton, B., & Galaway, B. (1989). *Social work processes*. Belmont, CA: Dorsey Press.

Council on Social Work Education. (1992). *Curriculum policy statement for baccalaureate and Master's degree programs in social work education*. Alexandria, VA: Author.

Council on Social Work Education. (2013). *Council on sexual orientation and gender expression*. Retrieved from http://www.cswe.org/About/governance/CommissionsCouncils/15550/15548.aspx

Crisp, C. (2006). The Gay Affirmative Practice Scale (GAP): A new measure for assessing cultural competence with gay and lesbian clients. *Social Work*, *52*, 115–126.

Crisp, C., Wayland, S., & Gordon, T. (2008). Older gay, lesbian, and bisexual adults: Tools for age-competent and gay affirmative practice. *Journal of Gay and Lesbian Social Services*, *20*(1–2), 5–29.

Davies, D. (1996). Toward a model of gay affirmative therapy. In D. Davies & C. Neal (Eds.), *Pink therapy: A guide for counselors and therapists working with lesbian, gay and bisexual clients* (pp. 24–40). Philadelphia, PA: Open University Press.

DeHart, D. (2008). Breast health behavior among lesbians: The role of health beliefs, heterosexism, and homophobia. *Women & Health*, *48*, 409–427.

Diaz, R. M, Ayala, G., Bein, E., Henne, J., & Marin, B. V. (2001). The impact of homophobia, poverty, and racism on the mental health of gay and bisexual Latino men: Findings from 3 US cities. *American Journal of Public Health*, *91*, 927–932.

Dinkel, S., Patzel, B., McGuire, M., Rolfs, E., & Purcell, K. (2007). Measures of homophobia among nursing students and faculty: A Midwestern perspective. *International Journal of Nursing Education Scholarship*, *4*(1), Article 24.

Drabble, L., Midanik, L. T., & Trocki, K. (2005). Reports of alcohol consumption and alcohol-related problems among homosexual, bisexual and heterosexual respondents: results from the 2000 National Alcohol Survey. *Journal of Studies on Alcohol*, *66*(1), 111–120.

Eisenbach, D. (2006). *Gay power: An American revolution*. New York, NY: Carroll and Graf.

Flaxman, N. (2001). Isolated and underserved: Reaching lesbian, gay, bisexual, and transgender seniors. *Marquette Elder's Advisor*, *3*, 39–42.

Fredriksen-Goldsen, K. I., Woodford, M. R., Luke, K. P., & Gutierrez, L. (2011). Support of sexual orientation and gender identity content in social work education: Results from national surveys of U.S. and Anglophone Canadian faculty. *Journal of Social Work Education*, *47*(1), 19–35.

Gay and Lesbian Medical Association. (2001). *Healthy people 2010: Companion document for lesbian, gay, bisexual and transgender (LGBT) health*. Retrieved from http://glma.org/_data/n_0001/resources/live/HealthyCompanionDoc3.pdf

Gay and Lesbian Medical Association. (2006). *Guidelines for care for lesbian, gay, bisexual and transgender patients.* Retrieved from http://glma.org/_data/n_0001/resources/live/GLMA%20guidelines%202006%20FINAL.pdf

Grossman, A. H. (2008). Conducting research among older lesbian, gay and bisexual adults. *Journal of Gay and Lesbian Social Services, 20*(1–2), 51–67.

Harris, M. B., Nightengale, J., & Owen, N. (1995). Health care professionals' experiences, knowledge, and attitudes concerning homosexuality. *Journal of Gay & Lesbian Social Services, 2,* 91–107.

Hart, M., Robach, H., Tittler, B., Weitz, L. Walston, B. A., & McKee, E. (1978). Psychological adjustment of non-patient homosexuals: Critical review of the research literature. *Journal of Clinical Psychiatry, 39,* 604–608.

Heck, J. E., Sell, R. L., & Gorin, S. S. (2006). Health care access among individuals involved in same-sex relationships. *American Journal of Public Health, 96,* 1111–1118.

Herek, G. M. (1992). The social context of hate crimes: Notes on cultural heterosexism. In G. M. Herek & K. T. Berrill (Eds.), *Hate crimes: Confronting violence against lesbians and gay men* (pp. 89–104). Newbury Park, CA: Sage.

Institute of Medicine. (2008). *Retooling for an aging America.* Washington, DC: National Academies Press.

Jackson, J. S., Brown, T. N., Williams, D. R., Torres, M., Sellers, S. L., & Brown, K. (1996). Racism and the physical and mental health status of African Americans: A thirteen-year national panel study. *Ethnicity & Disease, 6,* 132–147.

Jackson, N., Johnson, M., & Roberts, R. (2008). The potential impact of discrimination fears of older gays, lesbians, bisexuals and transgender individuals living in small- to moderate-sized cities on long-term health care. *Journal of Homosexuality, 54,* 325–339.

Jeyasingham, D. (2008). Knowledge/ignorance and the construction of sexuality in social work education. *Social Work Education, 27,* 138–151.

Johnson, C. V., Mimiaga, M. J., & Bradford, J. (2008). Health care issues among lesbian, gay, bisexual, transgender and intersex (LGBTI) populations in the United States: Introduction. *Journal of Homosexuality, 54,* 213–224.

Johnson, M. J., Jackson, N. C., Arnette, J. K., & Koffman, S. D. (2005). Gay and lesbian perceptions of discrimination in retirement care facilities. *Journal of Homosexuality, 49,* 83–102.

Kehoe, M. (1986). Lesbians over 65: A triple minority. *Journal of Homosexuality, 12,* 139–152.

Kimmel, D. C. (1978). Adult development and aging: A gay perspective. *Journal of Social Issues, 34,* 113–130.

King, S. (2009, February). Addressing the health needs of older gays and lesbians. *Liberty Press, 15*(6), 25, 28. Retrieved from GenderWatch (Document ID: 1646751781).

Knochel, K. A., Croghan, C. F., Moone, R. P., & Quam, J. K. (2012). Training, geography, and provision of aging services to lesbian, gay, bisexual, and transgender older adults. *Journal of Gerontological Social Work, 55,* 426–443.

Kochman, A. (1997). Gay and lesbian elderly: Historical overview and implications for social work practice. *Journal of Gay and Lesbian Social Services, 6*(1), 1–10.

Koerner, B. (2002, December 10). *What is sodomy?* Retrieved from http://www.slate.com/id/2075271/

Kramarow, E., Lubitz, J., Lentzner, H., & Gorina, Y. (2006). Trends in the health of older Americans, 1970–2005. *Health Affairs (Millwood)*, *26*, 1417–1425.

Krieger, N. (1990). Racial and gender discrimination: Risk factors for high blood pressure? *Social Science & Medicine*, *30*, 1273–1281.

Krieger, N., & Sidney, S. (1996). Racial discrimination and blood pressure: The CARDIA study of young black and white adults. *American Journal of Public Health*, *86*, 1370–1378.

Kuyper, L., & Fokkema, T. (2010). Loneliness among older lesbian, gay and bisexual adults: The role of minority stress. *Archives of Sexual Behavior*, *39*, 1171–1180.

LGBT Movement Advancement Project & SAGE. (2010). *Improving the lives of LGBT older adults*. New York, NY: Authors. Retrieved from http://safeusa.org/uploads/Advancing%20Equality%20for%20LGBT%20Elders%20[FINAL%20COMPRESSED].pdf

LGBT Organizations Fact Sheet Series. (2013). *After DOMA: What it means for you*. Retrieved from http://www.hrc.org/files/assets/resources/Post-DOMA_General_v4.pdf

Logie, C., Bridge, T. J., & Bridge, P. D. (2007). Evaluating the phobias, attitudes, and cultural competence of master of social work students toward the LGBT populations. *Journal of Homosexuality*, *53*, 201–221.

Longres, J., & Fredriksen, K. I. (2000). Issues in the work with gay and lesbian clients. In P. Allen-Meares & C. Garvin (Eds.), *Handbook of social work direct practice* (pp. 477–449). Thousand Oaks, CA: Sage.

Maril, R., & Estes, C. (2013). *Living outside the safety net: LGBT families and Social Security*. Human Rights Campaign and the National Committee to Preserve Social Security and Medicare Foundation. Retrieved from http://issuu.com/lgbtagingcenter/docs/livingoutsidesafetynet

Martin, J. I., Messinger, L., Kull, R., Holmes, J., Bermudez, F., & Sommer, S. (2009). *Council on Social Work Education-Lamba Legal Study of LGBT issues in social work*. Retrieved from http://www.lambdalegal.org/news/pr/va_20091102_cswe-and-lambda.html

Martinez, P. (2011). A modern conceptualization of sexual prejudice for social work educators. *Social Work Education*, *30*, 558–570.

Mayer, K. H., Bradford, J. B., Makadon, H. J., Stall, R., Goldhammer, H., & Landers, S. (2008). Sexual and gender minority health: What we know and what needs to be done. *American Journal of Public Health*, *98*, 989–995.

McFarland, P., & Sanders, S. (2003). A pilot study about the needs of older gays and lesbians: What social workers need to know. *Journal of Gerontological Social Work*, *40*(3), 67–80.

Meisner, B., & Hynie, M. (2009). Ageism with heterosexism: Self-perceptions, identity and psychological health in older gay and lesbian adults. *Gay and Lesbian Issues and Psychology Review*, *5*(1), 51–58. Retrieved from GenderWatch (GW). (Document ID: 1791869861).

MetLife Mature Market Institute. (2006). *Out and aging: The MetLife study of lesbian and gay baby boomers*. Westport, CT: Author.

Meyer, I. H. (2003). Prejudice, social stress, and mental health in lesbian, gay, and bisexual populations: Conceptual issues and research evidence. *Psychological Bulletin*, *129*, 674–697.

Morin, S. F., & Garfinkle, E. M. (1978). Male homophobia. *Journal of Social Issues,* *34,* 29–47.

Morrison, S., & Dinkel, S. (2012). Heterosexism and health care: A concept analysis. *Nursing Forum, 47,* 123–130.

Morrow, D. F. (2008). Older gays and lesbians. *Journal of Gay & Lesbian Social Services, 13*(1–2), 151–169.

Morrow, D. F., & Messinger, L. (2006). *Sexual orientation and gender expression in social work practice: Working with gay, lesbian, bisexual, and transgender people.* New York, NY: Columbia University Press.

National Association of Social Workers. (2013). *Diversity and cultural competence.* Retrieved from http://www.socialworkers.org/pressroom/features/issue/diversity.asp

National Gay and Lesbian Task Force. (2010). *FAQ sheet on LGBT elders and Outing Age 2010* [Data File]. Retrieved from: http://www.thetaskforce.org/downloads/release_materials/outing_age_2010_faq.pdf

National Research Council. (2006). *Examining the health disparities research plan of the National Institutes of Health: Unfinished business* [Executive summary]. Retrieved from http://fermat.nap.edu/execsumm_pdf/11602.pdf

National Senior Citizens Law Center in collaboration with Lambda Legal, National Center for Lesbian Rights, National Center for Transgender Equality, National Gay and Lesbian Task Force and Services and Advocacy for GLBT Elders (SAGE). (2011). *LGBT Older Adults in long-term care facilities: Stories from the field.* Retrieved from http://www.lgbtagingcenter.org/resources/resource.cfm?r=54

Newman, B. S., Dannenfelser, P. L., & Benishek, L. (2002). Assessing beginning social work and counseling students' acceptance of lesbians and gay men. *Journal of Social Work Education, 38,* 273–289.

Orel, N. (2006). Community needs assessment: Documenting the need for affirmative services for gay, lesbian, and bisexual elders. In D. Kimmel, T. Rose, & S. David (Eds.). *Lesbian, gay, bisexual, and transgender aging: Research and clinical perspectives* (pp. 321–346). New York, NY: Columbia University Press.

Orel, N. A. (2004). Gay, lesbian, and bisexual elders: Expressed needs and concerns across focus groups. *Journal of Gerontological Social Work, 43*(2–3), 55–77.

Phillips, J., & Marks, G. (2006). Coming out, coming in: How do dominant discourses around aged care facilities take into account the identities and needs of ageing lesbians? *Gay and Lesbian Issues and Psychology Review, 2*(2), 67–77.

Pugh, S. (2005). Assessing the cultural needs of older lesbians and gay men: Implications for practice. *Practice, 17,* 207–218.

Robison, J. (2002, October 8). *What percentage of the population is gay?* Retrieved from http://www.gallup.com/poll/6961/what-percentage-population-gay.aspx

Ryan, E. B., Meredith, S. D., MacLean, M. J., & Orange, J. B. (1995). Changing the way we talk with elders: Promoting health using the communication enhancement model. *International Journal of Aging and Human Development, 41*(2), 69–107.

Saghir, M., Robins, E., Walbran B., & Gentry, K. (1970). Homosexuality: Psychological disorders and disabilities in the female homosexual. *American Journal of Psychiatry, 127,* 147– 154.

Saghir, M. T., & Robins, E. (1973). *Male and female homosexuality: A comprehensive investigation*. Baltimore, MD: Williams and Wilkins.

Saulnier, C. F. (2002). Deciding who to see: Lesbians discuss their preferences in health and mental health care providers. *Social Work, 47*(4), 355–365.

Saunders, J. M., & Valente, S. M. (1987). Suicide risk among gay men and lesbians: A review. *Death Studies, 11*, 1–23.

Sebelius, K. (2011). *Repealing the health care law would be costly for LGBT Americans*. Retrieved from http://www.outinthemountains.org/2011/february/op-ed/index.html

Services and Advocacy for Gay, Lesbian, Bisexual and Transgender Elders. (SAGE). (2010). *Improving the lives of LGBT older adults*. Retrieved from http://sageusa.org/uploads/Abbreviated%20-%20Improving%20the%20Lives%20of%20LGBT%20Older%20Adults%20%5BFinal%5D

Siegelman, M. (1972). Adjustment of homosexual and heterosexual women. *British Journal of Psychiatry, 120*, 477–481.

Stein, G. L., Beckerman, N. L., & Sherman, P. A. (2010). Lesbian and gay elders and long term care: Identifying the unique psychosocial perspectives and challenges. *Journal of Gerontological Social Work, 53*, 421–435.

Stein, G. L., & Bonuck, K. A. (2001). Physician–patient relationships among the lesbian and gay community. *Journal of the Gay and Lesbian Medical Association, 5*(3), 87–93.

Swank, E., & Raiz, L. (2008). Attitudes toward lesbians of practicing social workers and social work students. *Journal of Baccalaureate Social Work, 13*(2), 55–67.

Wahler, J., & Gabbay, S. (1997). Gay male aging: A review of the literature. *Journal of Gay & Lesbian Social Services, 6*(3), 1–20.

Weinick, R., Zuvekas, S., & Drilea, S. (1997). *Access to health care—Sources and barriers* (MEPS Research Findings No. 3, AHCPS Pub. No. 98-0001). Rockville, MD: DHHS, Agency for Health Care Policy and Research.

Wolinsky, F. D., Callahan, C. M., Fitzgerald, J. F., & Johnson, R. J. (1992). The risk of nursing home placement and subsequent death among older adults. *Journal of Gerontology, 47*(4), S173–S182.

World Health Organization. (1984). Health promotion: A World Health Organization document on the concept and principles. *Canadian Public Health Association Digest, 8*(6), 101–102.

"They Just Don't Have a Clue": Transgender Aging and Implications for Social Work

ANNA SIVERSKOG

National Institute for the Study of Ageing and Later Life, Linköping University, Norrköping, Sweden

This article explores transgender aging, drawing from life story interviews with transgender adults aged 62–78. The analysis focuses on 3 themes: intersections of age and gender during the life course, lack of knowledge of transgender issues, and how previous experiences of accessing care and social services matter in later life. It illustrates how older transgendered adults carry physical and mental scars from previously encountered transphobia, which affect various aspects of later life. Implications for social work are discussed and client-centered care, with a biographical approach, is suggested to better meet the needs of transgendered older adults.

INTRODUCTION

The abbreviation *LGBT* (for lesbian, gay, bisexual, and transgender) is often described as *nonheterosexuality* or *concerning sexuality*. However, the *T* refers more to gender identity than it does to sexuality, and by being lumped together with the *L*, *G*, and *B* and described solely in terms of *nonheterosexuality*, transgender people and their experiences are made invisible. Although some transgender people class their sexuality as gay, lesbian, bisexual, or queer, there are also those who do not. It is crucial to develop a critical perspective of gender that reaches outside binary norms, and to widen knowledge about transgender identities within social work, so as to avoid discrimination and transphobic treatment of clients with nonconforming gender identities (Burdge, 2007; Burgess, 2000; Mizock & Lewis, 2008). Indeed, as Sally Hines argued, "Transgender communities largely exist as marginalized subcultures in terms of normative frameworks that guide social and welfare provision" (2007, p. 483). To understand the specific challenges, experiences, and concerns of aging transgender people, a focus on gender identity in relation to age is needed (Witten & Eyler, 2012).

Transgender aging is an underexplored field, with Fredriksen-Goldsen and Muraco (2010) describing older transgender adults as one of the most invisible and underrepresented populations in contemporary social research. The work that does exist on transgender aging is, to a large extent, based on quantitative studies (Fredriksen-Goldsen et al., 2011; MetLife Market Institute, 2010), or on literature reviews (Cook-Daniels, 2006; Persson, 2009). There seems to be a need for more empirical data regarding older transgender people, and specifically qualitative data. A key point in this article is to argue for a biographical approach to developing an understanding of the experiences of older transgender adults, as well as their needs within social services. This approach allows for an exploration of how individuals' lives are embedded and created within historical contexts and places, and how earlier life plays into experiences in later life. This project thus follows a narrative tradition where subjective experiences are valued rather than claims of truth and objectivity (Riessman, 2002).

The starting point for this article is in the life stories of older people—people who identify themselves as transgender or who have had previous transgender experiences during their lives. The empirical material consists of interviews conducted within a qualitative explorative project, with social gerontology, queer theory, and social work theory constituting the integrative theoretical frame. The aim of this article is to utilize a biographical approach to explore how earlier life experiences matter in later life, and how age and (nonconforming) gender identities can be understood in relation to one another. The analysis presented here explores experiences of transgender older adults within three themes: (a) intersections of age and gender during the course of life, (b) the lack of knowledge on transgender issues within different contexts, and (c) how previous experiences of accessing care and social services matter in later life and in relation to the future need for care. The article aims to contribute to the understanding of transgender adults' experiences, to discuss what implications they might have for social work and care professionals, and to offer suggestions for social work practice.

(Trans)Gender Identities

Transgender is an umbrella term for people who, in different ways, overstep society's gender norms relating to gender identity and expressions (Feinberg, 2006). *Trans*, used here synonymously with transgender, has different meanings in different times and places; communities, identities, cultures, and language are constantly recreated and renegotiated. A transgender person could be someone who is not comfortable with the legal gender that they were assigned at birth, or someone who has a gender identity that goes beyond those that are socially and legally available, namely *male* and *female*. Trans identities encompass a range of experiences: a feeling of being uncomfortable with gender expectations, to dress as a gender that is not expected from your legal gender (often referred to as cross-dressing, or in a Swedish context most often as transvestism), or to feel that one identifies themselves as a gender other than that assigned at birth. Indeed, the latter may well come with a desire to change the body with hormones and or surgeries (often referred to as transexualism). Trans identities may also lead to feeling an identification that goes beyond binary gender categories (often referred to as genderqueer). It can encompass a large number of identities, including bois, drag kings and queens, he-shes, etc. (Stryker, 2008). Some people who have transitioned and undergone sex reassignment surgeries may no longer identify themselves as trans (Witten & Eyler, 2012). The trans identity can be something that occupies parts of life, or something that is a life-long experience (Stryker, 2008).

The term *cisgender* refers to people who identify with the legal gender they were assigned with at birth. A more complex way to conceptualize this is the term *linear gender*, referring to when one's legal gender, body, and gender identity and expression follow a coherent line (Bremer, 2011). As queer theorist Judith Butler (1990) argued, a performance of gender as man or woman, based on a binary gender model, is necessary to be understood as a normal and intelligible subject. Gender is performed in relation to other power asymmetries, such as ethnicity, class, sexuality, and age. Certain expressions of femininity and masculinity acquire different meanings depending on the performing person's age (Twigg, 2004). The performance of gender, as well as the performance of age (Laz, 2003) is also dependent on the material body and its physical shapes (Butler, 2006).

The Swedish Context

All of the respondents interviewed in this article live in Sweden and, as such, it is relevant to provide a brief background summary regarding the legal and social situation for trans people in Sweden. According to Bremer (2011), queer bodies have, through history, been interpreted by the Swedish state as being in need of particular state intervention; something that still remains in Sweden, especially when it comes to trans people. Although transvestism was removed as a mental disorder in 2009, transsexualism still remains as such in Sweden—despite the change in the canonical *Diagnostic and Statistical Manual* (American Psychiatric Association, 2013) that resulted in its removal as a mental disorder. Because transsexualism legally constitutes a mental illness and requires a medical diagnosis, gender correction is covered by the national health insurance scheme in Sweden (Bremer, 2011). According to the Swedish law 1972:119, relating to the "assessment of gender identity in certain cases," it is clarified that people who have been diagnosed with transsexualism should have the right to transition, that is, to change their bodies with hormones and surgeries and change their legal gender (Svensk författningssamling, 1972). However, the law demands that for this to happen, the person in question must be over 18 years old and registered with the authorities in Sweden. Until the law changed in 2013, it was also a prerequisite that each potential patient be a Swedish citizen, unmarried and sterilized (Svensk författningssamling, 1972). However, in many countries within and outside the European Union, a legal change of gender is often tied to compulsory sterilization. These demands, as well as the need to adapt to narrow binary notions of gender to get the diagnosis, have been largely criticized by researchers, as well as trans organizations (Bremer, 2011; Engdahl, 2010).

METHOD

The interviews referred to in this article were conducted as part of a larger project in which 20 older LGBTQ identified adults were interviewed. Of these interviews, six were conducted with people who are, or during their life have previously been, trans identified. These six people were between 62 and 78 years old (born between 1933 and 1950) during the time of the interviews (which took place between 2010 and 2012). The informants were recruited via newspaper ads, snowball sampling, and through an online LGBT community. The informants had differing experiences with regards to how they related to their trans identities (see Table 1 for a brief presentation). Throughout the text, I use the pronouns preferred by the respondents: she, he or they.

The study was reviewed and approved by the Regional Ethic Committee in Sweden (Dnr 2010/29-31) following guidelines from the Swedish Research Council (2011). I conducted all interviews. I informed participants of the aim of the study, making sure to obtain their consent and to maintain anonymity. I use pseudonyms in the text to protect respondents' identities.

Because an important aspect of the research project is life course, life story interviews were conducted. During the interviews, participants were encouraged to talk freely about their lives, starting with when and where they were born. Depending on how detailed their stories were, they were asked questions to follow up from their stories, concerning their gender identities, social networks, relations, health, aging, and the body during different periods of their lives. The duration of the interviews was between 3 to 6 hr long, and they were all conducted in the informants' homes.

TABLE 1 Respondents

Name	Born	Trans Experiences and Present Living Situation
Lily	1945	Identifies as transsexual woman, came out in later life, got the diagnosis transsexual, but her health did not allow surgeries. On hormone treatment. Lives alone in a mid-sized city.
Lena	1945	Identifies as a transsexual woman, came out in later life, got the diagnosis transsexual, but her health did not allow surgeries. On hormone treatment. Lives alone in the countryside, children from previous marriage.
Sture	1935	Has identified as a woman during big periods of his life, but lays low with his trans practices during later life. He was in the transition process but didn't get the diagnosis, thus hasn't had access to trans care. He lives alone in a smaller village in the countryside.
Bengt	1933	Identifies as a man but has a female gender expression full time. He lives alone in a middle-sized city and has children and grandchildren from previous marriage.
Klas	1950	Identifies as a man with transsexual background. He was assigned female gender at birth and transitioned in his twenties. He lives alone in a mid-sized city.
Kjell	1946	Identifies as genderqueer and does not want to categorize themselves according to binary gender categories. Tried to get the diagnosis transsexual to get access to transcare, but wasn't diagnosed and then got breast implants at a private clinic and bought hormones abroad. Lives with their partner in a mid-sized city.

I used thematic analysis, which, according to Braun and Clarke (2006), is a method for "identifying, analyzing and reporting patterns (themes) within data" (2006, p. 79). Braun and Clarke argued that thematic analysis should be considered as a method in its own right, and that it can be applied across a range of theoretical and epistemological approaches, whilst still providing a flexible and useful research tool which can yield rich, detailed, and complex data. The recorded interviews were transcribed and coded in parallel with the process of conducting fieldwork. Thus, discoveries in the coding process could be implemented in future interviews for greater depth (Becker, 1998; Silverman, 2006). The initial coding was open and focused on feelings, repetitions, contradictions, turning points, etc. In the next step of the analysis, the codes were sorted into themes. These themes were a result of the empirical material, as well as the theoretical starting points and the research questions guiding the study (Ryan & Bernard, 2003).

The strength of this study lies in the qualitative life-story interview approach, which offers a complex understanding of transgender lives, and which also offers a life-course perspective in relation to experiences of aging. Thus, the aim of this approach is not to generalize findings to an entire trans population, but rather to contribute with empirical data to an understudied field within gerontology. The integrative theoretical framework allows for analysis, which in turn enables the researcher to capture intersectional understandings between age, gender, and social work practice. The limitations lie mainly in the small sample of the study. A bigger sample could have represented a greater variety of trans experiences. For example, it proved rather difficult to recruit people with trans-masculine identities as well, as those among the oldest old.

RESULTS

The result section is structured around three themes: (a) intersections of age and gender during the life course, (b) the lack of knowledge on transgender issues within different contexts, and (c) how previous experiences of accessing care and social services matter in later life and in relation to future need for care. These themes will be revisited in the discussion section so as to analyze and review their implications for social work.

Intersections of Age and Gender Throughout the Life Course

To understand the experiences of older transgender adults, it is crucial to understand their previous experiences of (trans)gender identities during life, and how these are intertwined with the historical context, which differs from the context in which younger transgender people are now growing up. This section focuses on how these people have experienced gender norms during life, and how this relates to age and historical context.

Narrow norms, closeting, and shame. Several of the respondents talked about how early on in life they wanted to dress in clothes that were not expected according to their legal gender, but that they also realized early on that this was not socially accepted:

> I wasn't old when I realized women's clothes were appealing to me; I was 3, 4 years old. And then I wore my mum's clothes and wore nightgowns and so on. But then I grew up and I realized that, damn, this is not good. Even in that age, you are kind of aware somehow that you just don't do like that. You should not wear girls' clothes.

This quote by Lena illustrates how there are expectations, based around the legal gender one is assigned at birth, of how to dress and act. Lena expressed this as something she just "realized" and was "kind of aware of," which indicated that this was knowledge internalized by norms, rather than someone outright telling her. The respondents talked about how trans identities and expressions were something invisible, and something they had never heard of at younger ages. Indeed, as Bengt stated; "It didn't exist; you didn't talk about this; you could not read about it; there was nothing. . . . It was something sick back then." The historical context, with few queer role models or images of trans people and where queer expressions relating to sexuality and gender identity were connected to something shameful, sick, or tragic, has resulted in limitations when it comes to relating to one's own feelings or experiences or being open. This has, in turn, led to long periods of being closeted and hiding one's gender identity from colleagues, partners, children, and friends. As Sture said:

> I was ashamed of this and I was scared, terrified that someone would reveal me. I had a box with things, shoes, sock, underwear, and things like that. And I was terrified that someone would open the box and wonder what that was.

Like Sture, several of the people confessed to having hidden clothes, but they had also burned them or thrown them away. The fears of being discovered were related to the potential reactions from one's surroundings and what people "would think." Gender norms and the expectations of following one's legal gender were described in terms of "a prison" and were experienced so rigidly that hiding appeared to be a better, or maybe the only, alternative. However, the risk of being exposed still remained a constant threat:

> It has been a threat level that someone would find out that I was interested in wearing women's clothes. So I kept away from that. I felt I would be completely estranged and left out if I did that. And that is something transvestites live with to a great extent, that you simply get pointed out and shamed. And I lived with this, and still do, as a limiting part.

This quote by Bengt illustrates how a step away from gender norms, based on a binary model, is perceived as carrying a risk of being pointed out, exposed, shamed, and left out. Trans identity here is connected to shame, and the threat of social reprisals plays a part in the extent to which people have been, and are, open with their trans identities. As Bengt's quote demonstrates, these feelings of shame and fear felt like scars; scars that he still lives with and that act as a limiting element, despite the changing social context.

The respondents also carried scars from consequences they encountered after being discovered. Sture talked about how, as a child, he was beaten up by his dad when he discovered him wearing his mother's clothes. Lena spoke about how she was exposed by her wife one day in their house, and about how her wife then went round the village where they lived "and told everyone what a scum I was, that I dressed in women's clothes." These narratives, among others, illustrate how people who cross gender norms may become subject to disciplining and social stigma. The feelings of shame also led to situations where people disciplined and limited themselves as well as their own behaviors.

Later life. There were both positive and negative experiences of coming-out processes, which emerged from the interviews. Although it had been rather unproblematic in many contexts for some, others had endured hard experiences with major social consequences. Bengt told how he came out in late life and then he went "straight out right away, I mean, when you waited that long you got nothing to lose." He had expected his friends to disappear, "but no one did; instead I just got more friends which was really nice". As mentioned, Sture and Lena had harder experiences when their trans identities were outed by others, and other difficult consequences stemming from coming out are illustrated throughout this article. What several of the respondents had in common was that they felt it was easier to come out in later life. Kjell said that this was connected to a different time era, but also to being in a different phase of life:

> I was a bit older. You don't have a career to think about anymore, you don't have to think about what the boss is going to say if I am this way, or what customers would think. You don't have to think about these issues, don't need to pay that regard. You don't have to be scared of that at least. I think that makes it easier.

The respondents' narratives illustrate how the time after retirement, when life is no longer occupied by work, can be perceived as a time where one is able, to a greater extent, to choose the social context one wants to be in. This can also mean more time to reflect on, among other things, gender identity and how one wants to express one's self. At the same time, there were people who chose to "go back in to the closet" in later life. Sture, who during his life had previously been open with his trans identity, chose to not be open when he moved to a smaller village. He said that he wanted to have peaceful relations with his neighbors, even if it was at the expense of being who he really is. Both Kjell's and Sture's narratives illustrate how space and place also matter when it comes to the possibility of being open.

Aging can also bring different possibilities when it comes to performing gender. Some felt that the body became more androgynous with age and others perceived bodily aging to be problematic for their possibilities of performing gender. Wrinkles, the inability to walk in high heels, and different shapes of the body were all mentioned as potential complications for gender performance. The aging body can also be something that limits one's ability to undergo sex reassignment surgery (SRS), which was the case both for Lily and Lena. Lily also experienced ageist attitudes during her process, with the welfare-officer questioning whether SRS was really necessary when she had "so little time left to live." This attitude left Lily feeling hurt and offended.

Several of the respondents also talked about how they had small social networks and few friends. When I asked Sture which relations were the most important for him, the answer was "none." For some, such as Klas, this was partly connected to starting a new life in a new place when he transitioned and came out, meaning that he no longer had his childhood friends. His work was the place where he met people; the weekends became "empty" from Friday night to Sunday morning if he did not go out on his own: "You know, going to a flee market or to a theater, you name it, it's so fun if you are two. Just a friend. I can miss that." For Lena, the loneliness was directly connected to the trans identity:

> It gets kind of lonely, because "normal" people, they don't invite Lena to their homes . . . for coffee, because what would the neighbors think? Then that norm comes into play again; it can sort of be contagious in a way. . . . Before I was over at people's houses to have coffee, but not after [coming out], not once. So, it has some social consequences.

Several of the respondents used the Internet as a way in which to meet lovers and friends, but expressed a frustration with that milieu, characterized by many "unserious" users, nonpersonal contact, and a focus on sex. Being lonely in later life can have effects on one's social well-being, as well as having material consequences for the lack of support and care from people who one trusts.

Using qualitative data, this section has offered a complex understanding of older transgender adults' experiences of gender norms in relation to age during the life course. It has illustrated how these people, in many cases, have lived with stigma as a central element during long periods of their lives. Earlier experiences of being closeted, shamed, and disciplined are something that one carries through life in the form of mental and physical scars, and that also have social and material consequences in later life. An understanding of these processes is important within social work with transgender older adults.

Lack of Knowledge About Trans Issues

One recurrent theme in the interviews was the lack of knowledge regarding trans issues that the respondents had encountered in various contexts. This lack of knowledge is something they had experienced in public discourses and care contexts, as well as within LGBT groups.

Lena had a feeling that: "People in general don't have an idea what this is, they don't." Klas also talked about public knowledge in relation to the recent years, and the explosion within mass media when it comes to information on trans issues: "We have been fed, fed, fed, who can have missed out on this? And still, they just don't have a clue." Lena and Sture talked about how they had experienced malicious portraits of trans identity that reduced trans people to something connected to drag, show, and comedy. On several occasions, the respondents had participated in news articles, documentaries, and TV shows with the aim of widening the knowledge of trans people. Some of the consequences of going public became brutal. Sture worked as a teacher when he participated in a documentary that was aired on national TV. Following this, he started to be harassed by Christian colleagues: "They used me as subject for the morning prayers, praying for me getting cured. . . . I experienced more and more opposition at work and then I got called up to my boss, who offered to retire me early." Several parents of the children in the school also called the principal and expressed worries for their children having contact with Sture, because they assumed he was gay. Even though Sture had not talked about his sexuality in the documentary, nonnormative sexuality was assumed to follow with nonnormative gender identity. The confusion around gender identity and sexuality is something that other participants attested to having experienced, as well. Lily thought that this confusion might have something to do with the term *transsexuality* and stated that another term would be preferable, "but it is so cemented today and then it is hard to change. But as I said, it does not have anything to do with sexuality, not at all." Kjell said:

> I think a lot of non-LGBT people believe that men that wear a dress are homosexual. I think that is a rather common prejudice. And because of this, I always point out that I am heterosexual when I speak to the general public. Even within RFSL [The Swedish Federation for Lesbian, Gay, Bisexual and Transgender Rights] there are many members that think that our common denominator is homosexuality, which it's not any longer. Today, the common denominator is this that you oppose what RFSL defines as heteronormativity.

Kjell continued by saying that they thought gays and lesbians would have knowledge about trans issues, but realized "of course that was not the case, but the lack of knowledge was as big there as in general in society." Thus, when the respondent's gender becomes something unintelligible for the general public, a queer sexuality is assumed. Kjell's quote regarding assumptions of homosexuality being the common denominator may offer an explanation. LGBT politics tend to put sexuality high on the agenda, and lesbian and gay rights are more discussed, politically formulated, and have gained greater knowledge than trans issues.

The participants also talked about how they had experienced a lack of knowledge regarding trans issues within care contexts. This has led to situations where they had to educate the doctors, care staff, and social workers. Lena talked about how she had been bringing information materials to the doctor when she had been seeking care. Even within the transition process, they had experienced this lack of knowledge among staff members who were supposed to work specifically with trans patients. Lily said that the welfare officer she met during the transition had "a little knowledge about trans people, but not very much." This was also the case with the speech therapist she met during her transition.

This section has focused on how the respondents experienced a lack of general knowledge among the general public, within care contexts, and even within the LGBT community. It has illustrated how a transgender identity may be tangled up with the risk of not being understood or seen as one desires, or of being harassed when going public with transgender identity. It has also demonstrated how the respondents repeatedly have to explain themselves, educate others, and dismantle misconceptions of what transgender means. This demonstrates the importance of enhanced knowledge regarding transgender issues within the care and social welfare sector.

How Previous Experiences of Care and Social Services Matter in Later Life

This section focuses on how people related to care in later life, how previous experiences of care in relation to one's trans identity matter, and about thoughts and worries regarding the need for care in the future.

Previous experiences of care. The respondents expressed a feeling that transgender care is not designed according to people's needs, but rather that people have to adjust to the expectations that are demanded to get the right to transgender care. As Sture said:

> And what can be established; the transsexual that managed to get their rights, these aren't any underachieving weak ones. You have to be quick and well-formulated. And you need a bit of fantasy. So it is not about being upright, but rather about going around it.

Both Sture and Kjell had experienced not fitting into the categories of a binary gender model and had been denied the right to transgender care, including hormone treatment and surgeries. Thus, they had experiences of not receiving the care they needed or felt they should be entitled to. Kjell, who was not able to get breast implants through public care because they were not diagnosed, had to finance the breast implants themselves. They contacted five different private plastic surgery clinics to check prices, of which two replied that they could not do this procedure because they considered Kjell to be a man. This does not only illustrate a lack of knowledge in these private clinics, but can also be interpreted as an active policing of gender and bodies, which is something that takes place within the private care sector, as well as the public care sector. Kjell chose to buy hormones while on a trip to France to start their own hormone treatment. This can pose a risk to one's health because it does not involve regular controls of one's hormone levels and how one's general health is affected.

Klas, who transitioned in the '70s, experienced a transition that was different to how it would be today. To get the diagnosis, he had to go to a gynecologist, which can be very difficult for someone not comfortable with their biological sex. He also had to be institutionalized in a mental hospital for one week, during which time he underwent many psychological tests. Lily, who transitioned in later life, expressed how she thought the process failed her. To get the diagnosis, she had to meet a welfare officer who asked her many personal questions. During this process, many thoughts and life experiences came up which she was left alone with;

> And I think this is a part within the process that they miss. They penetrate the person, and they discover a lot of things that are not taken care of if the person needs support. . . . Because when you get older, you have one life that you lived one way, and now you need to find another way.

What Lily expressed here was a feeling of the process being ultimately for the doctors. She felt "penetrated" by the welfare officer who asked her a lot of personal questions which he needed answered to be able to diagnose Lily. As illustrated, there is a consciousness about the need to adapt and say the right things to get the right to care. However, if the same questions stir up thoughts that can be hard to deal with, people are forced to cope with these issues on their own.

Sture talked about how one of the strongest reasons to come out in public was an urge for more public knowledge. This was related to how his friend experienced transphobic treatment at a hospital, which later made her commit suicide:

> I had a trans friend in Stockholm . . . whose car was hit by a drunk driver. She was not severely hurt, but was taken to the hospital in an ambulance. And that night, they took her temperature 40 times or so. And blood pressure just about many times. And everyone did this, from doctors to cleaners. She survived and she went home the day later. But 6 months later she went for the pills and she does not live any longer.

This quote illustrates how the nonlinear body was seen as something sensational, which made the care staff at the hospital cross boundaries at several levels.

Worries about the future. Something repeated in the interviews was a worry regarding having to move to an institution in the future where the staff would not have trans competence. Kjell expressed how they thought it is important to have more knowledge within welfare institutions and that it is important that the focus is not only on sexuality: "If they know something it is probably about homosexuals; trans people are, for most, rather unknown. Most people have not even met a trans person." Lena expressed how she fears the day when she will have to move to a nursing home and that she thinks about what will happen if she asks the staff to paint her toenails:

> And if they don't have any LGBT competence, then it's going to be a total brush-off. . . . As long as I live at home I think it will be alright, but then when you get older and maybe have to move to a nursing home . . . Yes, when it is time and they come here and see that it is a man in women's clothes, "God how disgusting; we don't want to go to that person again," you don't know right?

Lena expressed a fear that caregivers would see her as "disgusting" and refuse to give her care. Klas, who at the time of the interview worked within the care sector, was comforted by his own experiences of care-giving and that he knew that members of care staff usually don't care about the patients' personal lives. At the same time, he stated that it is another thing to be a care recipient. Because he was not out with his trans history in the city where he lived, he usually sought care in another city. However, he had a nurse who knew about his transition who helped him with the injection of testosterone. Because he has been going to her for the last 20 years, they had developed a good relationship: "And then I think like this, fuck—how is it going to be when she retires? Because I will need to continue with this the rest of my life. . . . I don't want to tell each and every one about this." This caused distress for Klas.

As illustrated earlier, several of the respondents also lived alone and had small social networks and few friends. This can add to worries about the future, when they would be left to public care.

This last section of the analysis has illustrated how the respondents have experiences of not getting the (transgender) care they need because this is often characterized by binary gender norms. It seems that care and social services were perceived as not being created for the clients, but rather created for a policing of genders and bodies. This led to a lack of trust in social welfare services, which in turn was reflected in fears and worries about future needs for care, where they were afraid of encountering transphobic attitudes.

Discussion and Implications

The biographical approach used in this study has allowed me to explore how previous life experiences affect later life experience. This has illustrated how, even though time and historical contexts change, one's previous life experiences are something that they carry through life, in the form of scars (both physical and emotional). In the first part of this section, I discuss the results from the study and relate them to the theoretical framework and previous studies within the field, following which I move on to discuss implications for social work in the last part of this section.

Gender norms throughout the life course. The article has demonstrated how older transgender adults often experienced narrow gender norms throughout their life course. These expectations were, based on the legal gender one was assigned at birth, of how to dress and act. This can be interpreted using Butler's (1990) theory on how a constant performance of femininity or masculinity that is coherent with one's legal gender is needed to pass as a normal and intelligible subject. There is an expected coherence following between one's legal gender, body, and gender expression (Bremer, 2011). Social discourses on trans identity and gender play an important role in the perceived possibilities of being open with one's trans practices. Time and place, along with age(ing), play into these experiences through historical and geographical contexts. It becomes clear how the discourses surrounding people have meanings for which identities and acts are available and possible (Burr, 2003, p. 31). Munt (2007, p. 3) pointed out how "groups that are shamed contain individuals who internalize the stigma of shame into the tapestry of their lives, each reproduce discrete, shamed subjectivities, all with their own specific pathologies." Several of the respondents in this study have experiences of being closeted for large parts of their lives. Although the social context has changed, feelings of shame and fear can remain in the respondents' lives. This corresponds with Fredriksen-Goldsen et al. (2011), who found, in their quantitative study with 2,560 LGBT adults aged 50 to 95, that older transgender people experience significantly higher levels of internalized stigma when compared with lesbians and gay men. There were also narratives in the interviews on how people who cross gender norms become subject to disciplining and social stigma from their surroundings. According to Burgess (2000), it is not unusual that gender expectations within families are often strong, and when these expectations are not met, interventions often occurred through discipline.

Several of the respondents felt that it was easier to come out in later life. This could be due to a different time era, but could also relate to being in a different phase of life. The time after retirement can offer possibilities to choose which context one wants to be in, and which people to have around, but can also provide more time during which to reflect on how one wants to express themselves. These factors can offer explanations as to why many older transgender people choose to come out in later life, after retirement (Witten & Eyler, 2012). However, coming out in later life can mean that it is too late to undergo SRS for those who wish to do it. Bodily aging can also affect the possibilities to perform one's preferred gender. Being unable to perform one's preferred gender can be a cause of personal and internal distress. It can also increase the external risks of not "passing" in gender performance, which may lead to a sense of diminished safety and fears of being harassed (Mizock & Lewis, 2008, pp. 337–338).

The results illustrated how several of the respondents had small networks and few friends. This is coherent with other studies where older transgender adults were less likely to have positive feelings about belonging to the LGBT community and would have significantly lower levels of social support then older cis-gendered adults (Fredriksen-Goldsen et al., 2011). Several researchers have pointed to the importance of the trans community as a source of support (Hines, 2007; Witten & Eyler, 2012); for those living in rural areas or in smaller cities, these networks are more often than not unavailable. Being lonely in later life can affect one's well-being, as well as having material consequences for the lack of support and care from people who the person trusts.

"They just don't have a clue"—The lack of knowledge. The title of this article, "They just don't have a clue," is a quote from one of the respondents, and represents a recurrent theme in the interviews, namely the lack of knowledge regarding trans issues that the respondents had encountered in various contexts. Despite trans people being present more often in Swedish mass media (Rydström, 2008) and trans issues being discussed more frequently, the respondents stated that people, in general, do not have knowledge on trans issues. When trans people are represented in the media, the respondents felt that it was often connected to drag, show, and comedy. They often encountered confusion around gender identity and sexuality, and when the respondents came out with their trans identities, people often assumed that they were homosexual. This might be due to the general lack of knowledge regarding trans issues, where people cannot grasp or make intelligible trans identities, but framing people as homosexual is something that reconstructs the noncongruence within a binary framework of heterosexual and homosexual, where only binary genders are possible (Stryker, 2006). Even within LGBTQ contexts, the respondents had encountered this lack of knowledge on trans issues, which, in turn, relates back to other studies where transgender people have less positive feelings about belonging to LGBT communities (Fredriksen-Goldsen et al., 2011).

The respondents also had experiences of lack of knowledge within care contexts, which had led to situations where they were forced to educate doctors, care staff members, and social workers on trans issues; something that happened even within transition processes. These experiences are confirmed by the Swedish National Board of Health and Welfare (2010), which claims that the knowledge on transsexualism within the care sector is small, especially within the outpatient care. As pointed out by Mizock and Lewis (2008, p. 347), the education of clinicians (and I add social workers here) should lie at the feet of the clinicians themselves and not be the responsibility of the clients who are there to receive care. As Donovan (2002) described, it can be stressful when meeting new doctors to answer the same questions over and over about one's gender identity. She claimed that this can lead to negative effects on one's mental stability.

Care and social services: Previous experiences and future worries. Previous care contexts during life can affect one's perceptions of care, especially encounters encompassing transphobic attitudes. Several of the respondents had experiences that involved not receiving the (transgender) care they should have been entitled to, because they were not considered to fit into the binary gender model. According to Bremer (2011), the Swedish transition processes are gender normative and aim to materialize bodies to female or male bodies. People whose gender identities do not fit into these categories are denied trans care. This is not something unique to Sweden. Indeed, Butler (2006) wrote about how an essential view on gender is represented and demanded to be able get the right to transgender care in the United States. This has, in turn, led to people arranging workshops for FTMs (female to male) who get the opportunity to train on adapting an essential view of gender before they apply for transition. The active policing of gender and bodies took place within the public sector, as well as in the private sector. There were also experiences of ageist attitudes in the transition process where a welfare officer questioned whether SRS was really necessary because the person had "so little time left to live." One respondent shared an experience where his trans-female friend had been in hospital and her body was seen as "sensational" and put on display by the staff. Donovan (2002) wrote about similar experiences; of becoming an embodied freak who can be put on display in medical contexts where the person is there to seek care.

When talking about the future, respondents seemed to refer back to a worry regarding having to move to an institution where the staff would not have trans competence and where they feared they would not be acknowledged as their preferred genders or be discriminated against because of gender identity. The respondents' fears can be interpreted as a fear of being in a situation characterized by a lack of agency where one is dependent on others in their personal sphere; people who one does not choose oneself (Twigg, 2004). These fears reappear in other studies of aging LGBT persons, with many fearing being discriminated against because of sexuality or gender identity (Fredriksen-Goldsen et al., 2011; Heaphy & Yip, 2006; Hughes, 2009). In some cases, this even means that people choose to go back into the closet in later life (as is the case with Sture), detransition, or even commit suicide (Witten & Eyler, 2012). Klas, who transitioned 40 years ago and, at the time of the interview, lived in a smaller city where he his trans history was not public knowledge, worried about what was going to happen when his nurse, who gave him his testosterone injections, retired. This situation caused distress for him, and also illustrates what Witten and Eyler (2012) have pointed out; that compared to older gay, lesbian, and bisexual adults who can choose whether they want to be open or not, trans people are more likely to be identifiable. In this case, it was Klas' hormone treatment, but in other contexts it can be a noncongruent body with scars or nonlinearity that reveals one's trans identity. The MetLife survey study with 1,200 LGBT boomers demonstrates how transgender respondents were almost twice as likely to feel vulnerable with health care providers and felt that seeking care was difficult compared to lesbians, bisexuals, and gay men (MetLife Market Institute, 2010).

Because several of the people interviewed lived alone and had small networks, they would be left having to rely on public care when in need of care and support in the future. Several studies point to the importance of networks and trans communities for support (Donovan, 2002; Hines, 2007; Witten & Eyler, 2012), but for people living in rural areas or who do not have access to these networks, the problems still remain. This is also an additional problem in a context where public care and social services are becoming increasingly privatized by Western governments, thus offloading responsibilities of public support onto local communities and families (Katz, 2005, p. 14).

Implications for Social Work

Even the relatively small sample of six people in this article illustrates the variety of transgender identities, as well as the different challenges and needs that follow. This, in itself, constitutes an important point; all transgender experiences are individual and different. This, in turn, means that it is impossible to learn about one right way to approach a transgender client. In contrast, I agree with Burdge (2007) in her argument that social workers "should reject a dichotomous understanding of gender in favor of more accurate and affirming conceptualizations of gender" (p. 243). She argues that a rejection of binary gender models is crucial because those are the foundation on which transgender oppression depends. This article has illustrated the great need for more knowledge and education on trans issues, and this education should take a starting point in a critique of heteronormativity including binary gender models. This will also prevent simplified assumptions and generalizations of trans people's identities and experiences whilst simultaneously opening up an acknowledgement of a variety of gender identities.

What may be the most crucial thing in supporting a transgender client is the right to self-definition. It is the client's right to define their gender identity, regardless of whether or not this gender is linear and coherent with one's legal gender, body, and gender expression. For the client to feel safe being open with their trans identity, the way in which they are approached, as well as the social context may be significant in terms of their perceived possibilities to do so. Does the atmosphere where social workers meet clients reflect views on binary gender norms, or can it be considered trans friendly? Do the formularies and intake forms allow for the client to list their preferred gender? Do social workers ask everybody for preferred gender identity and respect the answers they get? Are the bathroom genders neutral? As Mizock and Lewis (2008) argued, visual indicators and signs of trans-positive attitudes can make a difference. They mentioned LGBT-focused brochures in multiple languages, the posting of a nondiscrimination statement, and LGBT-related magazines as things which can be present in waiting rooms. They also suggest that the transgender community should be incorporated into all levels of service in healthcare settings that cater to this population. Several of the respondents in this study live in rural areas with no trans communities nearby, thus suggesting that education, curricula, and cooperation can also take place online via the internet.

For social workers to be equipped to meet the needs of older transgender adults, knowledge regarding the historical social and legal context in relation to trans identity is crucial. This article has illustrated how historical context, as well as age, play into one's trans experiences. This indicates that transgender people's lived experiences are important when it comes to understanding their present situation and needs.

Within client-centered care, life histories have been used to enable a more person-centered care (Medvene, Grosch, & Swink, 2006). A biographical approach could be useful in meetings with transgender clients, because an understanding of the life history and the arrival at one's gender identity is of great importance in terms of being able to meet the client's needs. As Nagoshi and Brzuzy (2010) purported, "The recognition of the importance of physical embodiment of intersecting identities and the understanding of how the narratives of lived experiences integrate the socially constructed, embodied and self-constructed aspects of identity are essential" (p. 437).

A strength of this approach is that it avoids the one right way to engage with transgender clients, but rather focuses on the individuals' experiences. However, although lived experiences are crucial for many, as this article has illustrated, certain older trans people who have transitioned earlier in life and have changed legal gender might not want to acknowledge their transgender past, and it is their right not to do so. Hence, people who do not want to speak about their transgender histories must be respected, and silences must be acknowledged as well.

Another important point to make is that client-centered care may work for moving the power in the meeting between client and health provider to the client, although this also has consequences in moving responsibilities to the client (Black, 2005). Because the interviews have demonstrated how the respondents feel that they must often play the role of educator, the biographical approach should be employed with the aim of reaching a better understanding between service provider and the individual client, rather than serving as a moment of education. Social workers must be educated on trans issues before they encounter the client. Thus, I advocate for LGBT competence training in social work that does focus on the T, that has a critical analysis of binary notions of gender, and that acknowledges the importance of individual lived experiences.

ACKNOWLEDGMENTS

This article was written during a guest visit at San Francisco State University. I thank Rita Melendez and Brian deVries who I worked with there. I also thank Håkan Jönson, the editor, and the anonymous reviewers for useful comments.

FUNDING

Financial support for this study was provided by grants from the Swedish Research Council for Health, Working Life and Welfare (2012-1062) and from the Solstickan Foundation. These grants made it possible for me to be a guest scholar at SFSU, where I wrote this article.

REFERENCES

American Psychiatric Association. (2013). *Diagnostic and statistical manual of mental disorders* (5th ed.). Arlington, VA: American Psychiatric Publishing.

Becker, H. S. (1998). *Tricks of the trade: How to think about your research while you're doing it*. Chicago, IL: University of Chicago Press.

Black, R. M. (2005). Intersections of care: An analysis of culturally competent care, client centered care, and the feminist ethic of care. *Work, 24*(4), 409–422.

Braun, V., & Clarke, V. (2006). Using thematic analysis in psychology. *Qualitative Research in Psychology, 3*(2), 77–101.

Bremer, S. (2011). *Kroppslinjer: kön, transsexualism och kropp i berättelser om könskorrigering* [Bodylines: Gender, transsexualism and embodiment in narratives on gender correction]. Göteborg, Sweden: Makadam.

Burdge, B. J. (2007). Bending gender, ending gender: Theoretical foundations for social work practice with the transgender community. *Social Work, 52*(3), 243–50.

Burgess, C. (2000). Internal and external stress factors associated with the identity development of transgendered youth. *Journal of Gay & Lesbian Social Services, 10*(3–4), 35–47.

Burr, V. (2003). *Social constructionism*. London, England: Routledge.

Butler, J. (1990). *Gender trouble: Feminism and the subversion of identity*. New York, NY: Routledge.

Butler, J. (2006). *Genus ogjort: kropp, begär och möjlig existens* [Undoing gender] (K. Lindeqvist, Trans.). Stockholm, Sweden: Norstedts akademiska förlag.

Cook-Daniels, L. (2006). Trans aging. In D. Kimmel, T. Rose, & S. David (Eds.), *Lesbian, gay, bisexual, and transgender aging: Research and clinical perspectives* (pp. 21–35). New York, NY: Columbia University Press.

Donovan, T. (2002). Being transgender and older. *Journal of Gay & Lesbian Social Services, 13*(4), 19–22.

Engdahl, U. (2010). *Att vara som/den "en" är: en etisk diskussion om begreppen rättvisa, erkännande och identitet i en trans*kontext* [To be as "one" is: An ethical discussion on the concepts of justice, acknowledgment and identity in a trans* context]. Linköping, Sweden: Linköpings Universitet, Institutionen för Tema.

Feinberg, L. (2006). Transgender liberation. A movement whose time has come. In S. Stryker & S. Whittle (Eds.), *The transgender studies reader* (pp. 205–220). New York, NY: Routledge.

Fredriksen-Goldsen, K. I., Kim, H.-J., Emlet, C. A., Muraco, A., Erosheva, E. A., Hoy-Ellis, C. P., . . . Petry, H. (2011). *The aging and health report: Disparities and resilience among lesbian, gay, bisexual, and transgender older adults.* Seattle, WA: Institute for Multigenerational Health.

Fredriksen-Goldsen, K. I., & Muraco, A. (2010). Aging and sexual orientation: A 25-year review of the literature. *Research on Aging, 32*(3), 372–413.

Heaphy, B., & Yip, A. K. T. (2006). Policy implications of ageing sexualities. *Social Policy and Society, 5*(4), 443–451.

Hines, S. (2007). Transgendering care: Practices of care within transgender communities. *Critical Social Policy, 27*(4), 462–486.

Hughes, M. (2009). Lesbian and gay people's concerns about ageing and accessing services. *Australian Social Work, 62*(2), 186–201.

Katz, S. (2005). *Cultural aging: Life course, lifestyle, and senior worlds.* Toronto, Canada: University of Toronto Press.

Laz, C. (2003). Age embodied. *Journal of Aging Studies, 17*(4), 503–519.

Medvene, L., Grosch, K., & Swink, N. (2006). Interpersonal complexity: A cognitive component of person-centered care. *Gerontologist, 46*(2), 220–226.

MetLife Market Institute. (2010). *Still out, still aging. The MetLife study of lesbian, gay, bisexual and transgender Baby Boomers.* Westport, CT: Mature Market Institute.

Mizock, L., & Lewis, T. K. (2008). Trauma in transgender populations: Risk, resilience, and clinical care. *Journal of Emotional Abuse, 8*(3), 335–354.

Munt, S. R. (2007). *Queer attachments: The cultural politics of shame.* Aldershot, England: Ashgate.

Nagoshi, J. L., & Brzuzy, S. (2010). Transgender theory: Embodying research and practice. *Affilia, 25*(4), 431–443.

Persson, D. I. (2009). Unique challenges of transgender aging: Implications from the literature. *Journal of Gerontological Social Work, 52*, 633–646.

Riessman, C. (2002). Analysis of personal narratives. In J. F. Gubrium & J. A. Holstein (Eds.), *Handbook of interview research* (pp. 695–710). Thousand Oaks, CA: Sage.

Ryan, G. W., & Bernard, H. R. (2003). Data management and analysis methods. In N. K. Denzin & Y. S. Lincoln (Eds.), *Colleting and interpreting qualitative materials* (pp. 259–309). Thousand Oaks, CA: Sage.

Rydström, J. (2008). Varför behövs transhistoria? [Why is transgender history needed?] *Lambda Nordica, 13*(1–2), 63–77.

Silverman, D. (2006). *Interpreting qualitative data: Methods for analyzing talk, text and interaction.* London, England: SAGE.

Swedish National Board of Health and Welfare. (2010). *Transsexuella och övriga personer med könsidentitetsstörningar – Rättsliga villkor för fastställelse av könstillhörighet samt vård och stöd* [Transsexuals and other people with gender identity disorders—Legal conditions for determination of gender, and care and support]. Stockholm, Sweden: Author.

Stryker, S. (2006). (De)subjugated knowledges: An introduction to transgender studies. In S. Stryker & S. Whittle (Eds.), *The transgender studies reader* (pp. 1–17). New York, NY: Routledge.

Stryker, S. (2008). *Transgender history*. Berkeley, CA: Seal Press.

Svensk författningssamling. (1972). *Lag (1972:119) om fastställande av könstillhörighet i vissa fall* [Law 1972:119 pertaining the approval of gender affinity in certain cases]. Retrieved from http://www.riksdagen.se/sv/Dokument-Lagar/Lagar/Svenskforfattningssamling/sfs_sfs-1972-119/

Swedish Research Council. (2011). *Good research practice*. Stockholm, Sweden: Swedish Research Council.

Twigg, J. (2004). The body, gender, and age: Feminist insights in social gerontology. *Journal of Aging Studies*, *18*(1), 59–73.

Witten, T. M., & Eyler, E. A. (2012). Transgender and aging: Beings and becomings. In T. M. Witten & E. A. Eyler (Eds.), *Gay, lesbian, bisexual and transgender aging: Challenges in research, practice and policy* (pp. 187–269). Baltimore, MD: John Hopkins University Press.

Brief Report

The National Resource Center on LGBT Aging Provides Critical Training to Aging Service Providers

HILARY MEYER and TIM R. JOHNSTON

Services and Advocacy for Gay, Lesbian, Bisexual and Transgender Elders (SAGE), New York, New York, USA

The National Resource Center on LGBT Aging was created in 2010 by Services & Advocacy for Gay, Lesbian, Bisexual and Transgender Elders (SAGE) with seed funding from the US Department of Health and Human Services. Three years into the project, thousands of aging and LGBT service providers have been reached with training and technical assistance; however, a great need, especially for cultural competency training, remains.

The National Resource Center on LGBT Aging was created in 2010 to improve the lives of lesbian, gay, bisexual, and transgender (LGBT) older adults. One of the primary objectives of the Center is to provide cultural competency training to aging service providers, to assist them in understanding the unique needs of this traditionally underserved population. Three years into the project, thousands of aging and LGBT service providers have been reached with training and technical assistance; however, a great need, especially for cultural competency training, remains.

BACKGROUND ON THE NRC'S CREATION

The Older Americans Act (OAA) was enacted by Congress in 1965 to assist older adults remain in their homes and communities as long as possible. The OAA directs the aging network (agencies and organizations providing services to older adults) to pay particular attention to serving populations with the "greatest social need" (Administration on Aging [AoA], n.d.-a). As such, the AoA, through the Administration on Community Living, has a history of funding national organizations through OAA funds to serve as technical assistance resource centers for specific minority populations, including Hispanic Americans, African Americans, Asian Americans, and Native Americans (AoA, n.d.-b). These resource centers were created to address the health disparities of marginalized groups by using innovative approaches.

Recent studies indicate that LGBT older adults are growing in population numbers and evidencing a number of health disparities (Conron, Mimiaga, & Landers, 2010; Dilley, Simmons, Boysun, Pizacani, & Stark, 2010; Fredriksen-Goldsen et al., 2010), in part due to LGBT older adults avoiding accessing services for fear of discrimination by providers (National Senior Citizens Law Center et al., 2011). In 2010, AoA took action by publicly recognizing that older LGBT individuals have unique needs that must be addressed. AoA published a Funding Opportunity Announcement for a 3-year grant to be awarded to an organization to establish the first technical assistance and training resource center for LGBT older adults (Grants.gov, 2009).

Services & Advocacy for Gay, Lesbian, Bisexual and Transgender Elders (SAGE) won the grant and, in March 2010, launched the National Resource Center on LGBT Aging (NRC) in partnership with ten other organizations—American Society on Aging; CenterLink; FORGE Transgender Aging Network; GRIOT Circle; Hunter College; The LGBT Aging Project; National Association of Area Agencies on Aging; National Council on Aging's National Institute of Senior Centers; Openhouse; and, PHI. As HHS Secretary Kathleen Sebelius stated, "Agencies that provide services to older individuals may be unfamiliar or uncomfortable with the needs of this underserved population. The Resource Center will provide information, assistance and resources for both mainstream aging organizations and LGBT organizations" (SAGE, 2010).

THE NRC TRAINING PROGRAM

One of the NRC's primary goals is to support mainstream aging service providers and LGBT organizations to better serve LGBT elders so as to ensure that they have the necessary services and support to successfully age in place. In support of this goal, the NRC created comprehensive training curricula for aging services providers and LGBT organizations entitled *Improving the Quality of Services and Supports Offered to LGBT Older Adults*. The curricula were developed in partnership with PHI and seven other organizations (LGBT Aging Project; Openhouse; GRIOT Circle; FORGE Transgender Aging Network; SAGE; CenterLink; and, evaluation partner Hunter College). The aging services providers curricula is the centerpiece of the NRC's training program, offering two 4-hr trainings geared specifically toward mainstream aging providers. The NRC also created and provides two 4-hr trainings geared specifically toward LGBT organizations.

Level I of the aging service providers training curriculum guides participants as they:

1. Learn about the culture, needs, and concerns of LGBT older adults;
2. Consider why LGBT older adults are less likely to access health and social services; and
3. Identify best practices for helping LGBT older adults to feel more included in aging network organizations.

The curriculum also provides tools and education to better serve the LGBT older adults who currently access, or are in need of, services.

Level II of the curriculum builds on Level I and guides participants to:

1. Identify health disparities between LGBT older adults and those who are not LGBT;
2. Explore judgments and assumptions, myths and misinformation about HIV and AIDS;
3. Recognize that individuals are entitled to their own diverse opinions and beliefs, and that their actions and behaviors must be consistent with workplace expectations in relation to inclusion and safety for LGBT constituents; and
4. Use role-plays to practice how to provide effective feedback to address bias from staff or other older adults, in order to create LGBT-welcoming environments.

The Level II training also builds in time to review policy and practice areas of participants' own agencies.

RESULTS OF THE TRAINING

As of April 15, 2013, over 2,400 providers in 26 states across the country completed the training (as measured by the number of providers who completed the posttest evaluation tool) and the evaluation results are promising. To examine changes in knowledge resulting from the training, one scale was used in both the pretest and posttest questionnaires. One set of questions tested knowledge of how to make an environment safe for LGBT older adults. The scale consisted of 8 true-or-false questions. The average score on this knowledge scale increased significantly from 6.65 (ranging from 1 to 8) correct on the pretest to 7.23 (ranging from 2 to) on the posttest as demonstrated by t-test analysis ($t = -12.44$, $p < .001$) comparing the mean pretest and posttest scores. Despite the high score on the pretest, which suggested that participants were well-informed about serving LGBT elders prior to the training, knowledge about how to make an environment more sensitive to LGBT elders still increased significantly. Additionally, to examine changes in attitudes as a result of the training, five questions were asked in the pre- and posttest questionnaires. Each question, in statement form, used a 5-point Likert scale for respondents to indicate the extent they agreed or disagreed with each statement. In three of the five items, attitudes changed significantly in the direction that was intended, as indicated by t-tests comparing mean scores on the Likert scale responses for each question.

In addition to measuring knowledge and attitude change directly after the training, the NRC has designed a follow-up assessment tool. In March 2013, the tool was distributed via an online link for the following reasons: (a) to pilot an instrument that would be used as an ongoing follow-up questionnaire 60 days after receiving the training, (b) to undertake a preliminary assessment of training participant knowledge and attitudes around serving LGBT elders; and (c) to solicit information on how training participants perceive the utility of the training and if they have changed their behaviors (individual or organizational) after participating in the NRC training. When introduced into the ongoing evaluation work of the NRC, the data will offer a better understanding of what happens 8 weeks after participants attend trainings. Information gained from the pilot test suggest that results of the training are sustained over time and that participants express continued interest in supporting culturally sensitive services for LGBT elders.

CHALLENGES AND OPPORTUNITIES REMAIN

Although the NRC has already made great strides in its 3 years of operation, substantial challenges and opportunities remain. For example, there is a tremendous need to reach providers, especially social workers, who may not have the time to be trained in-person for 4 or 8 hours. The NRC is attempting to meet this challenge by developing other training modalities that may be more conducive to agencies that need LGBT aging information but are unable to commit to 4 hr of training. There are also training needs for providers who are personally dedicated to understanding the unique needs of LGBT older adults but who do not have the organizational support to bring a trainer to their agency. In this case, the NRC is assisting on projects to create online learning tools that are accessible to individuals who can use self-directed learning tools. The NRC, along with a small number of other regional training organizations, offers a variety of training tools but the demand for accessible training options still remains. Social work education programs may also benefit from early training on these issues. The NRC has completed a number of trainings in undergraduate and graduate level programs, evidencing a fertile setting to teach cultural competency to students.

Although challenges of relatively scarce resources abound, the opportunity to create accessible learning tools and incorporate them into different environments where trainings are often eagerly sought, presents an exciting time for the fields of social work and gerontology.

FUNDING

The work of the National Resource Center on LGBT Aging is made possible through founding support from the United States Department of Health and Human Services through the Administration on Aging; as well as support from the Gill Foundation (grant #16139); H. van Ameringen Foundation; the Retirement Research Foundation (grant #2011-097); and generous individual donors.

REFERENCES

Administration on Aging. (n.d.-a). *Frequently asked questions*. Retrieved from http://www.aoa.gov/AOA_programs/OAA/resources/Faqs.aspx

Administration on Aging. (n.d.-b). *Information for professionals*. Retrieved from http://www.aoa.gov/AoARoot/Resource_Centers/Professionals.aspx#minority aging1

Conron, K. J., Mimiaga, M. J., & Landers, S. J. (2010). A population based study of sexual orientation identity and gender differences in adult health. *American Journal of Public Health, 100*, 1953–1960.

Dilley, J. A., Simmons, K.W., Boysun, M. J., Pizacani, B. A., & Stark, M. J. (2010). Demonstrating the importance and feasibility of including sexual orientation in public health surveys: health disparities in the Pacific Northwest. *American Journal of Public Health, 100*, 460–467.

Fredriksen-Goldsen, K. I., Kim, H.-J., Emlet, C. A., Muraco, A., Erosheva, E. A., Hoy-Ellis, C. P., . . . Petry, H. (2011). *The aging and health report: Disparities and resilience among lesbian, gay, bisexual, and transgender older adults*. Seattle, WA: Institute for Multigenerational Health.

Grants.gov. (2009). *HHS-2010-AOA-LG-1001. Technical Assistance Resource Center: Promoting appropriate long term care supports for LGBT elders*. Retrieved from http://www.grants.gov/search/search.do?oppId=50036&mode=VIEW

National Senior Citizens Law Center, Lambda Legal, National Center for Lesbian Rights, National Center for Transgender Equality, National Gay and Lesbian Task Force, & SAGE. (2011). *LGBT older adults in long-term care facilities: Stories from the field*. Retrieved from http://www.lgbtagingcenter.org/resources/resource.cfm?r=54

SAGE. (2010). *HHS awards major grant to SAGE to create first-ever national resource center for lesbian, gay, bisexual and transgender elders*. Retrieved from http://www.lgbtagingcenter.org/newsevents/pressArticle.cfm?p=4

Film Review

Transgender Tuesdays: A Clinic in the Tenderloin, by Mark Freeman. 2012, 60 min, $290.00 (DVD).

Transgender Tuesdays (http://www.transgendertuesdaysmovie.com) is a documentary about the pioneering work done at the first public health clinic in the United States for transgendered people. The Transgender Tuesdays clinic opened in 1993 at the Tom Waddell Health Center in San Francisco. This nighttime clinic was located in the Tenderloin, the red light district and the heart of the AIDS epidemic. Their groundbreaking work extended a harm-reduction model to treat transgendered people with respect and dignity, while providing access to high-quality health treatment.

As the film opens, viewers are asked to imagine looking in a mirror. The face looking back at them is not the right one. What is one to do? This question pulls viewers into the personal world of those who knew that something was not right at a very early age. Throughout the film, the stories of a dozen patients are shared. The first chapter of the film provides a glimpse into the past and what transgender people faced in earlier decades, beginning with the 1950s. Many of the patients from the clinic talked about growing up lacking role models and having no one they could talk to about how different they felt. Some became runaways, others were suicidal. Many fell into prostitution because they couldn't get a job and needed money to pay for their hormones. Substance abuse was common to cope with the stress and pain of their situation. Desperation made them vulnerable to medical quacks who would push black-market hormones and often sundry other drugs also. Unfortunately, the procedures of the quacks lacked exams, blood tests, or checkups to monitor their health. Their personal stories offer a compelling picture of the need for transgender healthcare and compassionate healthcare providers.

The second chapter of the film focuses on the history of the transgender clinic and its team—a first in the nation. In the early days of the clinic, many transgender patients were really sick—previously, there was no safe place for them to get health care, so they delayed seeking help until they were nearly at death's door. The clinic developed protocols for transgender care and made them widely available to anyone interested. Health care settings in other cities adopted the protocols; the ripples have subsequently spread across the country. Transgendered people felt that the clinic treated them like human beings—they felt safe, respected, and comfortable, rather than ashamed of who they were. Transgendered immigrants were common and often came with tremendous trauma and fear after being beaten up, tortured, called names, and having their life threatened in their country of origin.

The final chapter of the film focuses on the future and is hopeful. There are an estimated 1,000,000 transgendered individuals in the United States today, and increasingly children and young adults have an improved chance of being allowed to be who they are. However, transgendered people remain disadvantaged as the last minority lacking civil rights protections and basic but appropriate healthcare. It remains legal to fire someone for being transgendered in 33 states. At work, 90% of transgendered individuals experience harassment, mistreatment, or discrimination on the job and there is a 50% chance of losing one's job if one is outed. Since 1994, the Employment Non-Discrimination Act (ENDA), a civil rights bill to prohibit private employers with more than 15 employees from discrimination on the basis of sexual orientation or gender identity, has been introduced in nearly every United States Congress. In July 2013, ENDA (S. 815) passed through a Senate committee on a bipartisan vote and is now headed to the full Senate where it has a solid majority. In April 2013, an ENDA bill was introduced in the House (H.R. 1755) and has been referred and is in Committee.

This film conveys the personal traumas that transgender people experience in an openly hostile world where they lack basic civil rights accorded to other minority groups. It also suggests the courage it takes to endure while hiding one's gender identity—with family, at work, and at school. Substance abuse, prostitution, and homelessness are common themes. And yet, as Freeman notes, "Everyone knows a transgender person. They just may not know that they do." By reaching a general audience, this film helps viewers to see transgender people as an "us" rather than a "them".

Times are changing, but much remains to be done. Society continues to impose gender binaries on individuals who fall outside the male/female box and to limit legal protections and benefits. On several fronts, Canada remains ahead of the United States on LGBTQ issues, where gay marriage was legalized in 2005. The US Supreme Court overturned DOMA (Defense of Marriage Act) in June 2013, finally opening the doors for same-sex marriage. Up until this landmark legal decision, only 13 states recognized and permitted same-sex marriages. Sex reassignment surgery is covered in seven Canadian provinces—for 94% of Canadians. In the United States, some insurance companies cover transgender surgery, but most continue to exclude coverage of sex change surgery or any treatment of gender identity disorders.

Transgender people are no longer invisible and silent. The Canadian model, Jenna Talackova, made headlines when she waged a legal battle in 2012 to be allowed to compete in the Miss Universe Canada after being initially disqualified for being a transgendered woman. Sara Davis Buechner shared her personal story, in the *New York Times*, as an internationally known concert pianist who was born David Buechner. In 2002, no American insurer would approve payment for transgender surgery and so she underwent surgery in Thailand, which was so disfiguring that it required corrective procedures. Once she came out as Sara, she was no longer able to get bookings with top orchestras and was unable to find employment at any university. She moved to Canada, rebuilt her concert career, and is now a tenured professor in Vancouver, British Columbia.

In the United States, California has become a leader in efforts to ensure that transgender people have access to health care. Health care protections enacted in California in 2013 entitle transgender people to the same access to treatment as everyone else, including hormones. Unfortunately, in 47 other states individuals can still be denied insurance coverage because of their gender identity.

This film personalizes healthcare issues and the politics faced by transgendered people in a compelling narrative. Numerous educational films exist on topics related to LGBT issues—but none to date, that I am aware of, have addressed the unique health concerns of the transgender community. This film captures an important turning point in making health care accessible to the transgender community and will, hopefully, trigger discussion and reflection on broader LGBT issues among the public. The film will be useful in social work courses to enhance and strengthen student perspectives on the diversity of the LGBTQ community and the struggles they face to maintain their dignity and self-esteem when their rights are not acknowledged. The film emphasizes the importance of client-centered care and a strengths-based approach. I highly recommend this film, which points to the importance of continuing advocacy efforts and the possibilities for creating a society that accepts the LGBTQ community as full and equal members.

Debra Sheets, PhD, MSN
School of Nursing, University of Victoria
Victoria, Canada

Index

Note: Page numbers in **bold** type refer to figures
Page numbers in *italic* type refer to tables